THE
FAITH
FACTOR

THE
FAITH
FACTOR

☩

Proof of the Healing
Power of Prayer

DALE A. MATTHEWS, M.D.
WITH CONNIE CLARK

VIKING

VIKING
Published by the Penguin Group
Penguin Putnam Inc., 375 Hudson Street,
New York, New York 10014, U.S.A.
Penguin Books Ltd, 27 Wrights Lane, London W8 5TZ, England
Penguin Books Australia Ltd, Ringwood, Victoria, Australia
Penguin Books Canada Ltd, 10 Alcorn Avenue,
Toronto, Ontario, Canada M4V 3B2
Penguin Books (N.Z.) Ltd, 182–190 Wairau Road,
Auckland 10, New Zealand

Penguin Books Ltd, Registered Offices:
Harmondsworth, Middlesex, England

First published in 1998 by Viking Penguin,
a member of Penguin Putnam Inc.

1 3 5 7 9 10 8 6 4 2

All Biblical quotations are from the New Revised Standard Version,
except for those indicated as NIV (New International Version)
or KJV (King James Version).

The individual experiences recounted in this book are true. However, in
some instances, names and descriptive details have been altered to protect
the identities of the people involved. Certain cases are presented as
composites of more than one real person.

ISBN 0-670-87539-2

CIP data available.

This book is printed on acid-free paper.

Printed in the United States of America
Set in Galliard
Designed by Kathryn Parise

In loving memory of my grandfather,
the Rev. Dr. Louis B. Matthews, Sr.,
and my father, Dr. Louis B. Matthews, Jr.,
who "fought the good fight, finished the race,
and kept the faith."

(2 TIMOTHY 4:7)

ACKNOWLEDGMENTS

It is a formidable, humbling, yet deeply gratifying task to reflect on the dozens of individuals whose encouragement and wisdom have made this bookwriting adventure possible. Among the many to whom I am indebted, I would especially like to recognize publicly and thank warmly the following individuals for their invaluable contributions.

Those who taught and nurtured me in the faith: Jim Cavanaugh, Park Dickerson, Ernest Gordon, Ed Henegar, Dick Bauer, Lidabell Pollard, Steve Smallman, Butch Hardman.

Those who introduced me to the ministry of healing: Phil Zampino, Harold and Ann Hammond, Judith and Francis MacNutt, Norma Dearing.

Brave pioneers who first explored the boundaries of faith and medicine: Herb Benson, Larry Dossey, Morton Kelsey, Randy Byrd.

Fellow laborers in the research vineyard of faith: Harold Koenig, Jeff Levin, Dana King, Ken Olive, George Gallup, Margaret Poloma, the late Richard Friedman.

Former colleagues at the University of Connecticut Health Center who supported me in my initial and fledgling efforts to understand the relationship between faith and health: Peter Manu, Tom Lane, Tony Voytovich, Jim Freston.

Former and current colleagues at Georgetown University Medical Center for their advice and encouragement: John Eisenberg, Larry Beck, Ed Pellegrino, Zeses Roulidis, Dan Sulmasy.

Acknowledgments

Colleagues at the National Institute of Healthcare Research for their congeniality, enthusiasm, and partnership: Connie Barry, Renee Bergin, Vicki Lovett, Dan Kaufmann, Jim Collins, Rich Genter.

Dave Larson, who started this ball rolling in a big way, deserves a particular note of recognition and blessing. Thanks, Big Guy!

Colleagues at the Bayer Institute for Healthcare Communication who reinforced to me the central importance of the doctor-patient relationship in the healing process: Vaughn Keller, Greg Carroll, Dan O'Connell, Barbara Korsch.

Physicians who helped me to think and reason critically: Frank Davidoff, Alvan Feinstein, Tom Inui. Other physicians whose counsel and support I have valued: Tony Suchman, Dan Ford, Steve Booton, Carey Cottle, Walter Byrd.

Those who have modeled the integration of faith and medicine and who have helped me dream about what this integration might look like someday: David Stevens, Gene Rudd, Hal Habecker, David Allen, Lew Bird, George Simms, Dave Biebel.

Benefactors who have provided financial and moral support: John and Joe Gregory of Monarch Pharmaceuticals (a division of King); The Foundation for Spirituality and Medicine; and the officers of the John Templeton Foundation: Sir John Templeton, Jack Templeton, Chuck Harper, Fran Schapperle, Judy Marchand.

Other friends and colleagues who have supported me unconditionally in this work throughout the years: Sally Marlowe, David Earnhardt, Bruce Epperly, John Fletcher, Doug Kay, Ty Fabling, Marilyn Sousa.

My oldest and dearest friends in the world: Jamie Horton, Jim Sparks, Ed Campion.

Thinkers and writers who have influenced me: Paul of Tarsus, Blaise Pascal, Søren Kierkegaard, Paul Tillich, Paul Tournier, Jack Deere, John Wimber.

My patients, for their patience and generosity.

My agent, Gail Ross, for her perseverance, diligence, and chutzpah.

My editor, Mindy Werner, for her perspicacity, rigor, and discernment.

My mother, Dorothy, and my brothers, Paul and Skip, for a lifetime of love and support.

My wife, Demetra, for steadfast faithfulness and love. You've been everything: copy editor, companion, confidante, challenger, and champion; you've read every word, heard every talk, and knew what to say and write before I did: *Thanks!*

My children, Karen and Louis, who are my pride and joy, my blessing and legacy, the precious jewels and treasure of my life. May you always keep the faith and one day pass it along to your own children!

My Lord and Savior, the Name above all Names, to whom alone be the glory. *Thank you!*

—DALE A. MATTHEWS, M.D.

✠

I would like to acknowledge the valuable assistance of a number of people who provided information for this book: Sidney Van Nort, librarian, American Bible Society; Paul Walsh, president, Fellowship in Prayer; Jessica Fiorelli at the National Alliance of Breast Cancer Organizations; William C. Bryson for information on Alcoholics Anonymous; and Michael Lewallen for information on music therapy.

With a grateful heart, I would like to thank the individuals who have generously shared their stories for this book. I join Dale in recognizing with gratitude the excellent work of our agent, Gail Ross, and our editor, Mindy Werner. Thanks are due as well to Connie Wood and Tory Matthews for indispensable, intelligent research assistance. Connie and Tory join a host of others who deserve thanks for their prayer support of this project, including many members of my faith community, Grace Episcopal Church in Alexandria, Virginia, in particular Mary Blouin, who has prayed daily for this book. I want to thank Paul Hanley, Robert Malm, Rhoda Nary, and Karen Special for helping me chart a course through unknown waters. Thanks, too, to my dear friends Laura Akgulian, Drew Minter, and Brooke Russell, and to my cherished family members (too numerous to name!), for support and guidance.

My deep love and thanks go, as always, to my partner in life and work, Guy Lushin, for editorial insight, steadiness of soul, and great good humor.

—CONNIE CLARK

CONTENTS

✛

Contents

THE
FAITH
FACTOR

INTRODUCTION

In two decades of practicing medicine, I have been honored to participate in the healing process of thousands of patients suffering from all kinds of illnesses—heart disease, cancer, diabetes, depression, and more. Depending on each patient's particular problems, I have conducted examinations, provided counseling, prescribed medications, ordered tests, and made referrals to other practitioners, all according to prevailing standards of scientific medical practice. Many patients have benefited from my treatment; others have not. Some patients have had routine "textbook" recoveries from illness and surgery; in other instances, I have witnessed recoveries, even healings, that cannot be fully explained by science. In particular, I have frequently observed the power that faith and religious commitment can exert in maintaining health and in helping people recover from and cope with illness. I am not alone: many other physicians have made similar observations. Until recently, however, the medical profession has pondered these phenomena mostly in silence rather than making them the subject of scientific studies.

Today, that is changing. The lessons my patients and others have learned from personal experience are echoed in over three hundred clinical studies that demonstrate one simple fact: faith is good medicine. Indeed, the medical effect of religious commitment is not a matter of faith, but of science, and both doctors and patients are taking part in a revolutionary convergence of medicine and faith, which is transforming the way people seek healing.

The clinical emergence of "the faith factor" in medicine is an unexpected development for those of us trained in Western medical schools. For some of my colleagues, the idea of including spirituality in clinical care comes as a challenge, if not an outright shock. For me, however, the need to address patients' spiritual needs was not a surprise; rather, it grew naturally out of my deep-seated commitment to the doctor-patient relationship.

WHOLE-PERSON MEDICINE

On my first day of medical school, I learned what kind of doctor I did *not* want to be.

I walked into my first lecture at Duke University Medical School along with 109 other, equally nervous, first-year medical students. The lecture was given by a renowned scientist and professor of medicine. The professor's lecture focused on alkaptonuria, a metabolic disorder with a bizarre side effect: people who have it produce black urine. In order to make the effects of alkaptonuria real for us, the professor had asked a patient with the disease to come to the lecture. The patient sat in front of our dumbstruck class, accompanied by a big jar of his own black urine.

I don't remember anything being said during that entire hour about this patient as a human being. We did not address what it meant for him to have to urinate in public restrooms and face the frustration and humiliation of being different from everyone else. We did not hear his story of how he coped (or didn't) and his courage (or lack of it) in handling this problem. And when the lecture was over, he picked up his jar of urine and left the stage, never to be seen again . . . until next year, and another class of 110 students.

The lack of humanity in this introduction to medicine horrified me. But the day was just beginning! We went straight from the alkaptonuria lecture to the anatomy lab, where we began dissecting corpses without any kind of introduction or ceremony of transition. No mention was made of the former human being whose lifeless body lay exposed before us, reeking of formaldehyde. We did not honor her as someone who had had hopes and dreams and maybe children and grandchildren, an emo-

2

tional life, a sexual life, a spiritual life. We were just told to cut, and to keep on cutting.

I had gone into medicine hoping to learn and practice compassionate, person-centered doctoring. Yet here, on day one of my medical training, I ran headlong into a different world, one where the biochemistry of molecules was valued more highly than the pain of human beings.

Still, I wanted to learn everything I could about the human body and medical practice, even if the approach to the subject seemed cold and reductionist to me. I wanted to become a good scientist for the sake of my future patients. But for me, the science was secondary to the person, not the other way around.

I wanted to focus my energy on caring for people—*whole* people, not just their organs and tissues. From the beginning, I focused on the doctor-patient relationship, a unique aspect of medicine which in itself offers extraordinary opportunities for healing. Choosing internal medicine as my specialty, and choosing the doctor-patient relationship as one of my research topics, I had unknowingly selected a path that would lead me to discover the urgent need to restore the spiritual dimension of medicine.

In researching the doctor-patient relationship, I learned about the value of whole-person medicine as championed by Dr. George Engel in the 1950s. Dr. Engel established the "biopsychosocial model," a way of looking at and treating *all* aspects of patients—their psychological needs and social milieu as well as the biological perturbations accompanying diseases of the mind and body. Each patient should be treated as an individual, and each patient's concerns, expectations, fears, hopes, dreams, and worldview are worthy of the physician's attention. Dr. Engel stopped short of advocating that doctors address the spiritual dimension of patients' lives, but his whole-person model laid the foundation for the later inclusion of the spiritual dimension.

Building on Dr. Engel's work, a number of visionary physicians have brought us to a new era in medicine. Among the most notable of these thinkers are Dr. Herbert Benson, who has provided solid scientific evidence for the role of beliefs and meditative practice in human health, and Dr. Larry Dossey, who has been examining the healing power of prayer. Dr. Benson has demonstrated that beliefs—whether religious or otherwise—have a profound effect on physical and mental health. He has also documented the positive effects on health of "the Relaxation Response," a form of meditation involving the relaxation of the body and the focusing of the mind, which I will discuss at length in chapter 2. In reviewing the scientific literature on prayer's effects on human and nonhuman life, Dr. Dossey has proposed new models of prayer based on recent developments in quantum physics. When people pray for one another, he states in his book *Healing Words,* they participate in the unity of human and divine consciousness that transcends time and space. Through their research, speaking, and writing, Dr. Benson, Dr. Dossey, and a number of other scholars are helping to overcome the formerly staunch opposition by the medical and scientific community to *any* manifestation of spirituality in medical research or clinical care.

Religion may well be the final frontier to be explored in medicine, but patients are the pioneers of this frontier. According to polls commissioned in 1996 by *USA Today Weekend* and *Time,* four-fifths of patients surveyed believe in the healing power of prayer, and two-thirds want their doctors to address spiritual issues with them. A study by Dr. Dana King at East Carolina University in Greenville, North Carolina, showed that 48 percent of hospitalized patients want their doctors not just to talk about spiritual issues with them, but actually to *pray* with them. Yet how many physicians are prepared to do this? Dr. King found that doctors were praying with patients less than 1 percent of the time, and only rarely were doctors addressing spiritual needs. This is hardly surprising: our training as physicians has implicitly (and often explicitly) taught us to *avoid* the religious dimension in working with patients, and it certainly has not equipped us to address these issues in a sensitive, empowering manner.

I understand the hesitation many physicians feel about entering this realm with patients, because I have felt it myself.

LEARNING TO PRAY WITH PATIENTS

Though I have been a Christian since childhood, I did not begin my medical career with a clear awareness of the role of the spiritual dimension of medicine. Practicing my personal faith was, and is, a comfortable and comforting routine for me. But at first, praying with my patients and addressing their spiritual concerns did not come naturally. I had a great love for patients, a deep respect for the value of a close doctor-patient relationship, and an unwavering dedication to Dr. Engel's ideal of whole-person medicine. My concern with including spiritual issues as part of caring for patients gradually evolved from my interest and background in the doctor-patient relationship and my own deepening faith. It began to make logical sense to me that, as a proponent of true, whole-person medicine and as a person of faith seeking to live out my faith in a life of service to others, I should, and could, address *all* my patients' principal needs—physical, psychological, social, *and* spiritual. It did not make sense to exclude religion, which I knew was the most important influence in the lives of many patients, and call myself a whole-person doctor.

Slowly, without fanfare, but with trepidation, I began to ask patients about their spiritual lives when I took their medical histories. From the outset, I learned that some patients do not wish to address this aspect of their lives in my office, and that is perfectly acceptable to me as their physician. To continue such inquiries in an insensitive, offensive manner is a clear violation of the patient-physician bond needed for trust and healing: this realm should not be explored against the patient's will. But many patients have welcomed my inquiries. They know what many of us doctors are now just beginning to realize: faith and health are closely connected.

As I became more comfortable in exploring the spiritual lives of my patients, one patient responded by asking me to speak at her church. I was pleased to have the opportunity, and gave a talk on "Bearing the Cross of Suffering" for the church's Lenten education series. Word began to trickle out: "Dr. Matthews is a doctor who believes in God and will talk with patients about their faith!" Soon, patients were coming to me specifically because they wanted care for their spiritual problems as well as their medical ones.

Though I welcomed these new patients and the full range of their concerns, it still didn't occur to me to pray with them until, finally, one patient forced the issue into the open.

"I came to you because you're a Christian doctor," he said. "I would like you to pray with me."

Here I was, a doctor in a state-university teaching hospital, a "temple" of scientifically-based medicine, where religion was largely ignored, and where knowledge, not God, was worshiped. In this secular environment, I was asked to pray right now, right here, out loud, with a patient. I was uncomfortable with the idea, but, not wishing to offend the patient, I went through the motions, hoping to get the prayer over with quickly and return to more solid, medical ground—and hoping none of my colleagues would overhear me!

After this halting start, other patients began to ask for prayer. Through my care for them, I grew, and I expanded my method of practice and understanding of spirituality in the healing process. I realized that, as a person of faith, I no longer wanted to maintain a complete separation of my religious beliefs from my medical practice, particularly once I was convinced of the scientifically demonstrable value of prayer and religious commitment. Of course, there was never a question for me of imposing my religious beliefs and practices on patients who held different faiths or who had no interest in religion at all. But with patients who were yearning for exactly this kind of sharing, why should I resist?

Soon, praying with patients became a natural and satisfying task for me, and a helpful strategy for counseling patients. In addition to adjusting their medications and monitoring their lab tests, I began to share scripture verses with some of them, reading aloud from the Bible I keep in my office. I experienced the pleasure and joy of combining work and worship, and I began to see that, though addressing patients' needs is clearly the primary task of medicine, fulfilling my own desire for faith, connection, and meaning can be a welcome by-product. I also learned that, when my patients and I acknowledge God's presence, our doctor-patient relationship becomes a God-doctor-patient relationship. Each patient and I are partners with God and before God, asking him to place his anointing, his blessing, and his healing presence on the medical treatment and on us. With God's presence thus fully acknowledged, I don't have to try to "play God" any more. I can let God be God, and I can be the doctor.

Even today, this approach may seem revolutionary, and it is certainly quite different from my previous approach to medicine.

STANDING AT THE CONVERGENCE OF FAITH AND MEDICINE

Does praying with my patients make me less of a scientist? Definitely not. I have been thoroughly trained in the scientific method and I endorse its historic and continued value to medicine. As a doctor, medical-school professor, and clinical researcher, I trade in the coin of the realm: empirical evidence is the foundation, the gold standard, for all that we do. I am committed to the scientific basis of medicine, and I believe that progress in medicine is best made through careful observation and experimentation. That is why I am convinced that scientific validation of religion's healing effects is an essential first step toward incorporating spiritual approaches in traditional scientific medical care.

When it is confirmed by the knowledge and tools of medical science, I can wholeheartedly embrace the ancient, venerable power of faith in health and healing. Because of such scientific data, I now routinely ask my patients about the role of faith in their lives, and I tell them what many clinical studies clearly show—that regular attendance at church or synagogue is linked with better physical and mental health, greater life satisfaction, enhanced recovery from illness, and even increased life expectancy. If and when my patients want me to, I pray and share scripture with them. As a medical-school professor, I teach my students that the spiritual dimension is a sadly neglected aspect of medical care, and I urge them to acknowledge and respect the religious life of their patients. As a researcher, I am aware of the evidence presented in this book for the strong link between religious involvement and health.

In all these settings, I find myself in a unique role as a kind of "missionary to medicine." Though I never anticipated playing this role, it is not entirely surprising to find myself here.

A Heritage of Healing

My paternal grandfather, Louis B. Matthews, Sr., was the only one of twelve children in his family to graduate from high school. He went on to earn four degrees, including a Master's of Divinity and a Ph.D. Ordained as a minister in the Southern Baptist Convention, he quickly made plans to work in the field as a missionary. With his wife, Reka, he served four years in Buenos Aires, Argentina, before returning to the United States. Louis enjoyed a fruitful ministry in Tennessee and Indiana as a college professor, pastor, and acclaimed preacher.

My father, Louis Jr., remembers the one piece of career advice his father gave him: "Help people." It didn't really matter how; service to others was the point of living. My father chose medicine as his way of helping others. He practiced internal medicine for over thirty years, primarily at Mary Hitchcock Memorial Hospital and Dartmouth Medical School, in rural New Hampshire. My mother, Dorothy Watson, was also a medical professional—a nurse, who met my father on a hospital ward where they were both working.

Dorothy's family had also been influenced by medicine and illness. Her father, James A. Watson, the city architect for Yonkers, New York, lost his leg in an accident as a young man. While recovering from his crippling injury, he met a young nurse, Beatrice Adele Glover, who had emigrated from Russia. They fell in love and married, and my maternal grandfather persevered and thrived, maintaining a zest for life, pinochle, and cross-country travel despite his handicap.

Driven by his own faith and my grandfather's guiding words, my father gave of himself sacrificially through his medical practice. There was almost nothing he would not do to help a patient. No hours were too long, no distance was too far to travel to make a house call. He loved his patients, particularly the rural Yankee farmers, and they knew it and returned the sentiment gladly. Louis B. Matthews, Jr., M.D., was the best-beloved physician I've ever known, and deservedly so. As his son, I absorbed his way of practicing medicine by osmosis. I had often accompanied him as he made house calls in an old Volkswagen Beetle. And though my father did not pray with his patients, he sensed their spiritual needs and knew that the healing power of the physician was rooted not only in the medicines he prescribed, but, just as importantly, in his unconditional love and acceptance of them.

With this dual heritage, it is not surprising that, as a young man, I struggled over the choice between medicine and ministry. I chose medicine because I believed it would be a more practical way to live out my grandfather's motto. Today, however, as the gap between medicine and religion begins to narrow, the choice I made between medicine and ministry no longer seems so absolute. Fortunately for me, it is an auspicious era in which to be a doctor committed to understanding and invoking the spiritual dimensions of medicine. I can practice medicine as a form of ministry and serve people in need through medicine, hope, and prayer.

That service to others includes caring for and loving my patients and students as my father did. Today, as a medical-school professor, I see medical students experiencing what I did twenty years ago as I stood in the Seeley G. Mudd Library at Duke University School of Medicine, completely overwhelmed at the amount of information I needed to absorb, certain I could never know enough to be a good doctor. I tell my students what I have learned: "Knowledge of the human body is important. Knowledge of the human spirit is *more* important. Technique and skills for treating disease are important. Caring for human beings—love—is *more* important."

‡

How did I, a doctor trained in the critical, skeptical atmosphere and methods of twentieth-century science, come to believe that faith in God aids one's healing—that faith is good medicine?

The Wounded Healer Is Healed

Like many who want to help others, I am what the late Catholic priest and writer Henri Nouwen identified as a "wounded healer," one for whom

> . . . a deep understanding of his own pain makes it possible for him to convert his weakness into strength and to offer his own experience as a source of healing to those who are often lost in the darkness of their own misunderstood sufferings.

Through my own experiences in what theologian David Biebel calls "the University of Pain," I have grown in compassion, understanding, and the desire to serve others. I have had nagging physical problems, including migraines, neck, back, and knee pain. As a young man in medical school and postgraduate training, I struggled with bouts of depression and anxiety. But (as is true for so many of us) the pain that made me a wounded healer had its roots in my earliest years.

In many ways, my childhood was idyllic. Healthy and well loved, encouraged to learn and excel, I did well in school. In our home, great value was placed on the life of the mind. I have happy memories of my father giving me an "assignment" before leaving the house in the morning, telling me to find out about a historical figure, event, or concept that I could report on at dinner. I remember fondly the discussions and debates at the dinner table and the questions I'd pose to my mother while the dishes were being washed. When summer vacation came, my father would give me a five-dollar bill to buy as many books as I could to take on the family vacation trip. In those days, I could get ten paperbacks for that price, plenty of good material to digest on the beach or in the car. I loved the atmosphere of learning that pervaded our household.

But sadness lingered in our home as well. Before I was born, my older brother, Alan, died of pneumonia at the age of nine months. My parents' fourth son, Paul, born three years after me, developed chronic, disabling mental illness in early childhood.

The tragedies continued. As an infant, my youngest brother, Douglas, developed Wilms' tumor, a cancer of the kidney that was incurable at the time. One night when I was eleven years old, my parents sat my older brother, Skip, and me down to tell us that Doug was very sick—that things looked very bad, and that he either would not live, or would need dialysis for the rest of his life.

I loved my baby brother. I had seen his first smiles and laughs, watched him learn to crawl, played with him, fed him his bottle, and nurtured him as well as an eleven-year-old boy can. He could *not* die! After my parents' announcement, I bolted from the room, scrambling up to my bedroom on the third floor, where I knelt next to my bed and uttered the first authentic prayer of my life. I had mouthed the lines at church and when the family said grace before meals, but prayer hadn't yet made a big impact on me. This day, though, I lay crumpled beside my bed crying and earnestly begging God to save my brother's life.

My brother Doug died the next day, the day before his first birthday.

"He would have been so sick, Dale," my parents told me, "it's better this way." They meant that Doug's whole life would have been severely marred by illness even if he could have survived. Whereas they found some comfort in this line of reasoning, I did not understand. But I quickly learned to shelve my grief, just as I had done when my grandfather, the missionary, had died the year before, and my architect grandfather several years earlier. My parents were people of great discipline and dignity. By their example, they taught me that emotions were to be addressed in private, so my grief remained inside.

But though God did not spare my brother's life, he gave me a gift that would help me heal myself and others. Shortly after Doug's death, I became aware of a profound desire to read and understand the Bible. I began reading it every night. I did not always understand what I read, but I kindled a lifelong romance with this book, which I would later understand to be the Word of God. I see now that my passion for the Bible was both a primitive attempt to cope with the loss of my brother ("Maybe if I read the Bible regularly, God won't punish or kill me") *and* a spiritual gift from God, a desire to know him more fully. I understand now that God does not always say "yes" to our desperate prayers for healing, but he does not leave us comfortless, either. One of God's greatest gifts is the healing of grief after the loss of a loved one. My hunger and thirst for the scripture, I believe, was God's healing touch in my young life, the nourishment my soul sorely needed.

I have read the Bible almost daily since that time, and I believe that this practice has formed me as a Christian, as a husband and father, and as a doctor. Through Old and New Testament accounts of healings, I have learned to believe that God *does* heal. This knowledge and faith, given through the scripture, has been borne out in my patients' lives and in my own life. Out of this love for God's Word, my faith has grown.

I can vividly recall the pain of Doug's death and can easily witness the numbing effects of mental illness in my brother Paul's life, but I believe God has relieved me of profound grief. The brief episodes of depression and anxiety I experienced, which required counseling in my early years of medical training, have also been lifted. My migraines have been similarly healed, though my neck, knee, and back pains—reminders of old football injuries—persist, at lower levels. Having suffered these disorders, I have greater compassion for my patients, a gift that helps me serve them better. Having been healed of some of them, I can communicate firsthand the experience of healing from God available to all of us as his children. Continuing to suffer with other illnesses has allowed me to sympathize with my patients' ongoing struggles and encourage them to seek God's grace and presence in their suffering.

STEP INTO MY OFFICE

I am writing this book in answer to a simple question: "How can 'the faith factor' help you?" Whether you are healthy today or seeking healing, this book will guide you through the growing scientific evidence that religious involvement is good for your physical, emotional, and spiritual health. I will suggest ways you can put this information to work in your life, and I will share the experiences of many of my patients who have found greater health and well-being through prayer, worship, scripture study, and the support of a faith community. First and foremost as a doctor, I can understand that you may wish to seek healing for yourself or a loved one as you read this book. And although I write from a Christian perspective, having accepted Jesus Christ as my Lord and Savior and the Bible as Holy Scripture, I hope that this book will bring healing and encouragement to people who may not share my particular convictions. Prayer, worship, and community are universal forms of expression. The Bible, after all, is not only a sacred book for Jews and Christians, but is undeniably the most important book in Western civilization, the preeminent source and inspiration for Western architecture, art, music, literature, philosophy, and ethics over the centuries.

My hope and prayer in writing this book is that it will assist in your healing and your growth as a person of faith, whatever your tradition. The medical benefits of faith are not limited to any single tradition, but are open to all.

Now I want to invite you to step into my office. Let me tell you about the exciting scientific studies that are proving that religion is good for your health.

PART I

Science

CHAPTER 1

The Faith Factor

Imagine for a moment that you are visiting your trusted physician for a routine physical examination. You don't have any serious problems, just a few aches and pains—nothing to worry about. Your doctor gives you a clean bill of health and perhaps some advice or medication for the minor problems you've reported. And then he or she says:

"I want you to know that there's something else you can do that will improve your chances of staying healthy. It's readily available, accessible, and free. Would you like to know more about it?"

Now imagine you have a serious medical problem—chest pains, for example. Your doctor, after reviewing the results of an angiogram (an X-ray test of the heart), recommends bypass surgery, and describes the procedure.

In response to your inquiry about how best to prepare for surgery, the doctor says, "I just finished reading an article in a medical journal that described one factor that will lead to a better recovery. Would you like to know what it is?"

It's hard to imagine saying "no," isn't it?

Based on the research data we now have at hand, your doctor could—from a strictly scientific point of view—recommend religious involvement to improve your chances of being able to:

- stay healthy and avoid life-threatening and disabling diseases like cancer and heart disease
- recover faster and with fewer complications if you *do* develop a serious illness
- live longer
- encounter life-threatening and terminal illnesses with greater peacefulness and less pain
- avoid mental illnesses like depression and anxiety, and cope more effectively with stress
- steer clear of problems with alcohol, drugs, tobacco
- enjoy a happier marriage and family life
- find a greater sense of meaning and purpose in your life

These benefits of religious involvement have been well documented by scientific studies over the last three decades, studies published in authoritative, peer-reviewed medical journals like *American Journal of Public Health, Cancer, American Journal of Psychiatry, American Journal of Medicine, Heart and Lung,* and many others. Several years ago, I helped summarize these findings in a review called *The Faith Factor: An Annotated Bibliography of Clinical Research on Spiritual Subjects.* I was already convinced of the value of faith before undertaking the task of editing this four-volume bibliography, but the research findings made me a confirmed believer in the widespread benefits of the remarkable catalyst for health called "the faith factor."

Whereas certain epidemiological factors, such as socioeconomic status, diet, and exercise, have effects on human well-being, religious involvement seems unique in its breadth of influence; benefits have been demonstrated for most dimensions of human health, ranging from disease prevention and treatment to recovery and coping, from issues at the beginning of life (infertility and premature birth) to the end of life (alleviating death anxiety). Yet, because of a gaping chasm between modern medical science and religion, the faith factor has been woefully neglected in research and practice for centuries. Why has this significant health factor been overlooked for so long?

THE SEPARATION OF MEDICINE AND RELIGION,
THE TWIN TRADITIONS OF HEALING

At one time, medicine and religion were so thoroughly united that a medicine man was a priest. Many cultures throughout the world still regard their healers in just this way. In the West, religion and medicine remained closely linked until the end of the medieval period. The first hospitals were founded in monasteries; physicians of this era were usually monks. The link could also be seen in diagnosis: illnesses like the plague were attributed to spiritual causes (God's retribution for the sinful practices of humans).

With the advent of the Scientific Revolution, however, the twin healing traditions were separated. This revolution had its roots in the work of philosophers like Descartes, Hume, and Locke, who promoted a new method for seeking knowledge. Truth could be discerned, the seventeenth-century French philosopher Descartes insisted, *only* through the examination of empirical data and a rational, scientific method. Building upon this notion, remarkable investigators helped to create the Scientific Revolution, an unprecedented rise in knowledge in all scientific fields.

Overwhelmed by these extraordinary developments in experimental science, the church saw its formerly undisputed authority and command over truth crumble away. Since the experimental method could not be readily or confidently applied to God or to our experiences of God, religion was rooted out of science, including medicine. As adherents of the scientific method and worldview gained control over the intellectual life of the West, reputable doctors were left with only those medical techniques that stood up to scrutiny under the experimental method of modern science.

Today, centuries later, we see the unfortunate consequences of this split between religion and medicine. Doctors live in a world completely dominated by Cartesian philosophy, trained to think only in terms of what can be empirically proved in the laboratory. The prospect of discussing religion—particularly subjective spiritual experiences—makes many doctors feel uncomfortable. If doctors are asked to pray with patients—in the examining room, before surgery, or at the hospital bedside—most feel completely out of their "professional" realm. Yet many people urgently want to talk about their faith when they are sick. When illness brings patients into our offices, they seek relief of their physical symptoms, but many seek more. They want to know: "*Why* am I sick? Am I being punished? What does God have to do with this? Is it okay to ask God to heal me? Will it make any difference if I do?"

No doctor can answer these questions definitively, but I believe we can learn to listen openly and compassionately to our patients' spiritual concerns. If we are willing and the situation is appropriate, we can do more, perhaps pointing out a scripture verse, perhaps sharing a prayer or insights from our own faith journeys, or encouraging counsel with a member of the clergy.

Given the scientific evidence emerging today about religious involvement and health, even René Descartes would have to agree: doctors who want to help other human beings who suffer, doctors who want to be healers of whole persons, have an obligation to address the spiritual lives of their patients. In doing so, doctors will improve their bedside manner, but, even more important, they will help patients activate the healing power of belief in their lives.

Until recently, most people had not heard about the clinical evidence supporting the faith factor. That has started to change, thanks to the pioneering work of medical researchers like Herbert Benson, Larry Dossey, and others, and by increased coverage of this topic by the popular media. Since this is still new territory for most of us, I would like first to give you an overview of what the exciting evidence has to tell us—and how it can change your life.

In order to understand these data, however, we first need to understand two key ideas on which most of the research in this field is based. I will cover them in detail in later chapters; for now, a brief description will suffice.

1. *There is a difference between religion and spirituality.* Whereas the word "spirituality" connotes an individual's private search for meaning and connection, particularly his or her relationship with God, "religion" suggests the individual's adherence to an organized set of beliefs and practices endorsed by a community of fellow believers. One can be religious *and* spiritual; in fact, the evidence points to this combination as the ideal for enhancing health and well-being. But one does not *have* to be

religious in order to be spiritual, or vice versa. (See chapter 8 for more on the relationship between religion and spirituality.)

2. *Frequency of worship-service attendance is most often used as a way of measuring religious involvement.* This is not because such attendance is the only valid indicator of religiosity, but simply because attendance is easier to measure than most other indicators, particularly the more personal, idio-syncratic factors like one's perception of how God is working in one's life. In other words, it is easy to determine how often a subject in a scientific study attends worship services; it is far more difficult to determine how often, or in what way, that person feels close to God. Therefore, through-out this book you will frequently read about church or synagogue atten-dance as a "marker" or proxy for religious involvement, and you will see frequent worship attendance considered an indicator of "high religiosity." This is simply because worship attendance has been studied far more fre-quently than any other single religious or spiritual variable. As I discuss in chapter 11, there are reasons to believe that worship-service attendance *is,* in fact, a critical component of the faith factor, but it is not the only indi-cator of religiosity or spirituality, and future studies of the faith-health link will undoubtedly shed light on other, less studied behaviors, beliefs, and attitudes.

PHYSICAL HEALTH:
PREVENTION, RECOVERY, AND SURVIVAL

For many people, it makes sense that religion can benefit mental or emo-tional health. But what about killer diseases like cancer and cardiovascu-lar disorders? Or crippling illnesses like rheumatoid arthritis?

Here's the good news: scientific studies show that religious involve-ment helps people *prevent* illness, *recover* from illness, and—most remark-ably—*live longer.* The more religiously committed you are, the more likely you are to benefit.

Prevention of Disease

Let's turn our attention first to studies showing that the faith factor helps prevent disease. A classic 1972 study of 91,909 individuals living in Washington County, Maryland, found that those who attended church once or more a week had significantly lower death rates from the following:

coronary-artery disease (50-percent reduction)

emphysema (56-percent reduction)

cirrhosis of the liver (74-percent reduction)

suicide (53-percent reduction)

The survey respondents who attended church regularly also experienced a lower incidence of pulmonary tuberculosis, vaginal trichomoniasis (a sexually transmitted disease), and abnormal cervical cytologies (precancerous and cancer cells in the cervix). This study generated a series of hypotheses regarding possible mechanisms for the faith factor's effects. The reduction in emphysema and coronary-artery disease among churchgoers leads to the possibility that the religious population smokes less. The lower rate of cirrhosis may be caused by a parallel reduction in alcohol use; the lowered rates of sexually transmitted disease and suicide suggest corresponding changes in sexual behavior and enhancement in coping with life's problems.

This provocative study raised as many questions as it answered, drawing scientists' attention to a possible connection between religious involvement and health and defining areas for future inquiry. Since the study did not "control for," or eliminate the statistical importance of, factors such as smoking and alcohol consumption, investigators could not determine whether the lower incidences of cirrhosis, emphysema, and coronary-artery disease among churchgoers were linked to regular attendance alone, to lessened tobacco-and-alcohol use, or to both. As I discuss in the following chapter, the importance of religion in encouraging the maintenance of good health habits must not be underestimated, but healthy lifestyle is not the only factor that explains the positive impact of faith on health.

Clearly, maintaining a healthy lifestyle is crucial to good health. Consider the two major killers in our society, heart disease and cancer. We know that the risk of developing heart disease and many types of cancer (including cancers of the lip, oral cavity, pharynx, esophagus, stomach, larynx, lung, and bladder) can often be significantly reduced by abstinence from tobacco and alcohol and by participation in positive health habits, including a low-fat diet, regular exercise, and appropriate management of stress. Scientists have shown that religiously observant people are more likely than the nonobservant to embrace and maintain positive health habits. For example, in a 1991 study of 1,077 students at Northern Illinois University, the highly religious students (one-sixth of the total) had better overall health, less sickness, fewer doctor visits, and fewer injuries than their less religious or nonreligious cohorts. These students also had significantly lower rates of alcohol, tobacco, and drug use, and they exercised and used automobile seatbelts more regularly.

The importance of positive health habits has been demonstrated even more dramatically in National Cancer Institute–funded studies of members of the Church of the Latter-Day Saints (Mormons). Scientists J. W. Gardner and J. L. Lyon found that religious involvement among Mormons promotes a healthy lifestyle, which, in turn, appears to have a significant role in the prevention and treatment of cancer. Among the Mormons studied, those who were more religiously involved developed significantly fewer cases of cancer than their less observant peers. (Higher levels of religious involvement were defined as follows: For men, higher positions within the lay priesthood hierarchy, which are achieved by demonstrating greater adherence to church doctrines, including abstaining from alcohol, tobacco, coffee, and tea, and conformity to standards such as payment of tithes, moral cleanliness, honesty, and regular attendance at church meetings. For women, by frequency of attendance at worship services and other church activities.)

• Mormon women who were more involved with their church had less than half the rate of cancers of the digestive and respiratory systems than those who were less religiously involved.
• Mormon women experienced cervical cancer at a rate 45 percent lower than the national average.
• Mormon men at higher priesthood levels were significantly less likely to develop leukemias and cancers of the lip, oral cavity, pharynx, esophagus, stomach, larynx, lung, and bladder than were their less committed Mormon peers.

Studies of Seventh-Day Adventists (SDA) have also shown the faith factor's potency as a disease-preventing force. Like Mormons, Seventh-Day Adventists abstain from smoking and drinking alcohol for religious reasons; many Adventists also adhere to a strict vegetarian diet as part of their religious practice. No doubt these health habits contributed to the dramatic results of a 1983 study of Seventh-Day Adventists in the Netherlands; male Adventists were found to live an average of *nine years longer* than men in the general population, women four years longer. The SDA members got only half as many cancers as their non-SDA neighbors, and 59 percent fewer cases of cardiovascular disease. A 1983 study of male Seventh-Day Adventists and other alcohol abstainers in Denmark found that Seventh-Day Adventists developed malignancies at a much lower rate than the general population—69 percent of the expected incidence.

Are Mormons and Seventh-Day Adventists healthier than the average population simply because they have better health practices (less smoking and drinking, healthier diet), or because they are more religious? The answer is "both": these individuals adopt better health practices *because* of their religion. They choose to eat in a healthy way and to refrain from smoking, drinking, and using illegal drugs in their desire to live holy lives and to follow the tradition of their forebears. Those who avoid unhealthy substances or who follow a vegetarian diet do so not only because they want to be healthier, but because they believe it will bring them closer to God, a strong incentive for maintaining what for many is a difficult discipline. Thus, their markedly better overall health is not just the result of healthy practices; it can be traced back to their religious commitment, which encourages healthy practices.

But religious commitment can be effective in the absence of such practices. Frequent church attenders who do not abstain from cigarettes, alcohol, and high-fat diets can still benefit from the faith factor. Consider hypertension, the "silent killer" that leads to stroke and other cardiovascular problems. A 1978 study of 355 men in Evans County, Georgia, showed that those who attended church one or more times per week had significantly lower blood-pressure readings than individuals who attended church less often. The positive link between church attendance and lower blood pressure held up *even if the church attenders were smokers!*

A 1982 study of 2,754 men and women in Tecumseh, Michigan, found that women who attended church more frequently lived longer than those who attended less frequently. Unlike the Washington County study cited above, the Tecumseh County study controlled for other factors—such as age, history of heart disease and bronchitis, and degree of impairment on breathing tests—in assessing the impact of church attendance. In other words, the studies' results were adjusted statistically to "even out" the differences between subjects *except for* their frequency of church attendance. Such controls allow researchers to draw conclusions like the following: if Mary and Martha, two subjects in the study, are the same age and have a similar medical status, but Mary attends church weekly and Martha goes once a year, Mary is statistically likely to live longer.

Religious involvement has a strong positive impact on longevity, both because it promotes good health habits and for reasons unrelated to health behaviors, which I will discuss in chapter 2. Given these data, the prescription for a longer life includes refraining from destructive habits like smoking, engaging in healthy habits like regular exercise, *and* attending worship services on a weekly basis, if not more often.

Recovery from Illness

Though religious involvement appears to decrease your chances of getting sick, it does not eliminate them. Still, even when serious illness strikes, religion seems to boost the recovery process significantly. A study conducted in 1995 by Thomas Oxman, M.D., of Dartmouth Medical School, followed the progress of 232 elderly patients who underwent open-heart surgery. The overall death rate among these patients was 9 percent in the first six months after surgery. But for patients who said they attended church regularly, the death rate was only 5 percent; the death rate for non–church attenders was nearly three times what it was for churchgoers. More impressive still, within this group of believers, the thirty-seven patients who described themselves as obtaining significant "strength and comfort" from their beliefs *all* survived the six-month period.

When surveyed, many patients acknowledge the healing power of prayer. In a 1986 study, 586 residents of Richmond, Virginia, were randomly selected for telephone interviews in which they were asked, among other questions, "Have you ever experienced a healing of a serious disease or physical condition that you believed resulted from prayer or considered to be a divine healing?" Fourteen percent of the respondents answered "yes" to this question. The conditions healed ranged from colds and flu to cancer, back problems, fractures, and emotional problems. This, of course, is self-reported, anecdotal evidence without medical documentation, but the survey is one of a number indicating the strong beliefs among patients that prayer has a measurable healing effect. This finding has helped spark a new interest in reintroducing the spiritual dimension into clinical care.

MENTAL AND EMOTIONAL WELL-BEING

These and other studies have proved the value of prayer and religious involvement in the prevention of and recovery from physical illness, including life-threatening diseases like cancer and heart disease. But what is the impact of the faith factor on mental illness and addictions, which cause immeasurable and protracted suffering for patients, their families, and society as a whole? Until recently, mental illnesses like depression and anxiety remained intractable despite medical science's best efforts. Today, these illnesses are often successfully treated by pharmaceuticals and psychotherapy. Addictions to substances like alcohol, illegal drugs, and tobacco are still difficult to treat successfully. But just as the faith factor can make a significant difference in cardiovascular disease and cancer, it promises tremendous benefits for mental disorders and addictions. In fact, the unparalleled success of the spiritually oriented Twelve Step programs (Alcoholics Anonymous, Narcotics Anonymous, and others) demonstrates that the faith factor may be the best hope for the successful treatment of addictions.

Depression and Grief

Since I have personally experienced the pain of depression, I am particularly encouraged by the hope religious involvement offers in treating this disorder, which Winston Churchill called "the black dog." Quite distinct from "the blues" or "the blahs," which affect us all from time to time, clinical depression is a disease that affects over eleven million Americans annually. For unknown reasons, the rate of depression among women is twice the rate among men. In this regard, a study by Drs. D. Hertsgaard and H. Light from North Dakota State University in Fargo offers particular promise. In evaluating 760 Midwestern women, the researchers found that those with two or more children under age fourteen scored highest on depression and anxiety scales, and those with no children scored lowest. Sharing in decision-making about farm operations and visiting friends more than once a month helped women avoid anxiety and depression. In addition, women who attended church more than once a month experienced significantly less anxiety and depression than those who attended less frequently or not at all. These data may point to new ways to prevent depression among women and other populations prone to this painful condition.

The faith factor also seems to help men ward off depression. A 1990 study of 451 African-American men and women evaluated the impact of church attendance and other measures of religiosity on depression and found that people with higher levels of religious involvement reported significantly less depression. In fact, men with low levels of religiosity scored almost twice as high on the depression scale as their more religious counterparts.

Depression particularly threatens people in situations of high stress, such as the loss of a loved one. Bereavement is the most stressful event in life for many of us, as it was for my own family. Several studies show that religious involvement helps prevent depression at such times. In a 1983 study of ninety-two families who had lost a child between 1975 and 1979, 70 percent of the parents surveyed said their religious beliefs gave them comfort at the time of their child's funeral. A year later, 80 percent of the parents had found strength and solace in their religion. Though the illness and death of a child can be a severe test of faith, the study revealed that 40 percent of the parents felt that their religious commitment was actually stronger after the child's death. These parents had better psychological adjustment and fewer physical symptoms than those who did not experience strengthening of their religious beliefs during the bereavement period.

The death of a spouse also presents enormous challenges, not only emotionally but also through the increased possibility of physical illness. Christopher Rosik, Ph.D., surveyed 165 widows and widowers in Los Angeles and Ventura Counties, California, looking for a connection between religious commitment and bereavement. He found that widows and widowers with an authentic sense of a personal relationship with God cope better with the loss of their spouses than do their nonreligious peers or religious individuals who do not experience an active awareness of the presence of God in their lives. Other studies have illuminated this important reality: religious belief and practice, particularly when accompanied by a profound personal spirituality, ease the life-shattering effects of grief and help bereaved people face and adjust to their losses.

Can religion be helpful in treating severe mental illnesses like schizophrenia? Although we need more research in this area, one Missouri study of four hospitals and mental-health centers conducted in 1985 shows promise. Researchers C. C. Chu and H. E. Klein evaluated 275 African-American patients with schizophrenia who had been admitted to psychiatric-treatment centers, in an effort to determine which factors might influence the rate of rehospitalization for such patients. They found that religious affiliation was associated with a decreased risk of rehospitalization, particularly when the patient's family encouraged him or her to attend worship services while in the hospital. Though many people with psychotic illnesses like schizophrenia experience religious delusions and use religious language to express their distress, religion can also be a positive factor in the lives of those suffering from these terrible diseases. The Chu-Klein study points to the possibility that religion can provide a framework of meaning and a network of support which serve to anchor severely mentally ill patients.

Addictions

The success of Twelve Step programs like Alcoholics Anonymous has proved the value of a spiritual approach to recovery from addiction. This is underscored by the scientific data from studies of addiction. A 1981 study at the United States Public Health Service Hospital in Fort Worth, Texas, evaluated 248 men, 87 percent of whom were Mexican-American, with a mean history of eight years of opiate abuse (mostly heroin), comparing the effectiveness of religious and nonreligious drug-abuse treatment programs. The results were dramatic: patients attending the religious programs were *almost ten times as likely* as those attending nonreligious programs to remain abstinent from heroin use one year after the program ended. They were also far less likely to be on parole or probation.

Of course, the best strategy in reducing addiction is a preventive one, particularly among adolescents, where vulnerability to substance abuse is especially high. Religion can help with prevention, too, according to numerous studies. Religiously involved youngsters are markedly less likely to use tobacco, alcohol, and illegal drugs. A 1980 study of adult alcoholics suggested that religious involvement in adolescence may function as a "vaccine" against alcoholism. In this study, psychiatrist David Larson, president of the National Institute for Healthcare Research and a pioneer in the study of the faith factor, found that 89 percent of the alcoholics interviewed had lost interest in religion as an adolescent; only 20 percent of the nonalcoholics reported a similar history. Alcoholism expert Dr. William Miller believes that alcoholism drives out spirituality, and spirituality drives out alcoholism. This is based on a phrase from a letter written by Dr. Carl Jung to Alcoholics Anonymous founder Bill Wilson:

You see, alcohol in Latin is *spiritus* and you use the same word for the highest religious experience. . . . The helpful formula therefore is: *spiritus contra spiritum.*

In young people as well as older folks, the vacuum caused by an absence of religious involvement is too often filled by alcohol or drug abuse. But parents can take heart from numerous studies showing that family religious involvement has a strong preventive effect on substance abuse. The data from a 1984 study of six hundred public-high-school students in Atlanta are particularly revealing:

	% Likely to Use Drink Weekly	*% Likely to Use Marijuana*	*% Likely to Use Other Drugs*
Students rating religion as "extremely important"	8	5	7
Students rating religion as "not too important"	26	23	25

	% Likely to Use Drink Weekly	% Likely to Use Marijuana	% Likely to Use Other Drugs
Students who attended church frequently	5	11	12
Students who attended church seldom	20	15	21

Many other studies confirm these results, including a 1986 study of 16,130 high-school seniors that found that the students' religiosity was the strongest factor in determining drug and alcohol abstinence or abuse—stronger even than family-related factors, including whether or not the student lived with both parents. So, in addition to parental "sermons" against substance abuse, young people appear to benefit from hearing real sermons during regular worship attendance.

Addiction to tobacco results in 340,000 premature deaths annually and costs our society an estimated $13 billion in health-care expenses each year—in addition to immeasurable suffering. The faith factor holds great promise in helping people break tobacco's powerfully addictive hold. As we have seen, many individuals, including Seventh-Day Adventists and Mormons, avoid tobacco use out of religious conviction. The results of a startling study published in 1987 suggest that another aspect of the faith factor may also help break the bondage of nicotine addiction.

In this study, conducted by Drs. M. Gmur and A. Tschopp in Switzerland, a faith-healing practitioner laid his hands on the heads of 532 smokers. This was the only treatment the smokers received, yet 40 percent of them abstained from smoking for at least four months after the laying on of hands—a remarkable result! (Compare this result to an estimated 2 percent success rate for smokers using behavior-modification techniques to help them quit, or 13 percent for those using nicotine-replacement therapy.) After one year, 33 percent of patients in the Swiss study had stayed smoke-free; after five years, 20 percent. When participants were interviewed twelve years after the initial treatment, 16 percent were continuing to abstain from smoking.

Could one simple "treatment" alone—the laying on of hands—be solely responsible for such positive results? Future studies could help answer this question, but we do know that the long-term nonsmokers tended to be regular church attenders who had high expectations for the laying on of hands. In other words, their faith may have given them a meaningful context for this treatment, thus increasing its effectiveness. Because the long-term abstainers tended to consume less alcohol than their counterparts, they may also have benefited from lowered exposure to "social smoking" at cocktail parties and other venues where smoking and drinking are combined.

This intriguing study shows that we have much more to learn about the potential of faith in helping people recover from addictions. By remaining free of addictions' bondage, we safeguard our physical health and protect our overall happiness and contentment. Avoiding substance abuse, in fact, is a cornerstone of what researchers call "quality of life."

THE PURSUIT OF HAPPINESS

Do you want a happier marriage and a healthier family? A sense of purpose and zest for life? Greater peace of mind and contentment? In scores of studies, religious involvement appears greatly to enhance quality of life for people of all ages and in many walks of life. We can see this effect in the results of a 1992 study conducted by the National Opinion Research Center, designed to assess the personal impact of *losing* one's religion. The researchers administered detailed surveys to 26,011 individuals over the course of eighteen years. They found that religiously active people were significantly more likely than the "religious disaffiliates" to be happily married, to say that they were "very happy," to belong to community organizations, and to have voted in a recent election. The disaffiliates had experienced much more unemployment within the previous five years than their religious counterparts.

An earlier study examining the relationship between religious commitment and quality of life showed a strong linkage between religious involvement and a sense of life as being worthwhile. This 1978 study of 2,164 American adults assessed not only religion's role in quality of life, but also the importance of marital status, age, income, race, education, and health. Of all these variables, respondents' beliefs about religion's importance in their lives was found to be *the single strongest predictor for positive quality of life.* Of those who rated religion extremely important, 59 percent found their lives to be "very worthwhile," as opposed to the 35 percent of those who believed religion to be unimportant. Both regular worship attendance and church membership were also linked to a high quality of life. These findings held true for both men and women, and for respondents at all income levels.

"The family that prays together, stays together." Remember that old adage? Many scientific studies confirm its truth: marriage clearly benefits from the faith factor. A 1980 study of 7,029 individuals found that the frequency of church or synagogue attendance was a key factor in divorce rates:

Frequency of Worship Attendance	Divorce/Separation Rate
Less than once a year	34%
Once to several times yearly	27%
Once a month or more	18%

A study of 2,278 Americans of all faiths showed that frequency of attendance at religious services was the strongest predictor of marital happiness for both men and women—stronger than education, age, family income, occupation level, and number of children at home. In fact, worship-service attendance was the only such factor shared by both sexes.

Families weather children's adolescent years—the terrible teens—much more effectively when religion is an important part of family life. In addition to helping teens avoid substance abuse, religious involvement appears to help them stay away from high-risk sexual activity and delinquency. Researchers studying fourteen hundred tenth-graders in 1977 found that religious involvement was inversely related to seventeen delinquent behaviors, including driving a car without a license, carrying a knife or razor, running away from home, fighting, buying and drinking alcohol, selling and using narcotics, sniffing glue, and vandalizing property.

At a time when even one high-risk sexual encounter can result in HIV infection, parents will be glad to know that the faith factor can help reduce adolescent sexual activity. In a 1991 study, adolescents who attended church frequently were significantly less likely to engage in premarital sex, especially if they belonged to conservative denominations. Religion's protective effect extends to college students as well, according to several studies. Even among students attending a religiously affiliated school, greater levels of religious activity and personal spirituality are associated with reduced levels of sexual activity: 80 percent of students attending church three times a week were virgins, compared with 37 percent of those who attended less than once a week. Since only abstinence or mutual, lifelong monogamy confer complete protection from the sexual transmission of diseases like AIDS, gonorrhea, syphilis, and herpes, sexual abstinence among unmarried teenagers and young adults can be seen, from a medical point of view, as good for the students' health.

These data suggest a need to re-examine and re-emphasize the roles of family and religious involvement in curbing behaviors that threaten health and happiness. Given the many dire health risks facing our children today, it is critical to investigate and once again embrace these life-giving traditions of connection and meaning.

HANDLING LIFE'S HURTS

Religious involvement has many beneficial effects, but it cannot ward off all of life's crises. We each face bereavement and, ultimately, our own death; most people must meet a number of other challenges as well—job loss, divorce, and serious illness and disability, to name a few. Many studies have shown that religious involvement aids people in coping with a wide variety of crises, boosting our resilience, peace of mind, and endurance.

Few stressors can equal the stress of imprisonment. To assess whether religious involvement helps older men cope with life in prison, prominent gerontologist Dr. Harold Koenig of Duke University interviewed ninety-six inmates and found that 32 percent cited religion as their most helpful coping mechanism. Inmates who attended worship services weekly were much less likely to complain about physical symptoms than non-church-attending prisoners. Dr. Koenig and his colleagues also studied older male inpatients in a Veterans Administration hospital in Durham, North Carolina. In this population, too, those who frequently turned to religion as a method of coping were significantly less depressed than their nonreligious peers. Twenty-one percent of the men stated that religion was "the most important thing that keeps me going." Religious involvement in prison also appears to have life-changing potential, according to a 1997 study that showed that the inmates who most frequently attended Bible studies conducted by Prison Fellowship, a Christian ministry, were much less likely to be re-arrested than those who did not attend—14 percent versus 41 percent, a significant difference that offers new possibilities for dealing with recidivism.

Caring for chronically ill loved ones poses enormous physical and emotional challenges for the caregiver, but a 1994 study showed that the faith factor can offer help in this area as well. The study examined the relationship between religious participation and well-being by assessing these two factors in eighty-four elderly caregivers of Alzheimer's patients and eighty-one noncaregivers in the same age group. Not surprisingly, the caregivers reported a lower overall sense of well-being than the noncaregivers. But the caregivers who attended worship services regularly and said that their spiritual needs were being met experienced greater levels of well-being and lower levels of stress than caregivers who reported that their spiritual needs were not being met.

Aging is another significant life crisis, which presents a wide array of potential stressors, from disability to isolation to loss of purpose. Although a 1976 study of 272 patients (aged sixty to ninety-four) did not establish that religiously active older people lived longer than their nonreligious counterparts, it found that they *were* significantly happier and felt more useful. (Later studies have shown that religiously committed people live longer; see chapter 7 for more on this.) Among the 1,170 respondents to a 1982 survey, the older men and women who attended church regularly said they were *more* satisfied with their lives than they had been fifteen years earlier. Dr. Koenig, mentioned above, has conducted many studies of the link between religious involvement and positive quality of life in older Americans. In a 1988 study, he focused on the use of religion in coping among the aging, asking respondents how they handled life crises such as marital problems, injury or illness, business failure, or financial problems. By far the most popular coping mechanisms among the participants were religious in nature: placing one's trust in God, prayer, and finding help and strength from God, among others. Even support from family and friends was not as valuable as religious coping mechanisms to this group.

Serious physical illness also presents the prospect of loss and pain, but here again, the faith factor offers hope and help. A 1982 study examined the role of religious involvement in the lives of patients undergoing chronic hemodialysis, a stressful medical procedure which patients with kidney failure require several times weekly to stay alive. Patients needing hemodialysis struggle with illness *and* with the difficulty of their treatment, which can seriously disrupt work and family schedules. Researcher M. E. O'Brien found that hemodialysis patients who attended weekly worship services were more likely than nonreligious patients to comply with their medical regimen—an important factor in severe illness. The religious patients also reported less isolation and fewer feelings of powerlessness, had more satisfying social interactions, and credited their religion with helping them adjust to their illness.

These findings are echoed in a study of an even more severely impaired group of people—patients with spinal-cord injuries. Researcher Susan D. Decker, Ph.D., of the University of Portland School of Nursing, assessed the life satisfaction of a hundred paraplegics and quadriplegics over age forty, and found that the more religious individuals reported a significantly better quality of life than nonreligious patients.

Studies of patients with terminal cancer have also shown that religious involvement helps people deal with life's most difficult moments. A 1978 study of death anxiety among terminally ill patients found that dying patients with strong religious beliefs reported significantly lower levels of death anxiety than their nonreligious counterparts. In fact, religious involvement was more important to the dying patients' sense of well-being than low pain levels or close family support.

In another study of people with terminal cancer, researchers found that patients who regularly went to church had much less fear of death than those who did not attend worship services; religious patients also exhibited a higher degree of courage in dealing with their illness. Considering the benefits of religious involvement in facing death, we can easily see why "there are no atheists in foxholes." Human beings under threat of imminent death reflexively reach for the comfort and sustenance that faith offers. Given the findings of previously cited studies indicating lower anxiety and depression among religiously involved people, it appears that the dying person will maintain the greatest equanimity if he or she has developed a life of faith and religious practice over a number of years, rather than praying frantically to a little-known God at the moment of crisis.

A MEDICAL BREAKTHROUGH
OF UNPRECEDENTED PROPORTIONS?

As much as or more than any other factor measured by epidemiologists, religious involvement appears to promote health and well-being virtually from cradle to grave. Whatever life challenges we face, research shows that we will face them better if we have authentic religious belief and practice as cornerstones of our lives.

I've taken you on this "whirlwind tour" of the faith-factor scientific data to introduce you to these findings in their extraordinary scope. The tour is by no means inclusive; as you will see, the findings from many more remarkable clinical studies await you. In later chapters, I will go into each area—physical health and mortality, mental health, addictions, coping, and quality of life—in greater depth. I will examine the data in greater detail, share case histories of my patients (and myself), and suggest ways you might put the faith factor to work in your life.

For now, however, we must put the findings in context, and consider whether, from a scientific point of view, the re-emergence of the faith factor might truly be one of the most significant medical breakthroughs of this century or the next. There are many questions to be answered. Are the findings of all these studies truly valid, or mere flukes? If they *do* hold true (and I believe they do), other questions remain: *Why* does religion have such a strong effect on health and well-being? *How* does the faith factor literally bring about changes in our bodies? *Which* types of religious practice will be most effective? And, perhaps most troubling, we must look at those rare but important instances in which religious involvement *harms* people instead of healing them.

—————————— ✛ ——————————

CHAPTER 2

Too Good to Be True?
A Critical Look at the Faith Factor

"Okay," you may be saying to yourself, "let me get this straight. This doctor is telling me that having faith is good medicine? If I just pray, read scripture, and worship every week, I'll feel better, mentally, physically, and spiritually? And I'll live longer and better? *Right!* Sorry, Doc, but isn't this all too good to be true?"

Congratulations! Your skepticism is wise. It means you're looking out for yourself, and as a doctor I urge you to do exactly that—to take responsibility for your own health by making intelligent decisions and lifestyle choices. Asking questions about the data I've presented means you're not jumping onto the latest bandwagon just because it's headed your way. Fortunately, this time the bandwagon in health care is scientifically solid, despite some definite risks and possible negative effects of religion when it is misused, and I welcome the chance to address your questions and concerns. To place the benefits we outlined in the last chapter into proper perspective, let's examine together the reliability of the faith-factor data, and look as well at the occasional downside of religious involvement.

STORKS AND BABIES—AND THE FAITH FACTOR?

Once upon a time, in a faraway country, people witnessed the unfolding of a natural wonder. In a single year, the number of storks seemed to double or even triple. These big, gangly birds seemed to be everywhere you looked—in the trees, on ponds and rivers, and especially on rooftops in all the towns and cities. The government's chief naturalist undertook a stork census and pronounced that, indeed, the nation was swimming in storks, but no one, not even the chief naturalist, could explain why.

Later that year, the faraway country experienced another "bumper crop": an unprecedented number of babies were born. Obstetricians were called in from other nations just to manage the overflow. Hospitals were so crowded that women had babies on every floor, in every hallway. When the records were tallied, government statisticians confirmed what everybody already knew: the birthrate had risen dramatically in that particular year. Scholars and shopkeepers alike debated the causes of this baby boom. Was it the newly shortened work week? The increasingly explicit popular books and movies? Or the series of blizzards and squalls that had inundated the country the previous winter?

Finally, an eminent thinker from the nation's top university put the puzzle pieces together. He published an article that shook the academic community, proposing for the first time that the number of storks living in a country is directly related to the number of babies born in a given year. In fact, he said, storks *cause* the birth of babies, and there was good reason for further investigation into the mechanism of this previously unsuspected phenomenon.

A fable? Yes, but it serves as an example of how unrelated facts can be incorrectly linked, thus producing statistically significant—but invalid—scientific conclusions. Some critically thinking readers are doubtless wondering if the faith factor's effects on health might fall into the storks-and-babies category of "scientific" reasoning. Even people of faith who want to embrace the promising news about the health benefits of religious involvement may ask, "Are these studies genuine, or is all of this just wishful thinking? Can we really trust the 'faith-factor' data?"

Good news! By the standards of science, the faith-factor data are, in fact, quite reliable. We medical scientists are not jumping to conclusions when we say religion is good for your health. The studies I discuss in this book have met the standards of scientific inquiry, having been conducted according to its established guidelines, which include providing a careful description of the research methods (so the experiment can be repeated) and the complete disclosure of data for review by other scientists. Any scientific research may be influenced by researcher bias, but the soundness of the faith-factor data is confirmed by the replicability of these findings: in one review, over 75 percent of 325 studies of different types, undertaken by hundreds of different researchers, have produced findings indicating the benefit of religious involvement to health and well-being.

An *individual* study may have more or less scientific merit when subjected to close scrutiny. I have carefully reviewed the studies you will read about in this book to ensure that they meet the prevailing scientific standards of reliability and validity. However, considering the *cumulative* impact of the faith-factor studies, epidemiologists are obliged to address this relationship seriously in their studies.

To answer more definitively any questions you may have about the validity of the data, let me explain some factors in determining scientific credibility. Jeffrey S. Levin, Ph.D., M.P.H., an associate professor of family and community medicine at the Eastern Virginia Medical School faculty and a leading theoretician on the epidemiology of religion, has posed three crucial questions for consideration in reviewing the faith-factor data as a whole, a type of study known as a "meta-analysis":

Is there an association between religion and health? Yes, religious involvement is associated with positive effects on health in numerous studies of different designs, says Dr. Levin. He notes that more religiously strict groups, like Orthodox Jews, Latter-Day Saints (Mormons), and Seventh-Day Adventists, appear to enjoy greater health benefits because of their religious commitment and healthy lifestyle. Even when religiosity is measured in less strictly observing populations, data from multiple studies show "a trend toward better health and less morbidity and mortality, across the board, in the presence of higher levels of religiosity." The trend is observed in many denominations and for many aspects of physical and mental health.

Is the link between religion and medicine valid? This question is harder to answer. Scientists know that both chance and bias can influence a body of data. In every scientific experiment, observed results can be simply due to chance (random variation), in the same way that a flipped coin can turn up heads a few times in a row. But if we flip the coin a thousand times, it should turn up heads only 50 percent of the time (unless the coin has been altered). As Dr. Levin points out, chance is not likely to have played a major role in producing the faith-factor findings, because they have been identified in so many diverse settings, using such a variety of study designs, and because they produce positive results so commonly—with more than three-fourths of the published studies demonstrating the beneficial effects of religious involvement on health.

What about bias? To determine this, we must also look at what science calls *confounders,* or seeming linkages between a given factor and research results that are, in fact, spurious, usually because of a variable that has not been accounted for. To show what I mean, let's imagine that I have undertaken a study of sickle-cell anemia in two groups of people in the same city: members of the Bible Way Church and members of the Metropolitan Civic Association. I find that the incidence of sickle-cell anemia is dramatically higher among the Bible Way Church members, and I conclude that attending this church increases your chances for contracting the disease. A thoughtful critic might ask: What are the age, sex, ethnic, educational, and health-status comparisons between the groups? We then discover that the Bible Way Church is almost entirely African-American and the Metropolitan Civic Association is almost exclusively white.

Since we also know that sickle-cell anemia affects only African-Americans, we would now have to withdraw our invalid conclusion that church attendance causes this disease. Of course, if we did *not* know about this effect of ethnicity, we might reasonably hypothesize that religious involvement could be deadly.

Given that our scientific knowledge of human health is by no means perfect or complete, such confounders could easily arise as we evaluate the link between religion and health. For example, some have questioned the link between worship-service attendance and health, saying that people who are physically well enough to attend will naturally constitute a healthier group than those who are unable to attend for health reasons. In fact, however, according to researcher William J. Strawbridge of the Human Population Laboratory of the University of California, persons with physical disabilities are actually *more* likely to attend church. In addition, the effects of physical disability can be evaluated and controlled statistically. More carefully designed studies (including those discussed in this book) do control for these confounders in their statistical analyses, and most of these studies continue to show health benefits from religion.

Is it causal? Can we confidently say that religious involvement *causes* better physical and psychological health? In an influential article published in 1994 in the journal *Social Science and Medicine,* Dr. Levin says "maybe." To put his uncertainty into proper context, we must understand the rigors of the scientific definition of causality. For example, despite the existence of hundreds of studies showing an *association* between high blood cholesterol and heart disease, doctors cannot say unequivocally that high cholesterol is *the* cause of heart disease, because researchers have not yet determined exactly how the cholesterol acts to create coronary disease. Still, on the basis of the many studies showing a strong association between this factor and heart disease, medical science now firmly endorses the lowering of blood-cholesterol levels as a potentially life-saving preventive measure.

To demonstrate causality in medicine, research findings must be consistent, replicable, and unequivocal. This is most commonly seen in the case of diseases caused by infection or genetic factors. For example, all people who have AIDS have been previously infected with HIV; no one who has not first been infected with HIV has developed AIDS; there are no exceptions, no "gray areas." Therefore, we can safely conclude that HIV causes AIDS. A similar analysis can be made of individuals who have sickle-cell anemia: without the genetic abnormality that causes this disease, you cannot contract it; with it, you cannot avoid the illness.

Few other relationships between disease-causing agents and illness are so clear, however. In most cases, medical science works with probabilities. We know that disease-causing factors such as high blood cholesterol, diabetes, smoking, lack of exercise, and heredity make the development of coronary disease more probable. However, we cannot say that every person who is subject to one or more of these factors will develop heart disease.

In a similar way, we can conclude from the faith-factor data that religious involvement is a factor positively associated with greater longevity, prevention of certain diseases, faster recovery from some illnesses, and higher quality of life. In practical terms, this means there is a probability that a fifty-five-year-old African-American female who attends church weekly is more likely to live longer, avoid certain diseases, recover more quickly from some illness, and be happier than a fifty-five-year-old African-American woman who does *not* attend church at all. However, the faith factor's effects cannot be evaluated in binary terms—as either "yes" or "no," healthy or unhealthy. In no instance can you say that the total absence or presence of religion would eliminate all disease; we all know nonreligious people who are in great health and deeply devout people who are sick. Rather than looking for an all-or-nothing paradigm, we must consider religious involvement as a more fluid variable in the equation of health and well-being than other, binary variables, such as race, age, gender, smoking, and the like. The faith factor is one of many factors in a complex web, but this does not lessen its significance as a health-enhancing agent.

Until we have the results of many more carefully designed long-term studies of religious involvement, spiritual interventions, and health, scientists will not be able to answer "Is it causal?" with a definite "yes" or "no." But as we await new findings, the data we have today are strong enough from a scientific point of view to warrant the attention of scientists and physicians, even skeptics.

HOW RELIGION PROMOTES HEALTH: WHAT WE KNOW TODAY

As a person of faith, I believe God acts directly in our lives. To me, it is natural to assume that a loving God can and does answer our prayers for health and healing. However, this is a *theological* conclusion, a matter of faith, and I am writing this book first and foremost as a medical doctor, interested in matters and conclusions of science. Of course, we will never fully know how the faith factor works, because the transcendent dimension of life does not yield up all of its secrets to even the most skilled and aggressive researchers. By definition, the workings of an infinite, transcendent deity cannot be fully understood by finite human beings, no matter how excellent their science may appear to be. The results of studies of intercessory prayer in particular point to this transcendent dimension. This dimension's effects on human health can, to some extent, be measured, but they cannot be controlled or fully understood. Remembering that we can never fully plumb God's depths through research, we can still try to learn everything possible about how religious involvement affects health from a scientific point of view. As with other areas of medicine, ultimate mystery will always remain. A certain measure of faith, even in assessing the medical effects of religious involvement, is needed.

What can I tell you that we *do* know today about how religious involvement promotes health? The answer consists of a number of *subfactors* or *components*. Scientists have not pinpointed a specific health-enhancing chemical substance that is released into the bloodstream when people pray for themselves. A great deal of research must be conducted before such a mechanism is identified. Though we cannot point to a clearly established, single aspect of religious involvement that causes better health, my extensive review of the scientific literature reveals that religious involvement can be seen as a unique "combination agent" that efficiently delivers a series of powerful, interrelated ingredients promoting health and well-being. Some of the ingredients I have identified can be found in nonreligious settings, but they are more commonly found operating together in groups that endorse specific beliefs about the transcendent, or nonmaterial, dimension of existence and embrace practices related to those doctrines—in other words, religious organizations. (See chapter 8 for an extended discussion of religious involvement, particularly worship-service attendance, as the most efficient mechanism for delivering all of the faith-factor components.)

To help grasp the concept of the faith factor and its ingredients, I invite you to think of an old-fashioned doctor's bag, like the large beat-up black leather one my father carried on his house calls. I remember it in vivid

41

detail, not only because I was privileged to accompany him (and it!) on house calls, but because the bag was often left next to my chair in the kitchen, always at hand in case of an emergency.

As a youngster, I was in awe when Dad opened that bag and pulled out the right remedy for each patient—an injection to relieve a lady's nausea, some nitroglycerine for a farmer's chest pain, or some salve and sterile dressings for a girl's wound. It seemed to me there was something special for every sick person in that bag. Today, as a physician myself, I realize it wasn't just the individual remedy that made the patient better. All the elements—the reassurance of my father at the door with his bag, his gentle manner, the power of the treatment procedures, the "laying on of hands," and the faith of the patient—worked together to promote wellness.

Just as Dad brought to his patients many healing elements in his bag, I believe that the Divine Physician brings us healing elements in the inter-related and interdependent components of the faith factor I have identi-fied through my research and analysis. Please join me as we look through this "divine doctor's bag," examining the various remedies contained therein.

Remedy No. 1: Equanimity— Overcoming the Wear and Tear of Life

We live in a fast-paced society replete with threats to our safety. The nightly news chants a despairing litany of mayhem and disaster. Our schools and streets are no longer safe. Jobs we once thought of as secure vanish overnight, and financial disaster can quickly follow. We no longer share the sense of connectedness and purpose that once characterized neighborhoods, cities, and even nations. These stress-inducing factors leave us feeling out of control and anxious, and our increased stress levels seriously threaten our physical and emotional health.

But stress *can* be buffered; its wear and tear on our bodies and minds can be diminished. We can use methods of relaxation and meditation to clear our minds and free our bodies from the tension of contemporary liv-ing. Through his pioneering research, cardiologist Herbert Benson has identified a key method of stress buffering.

In a 1975 book, Dr. Benson explained the effects of stress on human physiology and how these effects can be countered through a simple form of meditation that elicits "the Relaxation Response." To evoke the Relaxation Response, we must take a series of steps (outlined in chapter 9), which include repeating a word, phrase, prayer, or sound, and passively disregarding distracting thoughts, returning to the focus word or phrase whenever these thoughts arise. Practiced regularly, the Relaxation Response has proved beneficial in the treatment of hypertension, irregularities in heart rhythm, chronic pain, insomnia, anxiety, depression, infertility, and the side effects of treatments for cancer and AIDS. Dr. Benson found that 80 percent of patients chose to use a prayer or religious phrase (such as "Heavenly Father," "Lord God," "Jesus," or "Mary") as their focus for eliciting the Relaxation Response, a finding that reflects the highly religious nature of Americans. To his surprise, this eminent cardiologist and scientist found himself teaching prayer.

Long before Dr. Benson identified the Relaxation Response, religious practitioners were bringing it about through prayer and meditation. As Dr. Benson writes:

> The Relaxation Response has always existed in the context of religious teachings. Its use has been most widespread in the Eastern cultures, where it has been an essential part of daily existence. But its physiology has only recently been defined. Religious prayers and related mental techniques have measurable, definable physiologic effects on the body. . . .

These effects include:

- a decreased heart rate
- a lower metabolic rate (the rate at which the body burns oxygen)
- a lower rate of breathing
- slowing of brain waves

You might say that, when people work to produce the Relaxation Response, they give their bodies a "time-out": a period of deep rest and relief from stress. Thus, any condition made worse by stress can be ameliorated by regular use of the Relaxation Response, whether it is brought about by Dr. Benson's technique, or by other methods, such as centering prayer, yoga, and Buddhist mindfulness practices like slow walking. In addition, relaxation has been associated with enhanced measures of immunity, including increased natural killer-cell activity and enhanced ability of the immune system to control virus replication.

The stress-buffering and immune-enhancing effects of meditative prayer techniques form one of the faith factor's most powerful components.

Remedy No. 2: Temperance— Honoring the Body as a Temple of the Spirit

As previously mentioned, some religious sects demand that adherents refrain from certain disease-inducing behaviors. We can see the roots of such recommendations in the dietary laws given to the Jews in the Old Testament and proscriptions against alcohol abuse in both the Old and New Testaments, some of which still hold up as medically excellent advice today.

Anyone, religious or not, who quits smoking, refrains from excessive drinking, or avoids a high-fat diet will reap health benefits. However, as we discussed above, some religious sects actively promote a healthy lifestyle as part of their doctrine, which seems to help people persevere with difficult disciplines such as maintaining a low-fat diet. In addition, deeply religious patients are more successful in avoiding unhealthy substances: their faith has provided both the motivation and the means for maintaining healthy habits. Although their main motivation is to grow in holiness, such believers often gain a secondary benefit: better health.

Remedy No. 3: Beauty— Appreciating Art and Nature

Have you ever felt exhilaration when you heard a glorious piece of music? Have you been moved to tears by the sight of a vivid sky at sunset? The human appreciation for beauty seems universal. We crave aesthetic pleasure on a deep level; we are enriched by our experiences of beauty, lifted up and refreshed, and a growing body of evidence indicates that aesthetic experience has demonstrable health benefits as well. Studies have shown that music, for example, can help improve the mobility of stroke or Parkinson's-disease patients, lift depression and anxiety, and even lessen the amount of anesthesia needed by women during childbirth. Many surgeons listen to music in the operating room: a fascinating study of fifty male surgeons showed that listening to music can reduce elevations in blood pressure and heart rate that often accompany performing tasks under pressure.

Visual pleasure, too, seems to be good for your health. In my own hospital, Georgetown University Medical Center, the televisions in patients' rooms offer an unusual sight on one channel: an uninterrupted view of the hospital chapel. Periodically, patients viewing this channel can watch a worship service take place; most of the time, they see only the camera's still view of the altar, but many patients choose to keep this channel on constantly. The chapel's pleasant tranquillity and its visual symbols of faith are reassuring and calming images.

Being present at worship services often provides a larger dose of aesthetic "medicine." In most places of worship, special efforts are made to provide beauty. Stained-glass windows, soaring architecture, floral arrangements all conspire to please the eye. Even the plainness of a Quaker meeting house gives us a sense of harmony and balance. Sacred music—whether ancient chant or contemporary praise songs, whether in Hebrew, Greek, Latin, or Old Church Slavonic—seems to soak into our very bones, carrying the message of God's glory and God's love deep into our beings. In some traditions, incense is used to represent our prayers wafting upward to God, and thus our sense of smell is stimulated.

Remedy No. 4: Adoration— *Worshiping with Our Whole Beings*

Christians who have memorized familiar hymns, Jews who have sung "Torah Ora" in temple when the Torah scroll is presented, and Buddhists who for years have chanted their prayers in the patterns of that ancient tradition know there's something special about participating in worship music. Singing allows us to engage our whole selves, body, mind, and spirit, as we express our feelings about our God and our lives. Active participation in music can deepen the health benefit of worshiping God.

Music deeply influences our memories as well. When you hear a favorite song from a particularly happy time in your life, it lifts your spirits; sometimes hearing music makes us feel transported back to another time and place. That powerful linkage of memories to music is captured in the familiar phrase, "They're playing our song." Personally, when I sing Christmas carols each year at my church's Christmas Eve service, the memories evoked—combined with the beauty of the hymns and the meaning of the holiday—bring tears to my eyes. I am fully engaged—physically, by the lusty activity of singing; mentally, as I read the carol texts and ponder their meaning; spiritually, as I pray through song; emotionally, as I am taken back like Ebenezer Scrooge to the images of earlier Christmases, of neighborhood carol sings, of midnight services, of hymnfests around the piano and the fireplace.

Movement used in worship also engages us on all levels of being, including the physical. We move to assume worship postures—kneeling, standing, bowing our heads, folding our hands, genuflecting, lifting our hands in praise. In some traditions, we also move to dance worshipfully.

Through worship, we turn our whole selves in love toward the Divine, activating, uniting, and reinvigorating body, mind, and spirit.

Remedy No. 5: Renewal— Confessing and Starting Over

Carrying the burden of guilty feelings can literally make us sick. As a physician, I have often witnessed patients' transformation once they have "confessed" a dark, long-held secret to me or to a trusted spiritual adviser. In both Judaism and Christianity, believers are urged to confess their sins and repent, and are given formal, regular opportunities to confess and to receive absolution, or assurance of forgiveness. The rhythm of regular confession and absolution, both in group and individual worship, allows us to recognize our mistakes, to share our painful feelings with God and with others, and to turn over a new leaf. Though guilt and regret certainly have their purposes, they can damage us mentally and physically if they are not released and resolved appropriately; confession and forgiveness within our religious traditions allow us to learn and to move on, rather than becoming unhealthfully preoccupied with our shortcomings.

Remedy No. 6: Community—
Bearing One Another's Burdens

It is a well-documented fact that, if you want to be as healthy as possible, it is important to maximize your social-support network—the group of family and friends who offer you practical help, emotional support, and spiritual encouragement in time of need. People who are isolated and lonely have poorer health than those who enjoy a network of caring people. Although there have been relatively few studies to date on intercessory prayer, or prayer said on behalf of another person, the faith-factor research to date indicates that your family's and friends' prayers for you may also have a powerful positive effect, as has been seen in a study by Dr. Randolph Byrd of patients in a hospital coronary care unit. (See chapter 9 for a detailed discussion of this study.)

Why is social support so important? Clearly, humans are social beings; we need each other in many ways. The mere presence of others may cause our brains to produce endorphins, the natural opiatelike substances that induce a feeling of well-being; the lack of human companionship has been linked to depression of the immune system. This is demonstrated by a study of medical students that found that lonelier students have lower natural killer-cell activity, and by a study showing that more isolated psychiatric patients have lower natural killer-cell activity, poorer immune responsiveness, and higher levels of stress hormones than others. On a more pragmatic level, friends bear one another's burdens, lightening the load of damaging stress. Social support lets us know we're not alone in facing life's difficulties, which can be a great consolation in times of stress. These advantages can be gleaned by social support in a nonreligious setting, but a number of studies indicate that social support in a religious context is even more beneficial, as I discuss in chapter 8.

Remedy No. 7: Unity—
Gaining Strength Through Shared Beliefs

People instinctively gravitate toward people who are like them; we know we have a better chance of connecting with individuals who share our point of view, whether in a secular setting like business, sports, or politics, or in our religious lives. Our comfort level rises as we learn of commonalities between members of a group, and the group that is unified around common values generates a kind of power that can achieve great things, whether it be the crowds of young people at Woodstock who ushered in the Age of Aquarius, or the clergy and volunteers who undergirded the civil-rights movement.

As a person of faith, when I attend worship, I enter into a community of persons who share common beliefs. I enjoy the comfort of "fitting in," being part of a group, even part of a long tradition of believers; I relax into a feeling of safety. My mind-set is deeply influenced by the principles and practices of my religion, which are reinforced by worship, teaching, and fellowship. If my faith flags momentarily, my spiritual brothers and sisters will remind me of God's promises and point me back to the tenets we hold in common. Sharing beliefs with fellow pilgrims can give us strength and relieve the isolation we so often encounter in our rootless, secular society.

Remedy No. 8: Ritual—
Taking Comfort in Familiar Activities

The effect of the aesthetic in religious experience and the power of religious singing and dancing are magnified by repetition. They become *rituals.* Our brains seem to be "hard-wired" to hold on to the experience of ritual. As Herbert Benson writes in *Timeless Healing:*

> . . . the brain retains a memory of the constellation of activities associated with the ritual, both the emotional content that allows the brain to weigh its importance and the nerve cell firings, interactions, and chemical releases that were first activated.

Most people already recognize the benefits of nonreligious ritual. Baseball players and golfers typically take the same number of practice swings in the same manner day after day. Children (and adults!) obtain benefit from bedtime rituals of reading or bath-taking that facilitate their transition to sleep. In certain cases, like patients with obsessive-compulsive disorder (OCD), rituals provide only temporary relief; a common example is washing one's hands hundreds of times a day. OCD patients begin by using rituals to reduce their anxiety. Unfortunately, as the disease progresses, the rituals' ability to ease anxiety dwindles.

We who engage in religious ritual also seek to allay anxiety, particularly over death. According to psychoanalytic theory, every person experiences a deep-seated death anxiety that motivates a number of behaviors, including the repetition of comforting words or gestures. When you repeat a prayer you have said hundreds of times before, when you sing a hymn you have known since childhood, when you kneel at the altar rail for communion for the thousandth time, you activate the calming power of ritual. To understand this power, we can simply reflect on the consternation that arises when worship rituals undergo change. Few initiatives cause greater division and pain in religious communities. Combined with the pleasure, comfort, and meaning we experience through the aesthetics of worship, ritual can give us a sense of security, assuring us that we have reached a safe harbor in our stormy world.

Remedy No. 9: Meaning— Finding a Purpose in Life

Human beings crave meaning. In fact, writes psychiatrist and Holocaust survivor Victor Frankl:

> Man's search for meaning is the primary motivation in his life. . . . This meaning is unique and specific in that it must and can be fulfilled by him alone; only then does it achieve a significance which will satisfy his own *will* to meaning.

This central search for meaning is accentuated in times of illness and disability. Again and again, my patients respond to illness by asking: "Why is this happening to me? Why now? What is the meaning of this illness in my life?" We create symbols, stories, systems of philosophy, transcendent works of art—all to make sense of our existence. Without a sense of purpose, we can literally wither and die. A good example of this phenomenon is the widow or widower who has spent years caring devotedly for a sick spouse. Shortly after the spouse dies, often within the year, the surviving mate, though apparently healthy, develops an illness and dies. Bereft of the sense of purpose provided by the task of caregiving, the individual cannot find a reason to meet the challenge of grief and find new purpose in life. Reacting to these emotions and to this mind-set, the immune system is overwhelmed and unable to respond properly, and disease follows.

Even in the midst of life's greatest difficulties, religion provides a framework of meaning that helps people find significance, thus alleviating the profound anxiety of meaninglessness. Our understanding and practice of faith give us the opportunity to live fully, knowing there is a reason we are here. As a consequence, we also enjoy better health.

Remedy No. 10: Trust— "Letting Go and Letting God"

In the Judeo-Christian tradition, our all-powerful Creator God is also *immanent,* present and involved in the minutiae of our daily lives. Veterans of Twelve Step groups express their willingness to invoke the immanence of a Higher Power through a familiar slogan: "Let go and let God." Our lives teach us that we have control over only a limited set of circumstances; we cannot solve all our problems through our own efforts. People of faith learn to turn their concerns over to God through prayer, asking for guidance, intervention, and strength. Just as confession and absolution offer relief from the crippling effects of guilt, "turning things over" allows us to acknowledge our relative powerlessness and to seek help from God. When we "let go and let God," we release our feverish attempts to control the uncontrollable, and our painful feelings of anxiety diminish.

Remedy No. 11: Transcendence— Connecting with Ultimate Hope

Often, our cares and concerns threaten to overwhelm us. We worry about work, finances, the IRS, our children, health, even our spiritual lives: "Am I good enough? Am I really pleasing God?" Important as these concerns may be, we need to remember that they are not *all-important.* Religion reminds us of the *transcendent dimension* of existence, teaching us about a God whose greatness and omnipotence reach far beyond our daily cares and woes, and inviting us to communicate with that great Holy One through prayer and worship.

Our religious traditions teach us to expect great things from God, thus setting in motion the health-boosting effect of positive expectancy— hope. In medicine, this dynamic is known as the *placebo effect,* a well- known phenomenon in which patients get better simply because they believe they will. Researchers have documented the placebo effect's amazing potency across the spectrum of illnesses. Through their work, we know that the brain can "set us up" to fulfill our expectations, positive *or* negative (the "nocebo" effect). We evoke the power of the placebo effect when we connect to a transcendent realm where our present wor- ries pale in comparison to the wonder of God's ultimate promises.

Religious involvement as examined in the faith-factor data gives us a framework in which to reach for the transcendent, thus activating our deepest hopes and setting in motion the power of positive expectancy. We also take ourselves out of our present situation, regaining a true sense of who we are by remembering our right relationship to the God who cre- ated us. Thus, we gain perspective and peace.

Remedy No. 12: Love— Caring and Being Cared For

The importance of love cannot be overstated. Without it, we risk losing our zest for life and our reason for being, and becoming more vulnerable to disease and other disorders.

At their best, religions evoke love in us and support its growth among us, as individuals and as communities of faith. Every great theological tra- dition focuses on the importance of loving God and loving our fellow human beings. It is our task as people of faith to grow in our capacity to do both. In the supportive environment of a religious congregation, rela- tionships can be forged and strengthened. Worship together allows us to fortify the ties of family and friendship. Many churches and temples also offer small-group fellowship opportunities in which the loving bonds between individuals can grow.

Healthy religious organizations focus on the primacy of love for others. The Bible tells us repeatedly to provide one another with the health-enhancing ingredient known as *agape,* a Greek word for uncondi- tional love used in the Christian scriptures. The world's great religious traditions all point to this kind of love as the basis for human belief and

behavior. When we abide in love, we live more deeply, fully, and health-
ily; we activate our highest potential as human beings. Love gladdens our
hearts and soothes our spirits. It is, according to the apostle Paul, the
highest of human qualities:

> If I speak in the tongues of mortals and of angels, but do not have love,
> I am a noisy gong or a clanging cymbal. And if I have prophetic pow-
> ers, and understand all mysteries and all knowledge, and if I have all
> faith, so as to remove mountains, but do not have love, I am nothing.
> If I give away all my possessions, and if I hand over my body so that I
> may boast, but do not have love, I gain nothing. . . . And now faith,
> hope, and love abide, these three; and the greatest of these is love.
> [1 Corinthians 13:1–3, 13.]

The twelve remedies that make up the faith factor are exponentially
effective: they combine to form a whole that is greater than the sum of its
parts. They do not have to occur simultaneously in order to be effective,
though I believe frequent worship attendance has been found to be a critically important variable, because it is within the context of worship that
all twelve components most frequently coexist (see chapter 8). We can't
definitively trace the way the faith factor works, as we can trace the role of
the influenza virus in creating influenza, but we do know this: the components of the faith factor seem to be powerfully effective agents in the
prevention of disease, the enhancement of recovery from illness, the
extension of life span, and the creation of well-being.

It is precisely because of the faith factor's powerful influence in people's lives that we must guard against the negative impact of certain religious behaviors and beliefs, which, though forming only a tiny minority
of religious experiences, have had dramatically deleterious effects on
human beings for centuries.

WHEN RELIGION'S IMPACT IS NEGATIVE

Religious involvement is like most any other healthful behavior: it can be
carried to extremes. An overweight woman might embark on a weight-

reducing diet and become obsessed with it; her obsession might develop into anorexia. An out-of-shape man might undertake an exercise program but start off too quickly and strenuously, risking ailments ranging from muscle strain to heart attack. It is also conceivable, of course, that a person might join a religious organization in a quest for wholeness and belonging, only to be caught up in a vortex of self-destructive behavior. To understand the potential dangers of religious involvement, one has only to consider the terrible loss of life at Jonestown, Guyana, in 1978, where 914 men, women, and children followed their leader, Jim Jones, drank poisoned Kool-Aid, and died. Or remember Waco, Texas, in 1993, where seventy-eight people perished in a fire that erupted when federal agents stormed the compound of the Branch Davidians, a group led by the highly charismatic David Koresh. Even when religious abuse does not result in direct bodily harm, it can be devastating, as we have seen in the cases of "faith healers" and other unscrupulous but charismatic individuals, who have bilked their followers of huge sums of money, only to vanish into thin air.

Judging the spiritual validity of any given sect is beyond my present task. I will, however, point to one key identifying factor that emerges in religious groups and proves to be dangerous to health: when leaders coerce or manipulate adherents to give up all personal autonomy, religious participation is likely to lead to *more*, not fewer, problems.

It is also troubling to me as a medical doctor when religious leaders urge adherents to avoid traditional medical care. To give just one example, researchers compared infant-mortality rates of the general population to those among members of the Faith Assembly, a fundamentalist sect whose members shun professional medical care. The infant-mortality rate among Faith Assembly women was three times greater than it was for the general population. Even more striking, the Faith Assembly experienced a maternal mortality rate that was almost a hundred times higher!

As a medical doctor, I believe our mental, physical, and spiritual health are best served when we enjoy the benefits of religious commitment *and* take advantage of the best that traditional medicine can offer us. Abstaining from medical care out of religious convictions seems to me an unnecessary and destructive "side effect" of religious involvement.

EXTRINSIC VERSUS INTRINSIC:
A CRITICAL DISTINCTION

A person's basic religious orientation can also evoke some of the negative effects of religiosity. For our purposes, there are two basic types of religious orientation, extrinsic and intrinsic, as put forth by Gordon W. Allport of Harvard University.

Extrinsics are people who, paraphrasing (and inverting) John F. Kennedy's memorable words, "ask not what they can do for their religion, but what their religion can do for them." Religion for extrinsics is a means to obtaining another end—health, security, status, power—even though they may not be consciously aware of their own ulterior motives. In recent years, several prominent televangelists have been revealed as essentially extrinsic in their religious activities. For them, the secondary gains of religious involvement—influence, money, sexual favors—mattered more than their religion's essential teachings. Extrinsically oriented people may even present convincing façades of religiosity: they may be among the most frequent attenders at worship services, the first to endorse the value of religiously inspired disciplines like dietary restrictions (although not necessarily the most faithful in following these rules!), and the most vocal in citing scripture or doctrine to support their views in a given situation. However, even if extrinsics work hard at fulfilling the more visible and measurable requirements of their given tradition, their hearts are not deeply engaged in a relationship with God. They may have failed to connect profoundly with their tradition's teachings for any number of reasons, some of which are discussed in chapter 8. Whatever the cause, their extrinsic orientation keeps them safely at arm's length from the more difficult requirements of authentic engagement with questions of faith. This may explain Dr. Allport's finding that extrinsics, despite their apparently proreligious stance, are more likely to show evidence of racial prejudice than nonreligious individuals.

People with an intrinsic religious orientation, on the other hand, ask not what their religion can do for them, but what they can do for their religion. Dr. Allport found intrinsics to be the least racially prejudiced of the three groups studied (extrinsics, intrinsics, and people who did not attend church at all). They have a deep-seated, authentic faith; they are religious because it reflects their underlying identity and character. Intrinsically religious people care less about social conformity than do their extrinsic brothers and sisters. They are God-oriented rather than self-oriented, and they are more likely to receive health benefits from religious involvement than those with an extrinsic orientation. Motivated by their love for God and their fellow men and women, intrinsics are often found doing the thankless and unglamorous work in religious communities—like tending the chronically ill or scrubbing the church basement—without looking for recognition. Though they tend not to talk about it, most intrinsics maintain a disciplined devotional life, praying and reading scripture every day. Characterized by humility and gentleness, intrinsics have a seamlessness about them: they "walk the walk" instead of just "talking the talk."

Paradoxically, many studies have shown that people who use religion merely as a tool to bring about benefits like power, prestige, or better health are less likely to reap the faith factor's health benefits. In a 1991 study assessing the role of extrinsic and intrinsic religiosity in depression, researchers found that depression levels went up among the subjects who scored as extrinsic on an inventory of religiosity traits. Conversely, those scoring as intrinsics were less likely to be depressed. In other words, people who are deeply and authentically religious ward off depression more effectively than those who are just "going through the motions." A 1989 study of bereavement among elderly widows and widowers also included a survey of intrinsic/extrinsic religiosity traits; extrinsic religiosity was found to be correlated with more grief and distress than intrinsic religiosity. Extrinsic religiosity, then, may actually bring negative health effects as well as preclude the faith factor's health benefits. This was also seen in a study of death anxiety, in which extrinsically religious people were found to have a significantly higher fear of death than their intrinsically religious and completely nonreligious counterparts. Given the characteristics of extrinsics and intrinsics cited above, we may speculate that this is because intrinsically religious people believe deeply in a trustworthy God and believe that they have a wonderful afterlife to look forward to, or at least that there is little to fear after death. Nonreligious people usually believe they will simply cease to exist after death, so there is nothing to look forward to *or* to fear. But extrinsically oriented people tend to view afterlife, heaven or hell, as a reward or punishment for how well they carried out their religious duties in life, so they have a great deal to be anxious about.

VIOLENCE IN THE NAME OF RELIGION

On a larger scale, people have demonstrated the negative potential of their religions—particularly the extrinsic type of religion—throughout history, claiming the right to persecute, oppress, and massacre others in the name of faith. One of history's grand ironies is that Jerusalem (whose name in Hebrew means "City of Peace"), a place of healing and miracles holy to the three great monotheistic religions (Judaism, Christianity, and Islam), has witnessed more wars than any other city. In battle after bloody battle, Egyptians, Israelites, Philistines, Babylonians, Greeks, Seleucids, Romans, Byzantines, Muslims, Crusaders, Mamluks, Ottomans, Englishmen, Jordanians, and Israelis have sequentially conquered this tiny piece of hillside, often claiming religion as their justification for conquest. Devout worship and pilgrimage have marked this city's life for nearly four thousand years, but so have conflagration and bloodshed growing out of the same religious beliefs that have inspired generosity, compassion, and cooperation.

As a doctor and a person of faith, of course, I deplore violence in the name of religion, but I recognize its pervasive presence throughout history. We can only hope and pray that the *positive* effects of religious involvement—not only health benefits but the benefits of altruism, peacefulness, and tolerance—will continue to outweigh its negative effects.

I am optimistic that this will indeed be the case. Given the significant health benefits of religious involvement, I believe religion's positive contributions will come to have an ever-greater influence on our society and on humanity as a whole. This surprisingly potent positive outcome of religious involvement may, in fact, prove to be one of the twentieth century's greatest medical breakthroughs, on a par with the development of antibiotics and advanced surgical techniques.

THE FAITH FACTOR: LATEST IN A SERIES OF UNEXPECTED DEVELOPMENTS IN MEDICINE?

Throughout medical history, some of the most important breakthroughs have come as surprises. Through observation, a doctor would develop a hypothesis that at first might seem highly unlikely or unconventional.

Often, these new findings generated significant controversy within the scientific community and the general public. But once their validity was proved, these seemingly controversial discoveries became cornerstones of medicine as we practice it today.

To cite one notable example from the nineteenth century: obstetrician Ignaz Semmelweis grappled with a puzzle involving childbed, or puerperal, fever, an infection of the female genital tract that often killed women who had recently given birth. Working in a prominent Viennese hospital, Semmelweis noticed that woman on one floor were contracting childbed fever at a dramatically lower rate than women on another floor. Women treated by midwives, he noticed, had fewer infections than those treated by medical students. Midwives were careful about cleanliness and were not allowed to do autopsies. But, Dr. Semmelweis observed, medical students did autopsies regularly and went to patients directly from the dissecting room without washing. The new mothers who were getting sick were being tended to by medical students just after they left the autopsy room. Noting that the students were not washing their hands, he hypothesized that neglect of handwashing might be responsible for the deaths of the new mothers. His hypothesis preceded Louis Pasteur's theory that the spread of bacteria caused disease, and the establishment of sterility as a primary requirement and common practice in treating patients.

To stop the spread of childbed fever, Dr. Semmelweis proposed something radical: he ordered all medical students working on the affected maternity ward to wash their hands in a solution of chlorinated lime before entering the ward. The rate of infection plummeted from 18 percent to 1.5 percent over several months. It dropped even further when Dr. Semmelweis extended his order to cover all students treating maternity patients, whether or not the students had previously been working in the autopsy room.

You might think Ignaz Semmelweis would have been lauded as a hero. Instead, his brilliant observations and courageous actions stirred up such controversy that he lost his position at the hospital and ended his career in disgrace at Budapest. He was eventually committed to an insane asylum and died of a blood infection, similar to the one he had prevented so successfully. This courageous doctor was vindicated in 1879, when the great scientist Louis Pasteur personally defended Semmelweis's theories at a meeting of the Academy of Medicine in Paris.

Today, of course, we accept the findings of scientists like Semmelweis as solid, irrefutable medical knowledge. Contemporary physicians pay scrupulous attention to maintaining sterile conditions in hospitals, offices, and laboratories. But when this concept first surfaced, it was viewed as misguided, even dangerous, by large segments of the medical establishment.

Semmelweis couldn't fully explain *how* or *why* his remedies worked. He only knew, through experimentation and observation, that they *did* work, and that lives could be saved if the proper measures were taken. The hows and whys could wait till later; in the meantime, morbidity and mortality rates would drop dramatically.

I believe the faith factor—neglected by many doctors for centuries, dismissed by some scientists as irrelevant—echoes the stories of medical pioneers like Semmelweis. Until recently, the small number of physicians and scientists who *did* take the faith factor seriously risked being labeled unscientific at best, deluded and dangerous at worst. Like Semmelweis, they risked losing prestigious appointments if they promoted their cause too fervently.

Researchers who have established the faith factor's benefits to health have forged ahead in spite of opposition, saying that the health of one's patients is more important than the health of one's career. We are using the scientific method to prove that the medical effects of religion are not just a matter of faith, but a matter of science. Truly, both doctors and patients are living on a new frontier of medical practice. Some caution is appropriate; after all, we are dealing with delicate matters of soul, conscience, and body, and significant practical and ethical issues arise, which I will discuss in later chapters. But I hope that both doctors and patients will not be dissuaded by excess caution. I hope we will embrace with all due speed the well-documented research findings that support the importance of the faith factor and the healthful practices it evokes.

It is entirely possible that, a century from now, people will look back at twentieth-century medicine and say, "Can you believe that those doctors never prayed with their patients? Just think how many lives could have been saved—if only they had set up intercessory-prayer teams in every hospital as we do today!" Will they be as stunned then that we didn't pray for our patients as we would be today if doctors didn't wash their hands before treating patients' wounds?

We *can* hasten the day when the faith factor receives the full recognition it deserves. As a doctor, scholar, and professor, I am attempting to do this in my practice, research, and teaching. As a patient, you can contribute, too, by telling your doctor how important the faith factor is to you, and enlisting his or her help as you seek healing for your whole person—body, mind, and soul—healing that is aided by the recognition and inclusion of the faith factor in your medical treatment.

CHAPTER 3

⊹

Healing the Body:
Restoring Our Physical Selves

Modern science has only recently begun to acknowledge the power of prayer and the faith factor in healing. But many sacred traditions tell us that people throughout the ages have perceived a relationship between spiritual practices and healing, long before the scientific method and our modern medicines came into being. In a world before prednisone and Prozac, there was prayer; people have been cured of arthritis, asthma, asthenia, and many other ailments by faith throughout recorded history. The recorded lives of the saints are a particularly useful resource in this regard. For example, we see evidence of dramatic healing in the life of St. Teresa of Avila, a sixteenth-century Spanish nun who was one of only two women to be accorded the title "Doctor of the Church." As a young woman, Teresa experienced a severe illness that forced her to leave the convent and return home to her family to be cared for. The medical care available at that time did nothing for her. Eventually she fell into a coma that lasted four days; although she came out of the coma, Teresa was weak, in great pain, and apparently paralyzed. Many people prayed for Teresa, including her family members and her sisters in the convent, but her condition did not improve quickly and she was not expected to live. She returned to the convent to meet her fate there. After eight months, she could move again; after two years, she could crawl. In what was

60

deemed a miraculous recovery, Teresa regained her mobility and resumed a full and active life.

Teresa's story is one of many unexplained healings to be found in the historical record. We cannot know the exact causes of her recovery, or even the precise nature of her illness. Certainly, we cannot extract a method or formula for healing from her story. What I believe we *can* discern from both historical and contemporary accounts of healing through prayer is this: the spiritual dimension of life is important to health in ways we do not fully understand, and physicians have a responsibility to address it.

In response to this emerging agenda, some doctors are forging a new synthesis of care, drawing on the wealth of knowledge available to us from experimental science, the wisdom garnered by patients from their personal experiences, and the insight we can glean from the great stories of the world's religious traditions. As we consider the evidence from modern science linking faith and healing, we will also examine the healing testimonies found in the Bible and other sacred texts. We will discuss scriptural stories of healing in chapter 10. To understand how patients combine faith's resources with medical treatment, we will listen to patients' narratives in their own words.

As we learn about people who have sought healing through medical and spiritual means, we find that their stories, though unique in many respects, can be grouped into several categories. Some people are not completely cured of their illnesses but learn to *cope with sickness* through prayer and other forms of religious involvement. For others, healing occurs in the form of *arresting the progression of illnesses* like cancer and heart disease. Still others experience *remission or complete healing of their illnesses* through the combination of prayer interventions and medical care. As a physician, I have found that the degree of healing that patients experience through the use of prayer, Bible study, community support, and the other components of the faith factor cannot be predicted or controlled. Of course, we know that the faith factor is not a panacea—the mortality rate for human beings still remains 100 percent. But even when physical healing does not occur, some degree of improvement almost always takes place, most often a sense of peace in facing serious illness or disability.

Let us begin our journey with the story of a contemporary woman who found a model and method for her own healing in the words of a sacred text.

✦

It was just a small lump in her neck, but it threatened everything: her own life, the future of her children (who were six, three, and one) and her husband. "It's probably thyroid cancer," the doctor had said to Barbara, a thirty-one-year-old wife and mother. "But we won't know until we've done hormone tests and surgery."

During that time of waiting, Barbara thought constantly about the fate of her family. "I was always anxious and afraid," she recalled. "What would the doctors find? What would happen to me? Would the man I love have to see me die and then raise our children alone? I began to get mild panic attacks where I had trouble breathing or sleeping."

Barbara had studied the history of the Bible and the early church intensively since she was a child. Given her intimate familiarity with the Christian Gospels, it is not surprising that she found a metaphor for her personal healing in a Bible passage. One Sunday, as Barbara was praying in church, the Gospel story of the woman with a hemorrhage kept coming into her mind:

Now there was a woman who had been suffering from hemorrhages for twelve years. She had endured much under many physicians, and had spent all that she had; and she was no better, but rather grew worse. She had heard about Jesus, and came up behind him in the crowd and touched his cloak, for she said, "If I but touch his clothes, I will be made well." Immediately her hemorrhage stopped; and she felt in her body that she was healed of her disease. Immediately aware that power had gone forth from him, Jesus turned about in the crowd and said, "Who touched my clothes?" And his disciples said to him, "You see the crowd pressing in on you; how can you say, 'Who touched me?' " He looked all around to see who had done it. But the woman, knowing what had happened to her, came in fear and trembling, fell down before him, and told him the whole truth. He said to her, "Daughter, your faith has made you well; go in peace, and be healed of your disease." [MARK 5:25–34.]

"She wanted to be healed but she didn't want to bother Jesus, so she approached him in a crowd and touched his robe," Barbara explained. "Of course, Jesus knew what happened and praised the woman for her faith. I wanted to be like that woman."

As Barbara prepared to go up to the altar for communion, she suddenly thought, "I *could* be like her." An Episcopalian, Barbara viewed the priest who was presiding at the Holy Eucharist as a "stand-in" for Jesus during the service. She decided she would touch the priest's robe when he gave her the communion wafer.

"I touched his robe, and he couldn't have known that I did, though he did know about my cancer," she remembered. "He did something in that moment that I had never seen him do before: he put down the paten with the communion wafers and came over to me; laying both hands on my head, he prayed for my healing."

After receiving the communion wine, Barbara stood up at the altar. "I was so overwhelmed with God's love that I knew I was healed," she said. "My healing wasn't physical at that point, but my heart was healed. I wasn't anxious or afraid or doubtful or sad at all. I had complete trust in God and his love, something he knew I needed far more than any other kind of healing at that moment." Her sense of serenity was not a fleeting, momentary experience: "During that difficult year of treatment for cancer, I maintained a peace and confidence that was a direct gift from God, impossible to mistake for anything else."

A few weeks after her healing at the altar rail, Barbara's surgery revealed that the lump was indeed thyroid cancer. She went through treatments then, and six months later for a recurrence. Somehow the medical treatment, too, seemed to be directly from God: "I felt that God had simply completed a healing he had started at the altar at church."

Today, Barbara is healthy and leads a full and prayerful life. Her youngest child is in college; the God-given sense of assurance she received in 1979 as the mother of three young children has been borne out in her life.

✝

According to the Bible, a supernatural force flowed from Jesus to the hemorrhaging woman, who probably was suffering from endometrial cancer or uterine fibroid tumors. Drawing on her knowledge of scripture,

Barbara reached out for that healing force just as the woman with hemorrhages had done almost two thousand years before. Like the woman in the Biblical story, Barbara acted in faith, demonstrating a persistent belief in God's ability to overcome illness, a belief that was instrumental in her seeking and receiving healing—both medical and spiritual. Barbara's cancer may not have been supernaturally healed; after all, she underwent medical treatment for the disease not just once, but twice. But she believes she felt God's healing touch that day at the altar rail. Her anxiety was lifted, her peace of mind restored. She was ready to deal with her illness, trusting in God to care for her and her family.

Did *God* heal Barbara's illness? That is not a question that science can answer. The question before us, rather, is this: does *belief in God* aid in healing? This *is* a scientific question, and from the evidence presented in this book, the answer appears to be "yes." In Barbara's story, we can clearly see that her faith helped her find peace in a time of great anxiety. We cannot prove whether it was God who healed her of cancer, the medical treatment, or both.

Barbara's story does show us how faith and medicine can work together in the lives of people with serious physical illnesses. Just as the resources of faith can help heal diseases that appear to have their basis in our psyches (like addiction and some mental illnesses), they also boost healing in cases of killer diseases like cardiovascular illness and cancer.

How do people employ the faith factor in their quest for physical healing? Let me introduce you to a number of my patients, colleagues, and acquaintances who have made journeys toward healing by embracing the resources of traditional medicine *and* faith.

COPING WITH ILLNESS

If I asked you to imagine a typical heart-disease patient, I'm sure you would never imagine Claire. This dynamic Italian-American woman in her late thirties was the picture of health, working out at the gym for an hour and a half daily, holding down a full-time job as a public-relations professional at a children's-advocacy organization, and going to school to complete a master's degree. Warm, outgoing, and highly motivated,

Claire had created a life full of achievement and activity. She truly "had it all"—but then, one December day, as she was planning to join her family for the holidays in New York City, her world came crashing down when she suddenly contracted a life-threatening illness, characterized by high fever, overwhelming exhaustion, shortness of breath, visual disturbances, weakness, and unusual skin rashes.

Claire was critically ill when I met her in the emergency room at the hospital where I work and teach, but fortunately she began to respond to vigorous treatment, including fluids and an extended course of intravenous antibiotics. She was diagnosed as having endocarditis, a severe bacterial infection of the lining of the heart, a condition that can be rapidly fatal if not diagnosed and treated promptly.

But Claire's initial hospitalization was just the beginning of a long, slow, and frustrating recovery that lasted for months. Clots of infected material passed from her heart to her brain, resulting in visual loss, and the infection damaged her heart valves, almost precipitating surgical repair.

"I was doing intravenous therapy at home every day for four to six weeks, so I had this thing in my chest and I was pumping myself full of stuff every day," she said. "I was just so weak and so tired and just really scared. I finally realized that I had almost died."

In her weakness, fear, and frustration, Claire reached out to God. Although raised a Catholic, Claire had stopped attending church years before and was no longer traditionally religious. She described herself as spiritual, not religious: "For me, when I need to relate to God, I go for a nice long walk in the woods."

I told Claire that illness can be an important opportunity for reflection and reordering of priorities. "You're on the go all the time, Claire," I said, "and sometimes the only time we get to look upward is when we're lying flat on our backs. Nobody wants to get sick, but sometimes we can find new ways of looking at the world when we have the opportunity to stop and reflect during illness. Is religion, or spirituality, an important part of your life?" I asked.

She shrugged. "I'm not much for organized religion, but I do believe in God. I'm not sure I'd fit into anybody's religious category, though, and I can't say I've done a lot of praying in recent years." Smiling, she added, "I guess I've been too busy for God."

"I'd like you to consider something," I said. "You don't have to be in anybody's religious category in order to start praying. Why don't you find a prayer in the Bible—maybe in one of the Psalms—or just make up your own short, simple prayer. Then, as you take your walk each day, repeat that prayer to yourself. Do you think that might work for you?"

"I'll give it a try, Doctor," Claire said.

On her next visit, Claire reported that she had been going outside ("where God is") to meditate, repeating her prayer verse according to the rhythm of her walking, as I had suggested.

"I feel so calm and centered after my prayer walks," Claire told me.

"Your prayer is actually bringing about the Relaxation Response, a way of reducing the stresses in your body," I told her. "Even after you've recovered from the infection, try to keep up this practice, because research shows it can help you stay healthy."

It was a long and difficult convalescence for Claire, but she has now resumed her active life, including more vigorous exercise. Claire's youth and basic good health, along with timely medical intervention and careful adherence to medical regimens (such as exercise), may be the only factors contributing to her recovery, but Claire believes her prayer walks helped, too, and her spiritual life continues to develop.

"I've learned that faith comes in a number of packages. You don't have to have a certain label or go to a certain church to feel the effects of it," Claire said recently. "If you're open to it, it's there. Before I got sick, I was looking heavenward mostly when things went wrong. That's definitely changed. Today, I say, 'I really thank you for letting me still be here, and I know you're with me, and please just stay with me so I don't get lost.' I spend a lot more time talking in my mind to God than I ever did before."

Like many sick people, Claire turned to God when life-threatening illness struck. This common response to illness suggests the possibility that human beings somehow *know* how critically important a link to God can be to the restoration of health. For Claire, illness became an opportunity to reexamine her priorities and to find a new way to approach her spiritual life.

✢

Feliciana is a naturalized American citizen, originally from Peru. She teaches Spanish to emotionally troubled high-school students in a multicultural environment and has a passion for her work.

"I will do anything for my students," she told me. "I am so concerned about them and their future. Somebody needs to get involved, to help them."

When she came to see me for the first time, Feliciana had suffered from severe, incapacitating migraine headaches for almost thirty years. While she had repeatedly sought medical treatment, Feliciana had found no relief from this debilitating disorder.

"My migraines were so bad I couldn't eat anything," she said. "I couldn't go to sleep. I would be awake the whole night, and often I couldn't work."

At her first visit, I examined Feliciana and talked with her about many aspects of her life, including her spirituality. I was impressed by her strong faith. Speaking with a conviction that surprised me, I felt compelled to tell her, "You have been sick for too long, and you won't have to be sick any more. I think God is going to provide a way for you to be healed." Knowing that prayer was an important part of her life, I asked Feliciana if she would like me to pray with her. She gladly agreed. We prayed together for healing of her disabling symptoms, and, drawing on recent pharmacological research on migraines, I prescribed a new medication for Feliciana—a medication that finally helped ease the migraines, unlike the scores of other prescriptions she had been given over the years.

"Without this medicine and without prayer, I could not be working," Feliciana told me.

As I continued to see Feliciana on a regular basis, I noticed that she was so involved with her students that she might be taking on their emotional pain, to her own emotional and physical detriment.

"Feliciana, do you take your work home with you each night? Do you worry about these youngsters even when you're not at school?" I asked her.

She sighed. "I certainly do!" she admitted. "I worry about them all the time. I even dream about them at night!"

"I'd like to share with you something I've learned as a doctor," I told Feliciana. "It's important to learn to be caring and sensitive to others without experiencing their problems as your own. Part of caring for others is learning to care for yourself. Could you try to leave your worries at school each day when you leave?"

"I don't know," Feliciana said. "I worry about the students because I love them. It's hard to put them out of my mind!"

"I know, Feliciana," I told her, "but, ultimately, taking care of these children is God's job, not yours. How about this: Could you say a prayer as you leave school each afternoon, turning the students over to God's care? Then, each evening, if you start worrying about them, remind yourself that they are in God's hands, and that you aren't going to worry about them until the next morning. Will you try that?"

"Yes, I think I could do that," Feliciana said. At her next visit, Feliciana told me she was finding comfort in this approach to her anxieties.

Daily scripture study has also been a helpful form of medicine for Feliciana; she frequently draws hope from two verses that I jotted down on a prescription pad for her:

"Come to me, all you that are weary and are carrying heavy burdens, and I will give you rest. Take my yoke upon you, and learn from me, for I am gentle and humble in heart, and you will find rest for your souls. For my yoke is easy, and my burden is light." [MATTHEW 11:28–30.]

I can do all things through Christ who strengthens me. [PHILIPPIANS 4:13.]

In better health today, largely but not completely free from the devastating disability of migraines, Feliciana teaches full-time and works with newly arrived Spanish-speaking immigrants, assisting them as they establish new lives in the United States. Feliciana credits medicine *and* prayer with her improvement, but I am aware that it could be the medicine alone that has made the difference. However, I have seen plenty of people with this condition who have become disabled and who have not been helped by medication alone. Looking at Feliciana's story from her perspective as well as my own, I believe she's right: it's probably the prayer and the medication together that have made her better.

ARRESTING THE PROGRESSION OF ILLNESS

How can faith help us when we receive a frightening diagnosis like cancer or severe heart disease? Often, such a diagnosis propels us into an endless series of harrowing decisions about treatment options and lifestyle changes. It may also entail learning to cope with lessened physical ability.

When she was forty-two, Leslie developed cardiomyopathy, a severe heart problem caused by a viral disease that attacks the lining of the heart. For years, Leslie could do little more than shuttle back and forth between doctors, hospitals, and even the National Institutes of Health, looking for a cure. At one university hospital, doctors evaluated Leslie for a heart transplant; at the time, they thought this dramatic step might be her only hope for survival.

Leslie's illness forced her to make an about-face in her lifestyle. Married to an airline pilot who is often out of town, Leslie loves to maintain her family's country home in the West Virginia mountains, treating it almost as a precious work of art. More than anything, this outgoing, vibrant woman wants to keep her home open to family and friends for frequent gatherings and celebrations. But when she contracted heart disease, she could no longer scrub the bathroom tiles on her hands and knees with a toothbrush every week, or meet the other stringent homemaking standards she had set for herself. Unable even to go up and down the stairs in her home, this "recovering perfectionist" whose house had to be "white-glove clean" struggled with her new weakness. Surviving an extremely serious illness, when doctors did not expect her to live, has helped her put her entire life in a new perspective.

Leslie and I often talk about her perfectionism. I remind her, "Only God is perfect. Sometimes we place more confidence in our abilities than in God's. Remember that God accepts us no matter what we accomplish. You're a human *being*, not a human *doing*."

Though Leslie had a strong faith, she often felt abandoned as she unsuccessfully sought treatment to make her well. At one point she remembers praying, "Lord, I think you've forgotten me. I'm not really going to get better."

Despite the heavy odds against her, Leslie *did* get better. Asking God for strength, she faithfully followed the medical regimes her doctors prescribed. She made difficult but crucial lifestyle changes, constantly turning in prayer to God for the ability to stay on a restricted diet and to take part in a cardiac-rehabilitation program that includes monitored exercise. A devout Christian before getting sick, Leslie says she prays even more today, and has received a great deal of intercessory prayer from members of her church, friends, and family.

When the cardiomyopathy was diagnosed, Leslie received a prognosis of two years' survival time. Instead, she has now lived fourteen years, and the pumping ability of her heart has doubled. Her cardiologist is baffled by her improvement and has no ready explanation. She may never again be able to scrub tile floors with a toothbrush, but she has learned important lessons from coping with her limited physical capacities, and she is at peace.

"Until I got sick, I was a person who was going morning, noon, and night, in the schools, church, everything—just continuously going. When I got sick, I couldn't accept the fact that somebody else had to do my work. But sometimes the Lord has to do something to get our attention. Having other people take care of me was a very humbling experience. Since I've slowed down, my priorities have changed. Now I know there isn't anything in the world as important as my grandchildren."

Leslie has learned to depend on others and to "let go and let God," rather than try to remain in tight control of her life and her environment. Though still partially disabled by the effects of her cardiomyopathy, Leslie is feeling better physically; recently, she told me that she was able to send out a batch of two hundred cards last Christmas—a cherished custom she had been forced by illness to put aside.

✢

Martha expected to be dead by now. At least, that's what her doctors told her would happen when she was diagnosed with a rare form of cancer in 1989. Adenoid cystic carcinoma, a cancer of the sinuses, threatened her life and sent her on a search for medical solutions. Doctors at renowned cancer centers across the country told her that her disease was terminal, and that the usual cancer treatments—surgery, radiation, and chemotherapy—would not help in her case.

A resourceful and determined person, Martha tried alternative healing methods, including an extremely restricted macrobiotic diet.

"I did that for seven months, went back in for an MRI [magnetic resonance imaging, a diagnostic test], and the tumor still sat there as big as life," Martha told me. "I decided to try mind control. I started going to Bernie Siegel's Exceptional Cancer Patient Clinic at Yale."

Martha found the clinic's program helpful emotionally, but the tumor remained. When her husband took another job, the couple moved to a small city in Maryland, and there Martha—previously not an actively religious person—started attending church. Something "clicked" for Martha, and soon she was meeting frequently with other church members for prayer and Bible study.

"I told the church members about my cancer and they started praying for me," she said. "I decided to go and have the tumor looked at again, because by this time two years had passed, and I thought, 'Maybe it isn't there any more, since I've had all these people praying for me.' "

But doctors at Johns Hopkins found the tumor still intact. They referred Martha to the University of Washington hospital in Seattle, which offered a new treatment for her form of cancer: neutron radiation.

The doctors warned Martha of the treatment's possible severe side effects, and indeed she did become very sick. After twelve treatment sessions out of a planned thirty-two, Martha left Seattle. "I told the doctors, 'You're killing me. I'm going to take my chances in the hands of the Lord.'"

Today, Martha is apparently in good health. The last MRI showed the tumor still in place, but Martha has no symptoms, and it has not grown.

"The doctors told me they had seen a hundred cases of this cancer, and every patient had died," Martha said. "The way I look at it is this: the Lord's got something he wants me to do. Otherwise, why am I alive? Why are all those other people dead?"

That strong sense of purpose in life has undoubtedly contributed to Martha's survival and to her sense of well-being. Even though the tumor remains, it is quiescent. There is no medical explanation for this. Why should Martha survive for years after diagnosis, whereas most patients with this kind of cancer do not? I do not know. Martha believes God has healed her. As a scientist, I say, "We cannot prove that *God* healed you, but it's clear that we have a lot more to learn about the effects of faith on health."

✢

A well-dressed, elegant, elderly woman named Dorothy came to my office for the first time complaining of shortness of breath. She reported that she was unable to maintain her usual level of activity. She had been an enthusiastic, vigorous walker, but difficulty in breathing had recently limited her walking to only one block, preventing her from participating in her most cherished activity: attending daily Mass. In my conversations with her, I noticed that she was carrying a prayer book and rosary beads.

Dorothy had gained over twenty-five pounds and had developed severe fatigue and sleep disturbance. On examination, she showed signs of overt congestive heart failure, including signs of fluid throughout her chest, an abnormal heart rhythm, and marked swelling of her ankles. I ordered an electrocardiogram, which revealed no evidence of irreversible damage, and a chest X-ray, which confirmed the presence of severe congestive heart failure.

I informed Dorothy of her diagnosis. "I'd like you to enter the hospital for treatment right away, Dorothy," I told her. "This condition is very serious."

But Dorothy grasped her prayer book and her rosary beads and said, quietly but firmly, "I am not going to go to the hospital. I want to go home and pray about this."

"I understand your desire to pray, and I will be glad to pray with you," I told her, "but you need to be admitted to the hospital today."

Dorothy insisted on going home and praying, however. Despite my insistence that immediate hospitalization was the best course for her, she only became more determined to make her own decision. Just as I cannot force anyone to take medicine, I could not force Dorothy to enter the hospital. She asked me to pray with her before leaving my office that day, so we prayed for healing for her congestive heart failure. I also gave her standard medical therapy, including three medications (digoxin, furosemide, and captopril) designed to strengthen the force of the contractions of her heart and to reduce excess fluids. She went home, took her medicines, and arranged for her priest, deacons, and church congregation to pray with and for her.

When Dorothy returned for an office visit one week later, I was astonished by her response. She had lost twenty-five pounds in one week, the swelling in her ankles had gone down, the fluid in her lungs could hardly be discerned, and she felt good again. This was a very dramatic response to treatment; though it was not completely outside the realm of medical possibility, it was much greater than I would have expected. Dorothy attributed her progress to prayer. Scientifically, this claim cannot be confirmed, but from a medical point of view, we can only say that the results of the treatment greatly exceeded our usual expectations.

Congestive heart failure patients have a high mortality rate over the course of five years. It's been four years for Dorothy, and she's doing very well. Was it the prayer, the pills, or both? Was it a miracle? I don't know, but her response was (and continues to be) impressive, for which she and I offered prayers of thanksgiving.

✥

As a doctor, I attempt to enter into each patient's way of looking at the world. If I want a good relationship with my patient, I must understand his or her worldview and incorporate his or her vocabulary and viewpoints into our discussions. So, when a patient like Dorothy attributes her progress to prayer, I ask to hear more about her beliefs and feelings. I do not debate with her about prayer's power to make her better. The same rules apply when I am treating a fellow physician, so when my colleague Dr. Mohammad Alijani told me that an angel came to him in a dream to tell him that he had cancer, I urged him to tell me about the angel.

On July 14, 1989, Dr. Alijani, who is also on the faculty at Georgetown University Medical School, became the first surgeon to perform a combined transplant of the kidney, pancreas, and small bowel. Through years of study, training, and experience, he developed and mastered this difficult and risky procedure, which is the only life-saving option for certain patients.

"I have the satisfaction of seeing bedridden individuals leaving the hospital functioning with multiple transplants," he said. "I am not just giving prescriptions for the common cold or dyspepsia—I do surgery that sometimes takes fourteen to sixteen hours, dealing with two groups: the dead and the near-dead."

A devout Muslim, Dr. Alijani finds support for his medical practice in his faith, and he believes that faith plays a significant role in his patients' well-being. "On the basis of my experience, the mind of the individual plays a major role in the healing process. What stands out above all is his or her faith. If you have faith, you will be a well-balanced, resilient person, prepared to resolve the problem." For Dr. Alijani, the link between health and spirituality is so strong that he sees prayer as a literal lifeline: "Just as my body needs water, carbohydrates, protein, and lipids, my mind needs Allah, and the only way to receive Allah is to pray."

In 1995, Dr. Alijani learned even more about the link between faith and health when he was diagnosed with lymphoma, a cancer of the lymphatic system. As he tells the tale, his spiritual life played a major role in the early discovery of the disease.

"I came back from an international meeting in June 1995. On Saturday, at midnight, I awoke, having just had a dream. I saw a physician standing on my right side with a white coat, examining me. Instead of examining my heart or asking me to take a deep breath, he was examining my leg. The experience of being examined was so vivid, I woke up and saw my own hand moving on my leg. I felt a lymph node there that I had never felt in my body.

"I washed my face, said my prayers, and went back to bed. At breakfast, I explained to my wife and a friend who was staying with us, 'It looks like I have lymphoma.' "

Dr. Alijani reported his suspicion to the physician he was seeing at the time. "He said, 'Don't worry, I'll see you in a few months.' But because of my dream, I became stubborn and told my colleague: 'Take this lymph node out of my body!' The lymph node was excised, and it was diagnosed as being lymphoma. For three weeks, I went through thorough examinations, looking for any spread of the tumor. All the tests came back negative.

"I believe the dream was given to me by Allah so that the cancer would be caught at the earliest possible stage, Stage I," Dr. Alijani said. After a course of radiation therapy, Dr. Alijani remains cancer-free, but the experience has had a profound effect on his life.

"I consider it was a death prior to the real one," he told me, "because, if the lymphoma had been a Stage IV instead of Stage I, survival would be only nine to twelve months. The doctor in the dream was an angel sent to help me."

Today, Dr. Alijani continues to be healthy. He maintains a rigorous schedule, having trained himself to sleep only four hours per night in order to keep up with the demands of his profession and to have time for the five daily prayers prescribed in Islam. He often prays for his patients in the wee hours of the morning. Through his prayer for himself and others, he has gained an equanimity that allows him to deal with his cancer diagnosis without fear.

"When I learned I had cancer, I prayed: 'Whatever you think is good for me, whatever you think I should go through, please do it,' " said Dr. Alijani.

Prayerful Healing Interventions, Remarkable Results

We have looked at the role of faith in helping people cope with and recover from illness. But what about the unexplained, spontaneous healings that sometimes occur when people seek direct intercessory prayers for healing and, particularly in the Christian tradition, anointing with oil and the laying on of hands?

Medical science has only begun to define the workings of the faith factor—including the effectiveness of such components as the Relaxation Response, social support, shared beliefs, and transcendence—but it has not even begun to discern how sacramental healing works. Several studies have shown that this approach does, in fact, have notable effects. I mentioned previously the Swiss study in which smokers received the laying on of hands by a faith healer: 40 percent of the smokers stopped smoking for at least four months, and 16 percent stopped for twelve years, astonishing results in view of the difficulty of kicking the nicotine habit.

Prayer for healing was also proved effective in a 1988 study in the Netherlands, which evaluated the effect of laying on of hands in three groups of patients with hypertension. One group received laying on of hands weekly for fifteen weeks from healers trained in this procedure. The second group received weekly "positive intentions" (thoughts directed at healing) from healers located in a room adjacent to the experimental laboratory. The third group, the so-called control group, did not receive any interventions. All of the patients were told they might be prayed for. Similar reductions in blood pressure were seen in each of the groups, but the group that received the laying on of hands reported a significantly greater sense of well-being. This study suggests that the power of touch, linked with prayer, could increase the effectiveness of spiritual healing efforts, not only by evoking physical healing, but also by increasing the patient's feelings of well-being.

In chapter 1, I mentioned several other dramatic findings about the power of direct healing prayer and intercessory prayer, but there are still relatively few scientific studies of these phenomena. We do know that many Americans pray for healing. A 1991 telephone survey of 325 Midwesterns found that 30 percent regularly prayed for healing and to maintain good health. Twenty-one percent of respondents in a 1988 North Carolina study reported having attended a faith-healing service, and over half had watched faith healers on television; 6 percent said they had been healed by faith healers, and 15 percent said they knew someone who had been healed in this way. Since there was no independent observation of the healings reported by the patients, we cannot conclude that healings *did* occur, but the study tells us that a significant number of the patients interviewed *believed* they had experienced faith healing and wished to pursue spiritual healing methods as well as traditional medical approaches. The study did not, and could not, tell us if the healings actually happened; we are only at the threshold of understanding scientifically if, how, and when faith healing works.

THE CLEARWATER RHEUMATOID ARTHRITIS STUDY

In 1996, I received funding from the Foundation for Medicine and Spirituality and the John Templeton Foundation to conduct a study in Clearwater, Florida, on the effects of intercessory prayer on patients with rheumatoid arthritis. To set up the intercessory-prayer teams for the study, I turned to Francis and Judith MacNutt, well-known healers, authors, and founders of Christian Healing Ministries in Jacksonville, Florida. I had read Francis MacNutt's book, *Healing,* which sold over one million copies in the 1970s, and was familiar with the couple's work. I asked Francis if he would be interested in participating in a scientific study of prayer and outlined my ideas.

"I've been waiting thirty years to do a study like this," he replied. "I would be pleased and honored to participate."

Francis, Judith, and their teams of trained prayer ministers spent approximately twelve hours, over a three-day period, praying for each patient and teaching the patients about the Christian healing tradition. Though the study results are not yet complete, I want to share with you two stories from patients in the Clearwater study. Perhaps the best way to understand the healing power of faith is to hear from those who have experienced it.

Rita: Dancing for Joy

Rita came to Clearwater without a great deal of hope. "I'm really completely handicapped," she said on the first day of intercessory prayer. "I'm on prednisone and painkillers. That lets me have some kind of a life, get up and have my breakfast, get dressed—not much. I really couldn't get involved in anything."

For Rita, always an outgoing and dynamic person, rheumatoid arthritis was eroding her life's meaning. "I'm living my life not for anybody else, just for me. It's selfish. I like to do for others. Thank God I'm able to do for myself, that I'm not having somebody else come in to care for me."

Rita had sought the best available medical care, and she had prayed for her recovery on her own. "I rub my body with cream and I pray. I believe, and that's the only way I can live, even if I don't feel God's presence."

But Rita began to feel better—and to experience God's presence— after just a few prayer sessions conducted by intercessors from Christian Healing Ministries. The prayer-study protocol included several sessions each day of "soaking prayer," or intensive, hour-long periods of laying on of hands and prayer by two prayer ministers with each patient, as well as teaching sessions about the nature of spiritual healing. Prayer-team member Bobby Fallon asked Rita to assess her pain level after the first prayer session:

"At this time, now that we've prayed with you, on a scale of zero percent to one hundred percent, with one hundred percent being maximal healing and zero percent being no healing, where would you say the prayer took you?"

Rita considered for a few minutes before answering: "I would say 40 percent—but it's really more. Look at how I can get up from the chair!" She bounced up to a standing position like a flexible young girl. "Usually I would have to concentrate, and pray, 'Please God, give me the strength to get up, then slowly I would count one, two, three, and push up.' Not now!"

Rita experienced a spiritual sensation during the team's prayers for her: "I felt like I was breathing God's presence in, that I was breathing light in. Most of the time I feel heavy and I can't move. After the prayer, I felt good. I wanted to get up and walk and bounce and dance!"

In fact, that day Rita felt so good that she danced a modified version of the Macarena, which she had seen but never been able to attempt herself. "I can't do the wiggle at the end," she said, but then, with a delighted smile, she managed it!

Six months after the initial prayer sessions, Rita continues to do better. She felt very well the first month after the Clearwater gathering, then experienced a setback, needing to use a walker for the first time. Spiritually strengthened by her experiences with the prayer ministers, Rita reports that she "dared to demand a miracle of God." Soon, her condition improved markedly again, and she was able to leave the walker behind. Pain and joint stiffness still remain problems for her, but she is definitely doing better than before the study.

Mike: "There's Something Weird Going On Here, and I Love It!"

Mike, a sixty-five-year-old man, was diagnosed with rheumatoid arthritis when he was in his twenties. In the intervening decades, he had been through a great deal of pain, suffering, and medical treatment. Like many rheumatoid-arthritis patients, Mike can describe a history of treatment with strong medications, from prednisone to Cytoxan to methotreate; repeated surgeries and courses of physical therapy; and periods of remission, then relapse.

Mike walked stiffly with a cane at the beginning of the four-day session. He had severe pain in his hands, which had been operated on a number of times. After receiving many hours of prayer and laying on of hands for healing, Mike reported dramatic results.

"Look, no cane today!" he said. "I couldn't have walked without it yesterday or the day before. I had come to rely on the cane, especially since I've been out of remission. My feet are in good shape today. I'm able to walk a pretty good distance, and I couldn't have done this a night or two ago."

Like many patients in the study, Mike also noticed improved flexibility and reduced pain in his hands: "I was preoccupied with the pain in my hands. Lynn [a member of the healing-prayer team] prayed with me and held my hands, and I had a warming sensation, almost like energy vibrating down my hands, and my hands don't hurt nearly so bad. I ate dinner today and was able to handle a cup and a glass. Usually with those cups that have dainty little handles, I spill them immediately. And glasses take two hands. But I did all right today!"

Though Mike describes himself as a spiritual person and frequent churchgoer, he had come to the study not knowing what to expect. Grinning, he said, "There's something weird going on here, and I love it!"

Relieved of the pain and disability his rheumatoid arthritis has caused, Mike is now living a full and active life. To take care of himself, he does water-exercise therapy three times a week. Recently, he started a carefully monitored weight-lifting program.

"I try to laugh at myself at least three times every day before dinner," Mike said. "That's not easy to do, especially living alone. So I have to think of something to laugh at myself about. I used to take myself so seriously. I had more pain then."

Ten months after the first healing-prayer sessions, Mike continues to report a remarkable improvement. He is, in fact, pain-free and able to go without medication of any kind for his arthritis. Mike loves to dance, but for many years he had to ask for a cortisone shot in order to go dancing even for a couple of hours. Today, he goes dancing without the cortisone—and without pain. He says he feels better today than ever before in his life.

✢

I look forward to compiling the final results of the Clearwater prayer study with great hope—hope that intercessory prayer in conjunction with medical treatment can provide a valuable means for enhancing healing in patients with rheumatoid arthritis, a crippling and painful disease whose sufferers often cannot find complete relief through medical approaches available to us at this time.

Rita's and Mike's stories are dramatic indeed. But prayer for healing does not have to take place in unusual settings like a scientific study. When people believe in the power of healing prayer, it can happen anywhere, any time—and the apparent results are sometimes striking.

COMPLETE HEALING THROUGH PRAYER

As just one example of the power of healing prayer, let me share with you the story of Kathy, who is human-resources manager at a nonprofit research institute. In 1996, Kathy underwent a routine mammogram that revealed a lump. Surgeons recommended that she proceed with a biopsy. Like most women in this situation, Kathy was scared and upset. She turned to prayer to help her through her ordeal. Two co-workers offered to pray for Kathy one afternoon in her office. They followed the ancient Christian healing practice of laying hands on Kathy and praying intently for the healing of the breast lump.

As Kathy remembered it, "They just prayed and prayed and prayed, and I was praying to myself. It was powerful!" On the day of the biopsy, unbeknownst to Kathy, a group of friends from church prayed for her throughout the morning, and an elder from her church met her at the hospital, where he led Kathy, her husband, and her mother in prayer.

"I was hoping the lump would be gone," Kathy said, "but I had also accepted the fact that, whatever God decided, it was his plan. I thought, 'So far, God has been so wonderful to me, I'm just going to 'go with the flow' and thank him.' "

The doctors started the biopsy procedure with another mammogram to locate the breast lump, but there was no lump visible on the X-ray. Kathy recounted the moment with wonder:

"They had two more sets of X-rays, done by two different radiologists, and they kept comparing them to the former X-rays, which showed the lump, and it was gone." Puzzled, her radiologist decided to go ahead with the procedure, injecting dye and inserting the biopsy needle, in hopes of finding the lump. Still no lump could be found.

"It became very comical," Kathy said, "because I was thinking, 'Thank the Lord!' and the doctors kept on matching up the X-ray with the earlier X-rays, matching veins, trying to find the lump, and they couldn't."

"Do you believe in the power of prayer?" the technician asked Kathy.

"Do I ever!" she answered.

Throughout her ordeal, Kathy found reassurance and hope in the scripture verse she refers to as "my" verse: "I can do all things through Christ who strengthens me" (Philippians 4:13). Whether or not she had received a cancer diagnosis, Kathy was ready to accept God's plan for her. This time, though, an unexplained healing occurred.

Physical Healing: Mystery and Potential

Cancer and heart disease (our nation's two top killers) plus hypertension, diabetes, migraines, rheumatoid arthritis, and more—I have seen my patients get better faster, get better unexpectedly, and cope better with remaining symptoms when the resources of faith are linked with the resources of medicine. What can we conclude from the stories in this chapter?

First, we have seen a *broad spectrum of healing experiences* influenced by religious practice and spirituality. They range from an early diagnosis, as in the case of Dr. Alijani, to improved coping with illness (Claire, Feliciana, Rita, and Mike), to arresting the progression of disease (Leslie, Martha, and Dorothy), to what may be complete healing of Kathy's breast lump.

Second, we observe that patients participate in a *wide range of spiritual-healing practices,* including praying and meditating, attending worship services, reading scripture, and seeking the social and prayer support of friends in the faith community. They tap into the resources that evoke the twelve remedies making up the faith factor, from "letting go and letting God" to improving their lifestyles through proper diet, exercise, and stress-reduction techniques.

Third, we understand that *the type and degree of healing through spiritual means are not within our control.* There is no evidence that Kathy prayed "harder" or "better" than did Martha, yet Kathy's mass disappeared and Martha's did not. Does this mean that Kathy "did it right," whereas Martha fell short of the mark? Not at all. If we believe that God is the source of healing, we can keep in proper perspective the degree of power we wield in seeking healing through spiritual practices. As Dr. Alijani so eloquently put it: "When I learned I had cancer, I prayed: 'Whatever you think is good for me, whatever you think I should go through, please do it.'" For him, it is more important to seek God's presence and to draw close to God than to achieve a particular level of healing. At the same time, from the evidence presented in my patients' stories, we have every reason to hope that healing may occur, in some manner, to some degree, when we join the promise of faith to the procedures of medicine.

I am excited to be a part of the research now under way to determine exactly how this dynamic works. However, having witnessed the faith factor's benefits, I am not waiting until every possible fact is in before taking advantage of these effects. Of course, patients should not—indeed, cannot—be forced to follow "doctor's orders" when it comes to issues of faith and spirituality, any more than Dorothy could be forced to follow my medical recommendations. Individuals must choose whether to look to faith and religious practice as a source of healing for physical problems. If they choose to incorporate the spiritual dimension in their quest for wellness, they can look to religious and spiritual traditions for resources in addition to seeking medical treatment. We will look at some of the many approaches to spiritual healing in later chapters. For now, let us continue to trace the positive effects of the faith factor in another kind of disorder—mental illness.

CHAPTER 4

———————— ✥ ————————

Healing the Mind:
Finding a Lasting Peace

According to the National Institute of Mental Health's Depression/ Awareness, Recognition, and Treatment (D/ART) program, approximately 17.6 million Americans suffer from depression in a given year. The economic cost of depression to our nation was estimated to be between $30 and $44 billion annually, with an estimated two hundred million workdays lost each year to the disease. Depressive disorders, once dismissed merely as "the blues" or even as a moral failing, plague men and women of all ages, but are most commonly seen among women in their twenties and thirties. The typical symptoms of depression, in addition to the mood problems, include sleep, appetite, and weight disturbance; overwhelming guilt; fatigue; impairments in thinking, concentration, and behavior; and lack of interest in usual hobbies and activities. Untreated, depression can lead to suicide, but even without such a drastic outcome, depression robs people of the joy of living.

Anxiety disorders, too, diminish the quality of life for many people. According to figures from the National Institute of Mental Health, more than twenty-three million Americans suffer from these illnesses, which are even more common than depressive disorders. Ranging from heart palpitations, shortness of breath, dizziness, diarrhea, and insomnia to full-blown phobias and panic attacks, anxiety disorders go far beyond simple feelings of nervousness. In some cases, what appears to others to be an irrational fear can force patients into living like recluses, terrified even of leaving their homes.

Depression and anxiety are not "just in your head"; they are real diseases, with physical, emotional, and spiritual pain accompanying well-defined changes in brain chemistry. Because both disorders can cause a variety of physical symptoms in addition to emotional problems, they can masquerade as many other illnesses; treating them properly requires skillful diagnosis. Today, in addition to psychotherapeutic approaches, doctors can choose from a wide array of potent pharmaceuticals to treat depressive and anxiety disorders. New antidepressant medications like the serotonin-enhancing Prozac, Zoloft, and Paxil, and antianxiety drugs like Xanax and Klonopin have made these illnesses much easier to treat. As with most illnesses, good nutrition and regular physical exercise help significantly in recovery.

The faith factor, too, can make an enormous difference for sufferers from depressive and anxiety disorders. In the first place, studies show that people of faith are less likely to become depressed and anxious than their nonreligious counterparts. The study of anxiety and depression among women in the rural Midwest mentioned in chapter 1 found that frequent churchgoing was associated with lower levels of anxiety and depression. (This study looked at the role of social networks *and* religious involvement as factors in anxiety and depression, but there is a difference between the two factors; please see chapter 11 for a detailed discussion of both.)

These findings were echoed for women *and* men in a national study of the causes of psychiatric illnesses; the study found that, in 2,679 baby-boom-generation participants, the rates of psychopathology, including depression and other mental illnesses, among frequent church attenders was half that among infrequent attenders (18 percent versus 34 percent). This finding was true across denominational lines among the Protestants surveyed, regardless of whether they belonged to Pentecostal, conservative, or main-line churches.

What about people of different faiths? Few comparative studies have been done. In a study of Christian and Hindu patients in India, the psychological well-being of the patients was carefully evaluated, with factors such as mood, sleep, and cognitive impairment being assessed. For Christian men and women, and for Hindu women, frequent attendance at worship was correlated with fewer psychological problems. (For unknown reasons, this effect did not hold true for Hindu men.) There was no over-all statistical difference between the Christian and Hindu groups, suggest-ing that the faith factor may be equally beneficial regardless of religious affiliation.

The faith factor's protective effect was also demonstrated in a 1992 study of 1,110 elderly male patients in a Veterans Administration hospi-tal. The men who spontaneously reported, in answers to open-ended questions about what helped them handle their problems, that religion helped them cope were much less likely to suffer from depression than those who did not mention using religion to cope. This finding held true even after statistical adjustments were made to control for factors such as alcohol use, history of psychiatric problems, age, race, social support, and health status. In a study that assessed the psychological health of mem-bers of a Pentecostal church in Newfoundland, church members who took part in healing rituals and participated more actively in all church activities reported significantly fewer symptoms of psychological distress than those who participated less in such activities. This study featured an unusual methodology: the investigators personally participated in all church activities for twelve months, so they were able to make direct observation of the subjects' behavior. Both the observers' reports and the subjects' self-reports supported the correlation between higher levels of church activity and lower levels of psychological distress.

These studies show that religious involvement can protect against psy-chological problems. Now let us look at another group of studies, showing that people who *do* suffer from significant mental illnesses like depression and anxiety are less likely to be religiously involved than individuals who are psychologically well. In a study of a hundred outpatients at a mental-health clinic and a hundred controls without mental illness, researcher Rodney Stark found that 16 percent of the mentally ill claimed no religious affiliation, versus only 3 percent of the non–mentally ill patients. The men-tally ill patients were also less likely to say that religion was important to them, and their church attendance rates were lower than the non–mentally ill subjects.

Suicide is the most severe outcome of mental illness. Here, too, faith makes a positive difference. In a 1974 study of suicidal feelings among 720 members of the general population in Connecticut, researchers found that individuals reporting suicidal feelings were less likely than their nonsuicidal peers to belong to a religious organization, to attend religious services, or to pray. A large 1972 community-based study found that people who attend church once a week or more are only half as likely to attempt suicide as others. And researchers J. B. Ellis and P. C. Smith found in a 1991 study that, among one hundred college-student subjects, those with a strong sense of religious well-being were less likely to commit suicide than those who did not derive peace and satisfaction from religious involvement.

Of course, even if they are less likely to suffer from mental illness, religious people are not immune. Once such a malady strikes, however, the resources of faith can enhance the healing process. The stories of people recovering from anxiety and depression illuminate how the faith factor helps lift the burden of these debilitating illnesses. Let's look first at depression, the experience of which was described aptly by the poet John Keats in a letter to a friend: "I am in that temper that if I were under Water I would scarcely kick to come to the top."

DEFEATING DEPRESSION

Though it often occurs in the wake of significant stress, depression can appear in a person's life without warning or precedent, as if a terrible fog had dropped over one's mind, moods, and body. Researchers have found that the resources of religious faith can help patients with depression recover. A 1980 study measured the results of different approaches to group therapy, including therapy using religious imagery and therapy without religious imagery. The study's subjects were undergraduate patients with depression who scored high on standardized tests of religiosity. At the study's conclusion, just 14 percent of patients in the religious-imagery group remained depressed, as compared with 60 percent of patients in groups not using religious imagery. Interestingly, the two therapists conducting the religious-imagery groups were not themselves religious, but were able to help patients draw on the hope and assurance of their faith by encouraging them to use religious images (e.g., "I can visualize Christ going with me into that difficult situation in the future as I try to cope").

PRAYER AND PROZAC

I call upon personal faith resources (my patients' and my own), as well as medical knowledge and skill, in working with religious individuals who suffer from depression, such as Sarah, a thirty-five-year-old mother, nurse, and church musician, who had always been an upbeat, high-achieving person. More than anything, she loved to glorify God in her music, directing the choir, playing the organ, and singing. But when depression came, music no longer brought joy; she felt as if she were merely playing scales.

Sarah suffered not only from depression but also from chronic fatigue syndrome. She went through bouts of exhaustion, joint and muscle aches, fevers, and chills. She had nearly lost hope by the time she came to see me. I prescribed an antidepressant, Prozac, and recommended that she seek counseling.

In typical fashion, Sarah did not immediately respond to treatment; as we waited for the medication to take effect, her moods got even bleaker.

"I remember going through a period of time when I would dream about the scalpels at work, dream about bringing them home and slitting my throat," she told me recently, as we reflected together on her illness. "I had never had thoughts like that in my life! But that's just how low I was."

One day during that time, Sarah called me and said, "I just feel so hopeless."

"Sarah," I said gently, "I have enough hope for both of us." After ascertaining that she was not actively suicidal and did not require immediate hospitalization, I urged her to schedule an appointment as soon as possible. When we met, I continued to encourage her use of medication and counseling, but I also kept exploring with her the possibility of using prayer and meditation quite consciously as part of her healing regime.

"I should have thought of that myself," Sarah said, "but I've been in too much pain to think straight."

"I believe that, once the medication takes full effect, you'll start to feel better and think more clearly," I told Sarah. "In the meantime, I'd like to suggest some Bible verses to meditate on that I think will help you."

Taking out my prescription pad, I wrote down two verses for Sarah: "You will be transformed by the renewing of your mind" (Romans 12:2) and "There is no fear in love; perfect love casts out fear" (1 John 4:18).

I tore off the prescription blank and handed it to her. "Think about praying these scripture verses when you feel down," I suggested. "Keep them with you and use them in prayer whenever you need them, and let me know next time how you're coming along."

At her next visit, Sarah was noticeably less depressed. Within several months, she had made a dramatic improvement. Looking back on her experience of depression today, Sarah gives thanks to God for the ability to pray with those two hope-filled Bible verses.

"That's what got me through," Sarah said. "I just clung to that hope."

Four years have passed since Sarah began medical treatment, and she is much better. To cut down on stress in her life, she has reduced her work schedule and her church involvement. "I still am helpful to others and to the church, but as far as extending myself, I've cut back a lot," she said. "I need more time for me, and more time with God."

It took Sarah months to realize that she needed treatment for depression—months when her faith did not seem to help at all. Even after her depression was diagnosed, it took several more months for the treatment—which we called "prayer and Prozac" (plus counseling)—to take effect. The depression did not lift instantly once treatment began, and I continue to monitor her closely to ensure that she stays well—relapse is not uncommon in patients with depression.

As Sarah recovered from her depression, music returned as a source of joy and inspiration.

✝

Despite the remarkable strides made by psychopharmacological research in recent decades, many people with depression and anxiety resist taking medication for their illness. Unfortunately, there is still a stigma associated with mental illness of any kind; people believe they should be able to overcome these problems through will power or mind control. Individuals with a strong religious orientation may feel this resistance even more strongly, insisting that they *must not* feel anxious or depressed, because they believe in God, or demanding that God heal them without medication. They can fall into a trap of thinking, "I wouldn't be depressed if I had enough faith." The fact is, depression and anxiety can strike *anyone*, regardless of his or her faith commitment. To date, studies have not been undertaken to measure brain-chemical levels among religious and nonreligious individuals, so we cannot know the degree of influence religious activity may have on the levels of neurotransmitters like serotonin. But we *do* know that medications that favorably alter the brain's balance of neurotransmitters can lead to significant improvements in mood and overall function, which, in turn, may serve to renew spiritual aspects of life that have lain dormant from depression.

I have found some Biblical answers to the objection against using medicine, which I used to help my patient Ron come to terms with his illness. Ron, age fifty-five, was a deacon in his church and a devout Christian since his conversion experience twenty-five years before. When he came to see me, he complained of feeling "washed out," tired, and achy. He was having trouble sleeping and concentrating on his work, his interest in his hobbies—woodworking and playing bass guitar in a country-music band—had waned, and his formerly robust appetite had dwindled.

"I don't know what it is, Doctor," he said. "I just don't feel like doing the things I normally do. It's like I'm only half alive or something."

After listening intently to Ron and running some tests, I made a diagnosis of clinical depression. But when I mentioned the term "depression," Ron froze.

"Dr. Matthews, I can't be depressed!" he said emphatically. "A lot of people look up to me at church and in my community. I'm a Christian! There's no way I can be depressed!"

I reminded Ron of the great men of faith in the Bible who became depressed: the prophets Elijah (1 Kings 19:3–5), Jeremiah (Jeremiah 4:19–20), Jonah (Jonah 4:1–3), and King Saul (1 Samuel 16:14–16). I assured him that depression was not due to a lack of faith, nor was it caused by a moral defect, weakness, or lack of will power on his part. Going into some depth about the physical basis of clinical depression, I explained that depression can be caused by a chemical imbalance in the brain, and that God had given medical professionals the knowledge and expertise to understand this illness more fully.

"Ron, today we have some excellent medications and therapies, including psychotherapy and spiritual counseling, to treat depression," I told him. "By restoring an important brain chemical, serotonin, to its proper level, we can relieve your depression."

"I don't know, Doctor," Ron said. "I feel awfully funny about taking a drug to fix my state of mind. I just need more faith and to pray more." I told Ron that Jesus himself had used medicines to cure people. Turning to the Bible that I keep in my office, I read to him two stories from the Gospel of Mark (7:31–37 and 8:22–26), in which Jesus healed a blind man and a deaf-mute man by using saliva, which was considered to have medicinal properties in those days. I then said, "The District of Columbia Department of Health won't allow me to use saliva, but they *will* allow me to use Prozac!" I also read him the following passage:

> And whatever you do, in word or deed, do everything in the name of the Lord Jesus, giving thanks to God the Father through him. [COLOSSIANS 3:17.]

"Ron," I explained, "that means *whatever* you do, whether you're at work, taking a shower, flossing your teeth, or even taking medicine for your depression. Whatever you do, pray and give thanks for all things. Pray as you're taking your medicine!"

Because I presented an argument for medicine based on Biblical passages, Ron consented to taking an antidepressant medication. He prays in thanksgiving each time he takes it, and his depression has abated.

✢

My patient Frank also initially resisted the use of antidepressant medication. In his late thirties, Frank felt as though he was falling apart. He had always been a hard-driving, ambitious person, a sales-and-marketing executive who climbed the corporate ladder of a regional retail chain with alacrity. Suddenly, however, he started to experience strange symptoms, including ringing in his ears, aches, pains, and exhaustion. Dark moods plagued him, and he spent whole days in bed, unable to work. A Presbyterian active in his church community, Frank looked for help there but at first found little understanding.

"People at church were attempting to minister to me in ways that really didn't help, just slapping me on the back and saying, 'Prop yourself up,' 'Pull yourself out of it,' " he recalled. "That did not help."

Frank looked for physical causes for his problems, casting about for reasons. He said to himself, "Let's see, maybe it's that operation I had on my inner ear when I was a kid." Looking back, Frank later concluded that everything he tried to do to "fix" his depression only led him deeper into the darkness. Finally, he came to me for a physical examination. After examining Frank, running tests, and talking with him, I told him that my diagnosis was depression and that I would like to prescribe an antidepressant.

At first, Frank rejected the idea that he needed a medication for his mind. I explained how antidepressants work, restoring the brain's neurotransmitters to normal levels, and I told him how he would probably feel once he began the drug therapy.

"It will be a little bit like running with ankle weights for a while," I explained, using a metaphor that this former marathon-runner could relate to. "Then it will feel like you've taken them off and you can run freely and easily again."

Frank agreed to try the medicine. Over the course of the next few weeks, some of his symptoms began to abate; the ringing in his ears, which is a classic symptom of anxiety, disappeared. In addition to the medication and counseling I was providing, I urged Frank to seek once again the help he needed from his church, possibly in the form of a men's prayer group. Because he had been so disappointed by the earlier response of his fellow church members, Frank was afraid to try again.

"They told me to 'buck up,' and I couldn't," he told me. "What would they think if they knew I was on medication? They'd probably think I was crazy!"

"You don't have to tell them about the medication unless you decide you trust them," I replied. "I know it can be difficult to open up to people about your problems. If there are regular men's-prayer and Bible-study groups meeting at your church, I'd suggest you join one of them right away."

Just as I had urged Frank to take antidepressants, now I was insistent about his need for the support and accountability provided by a small fellowship group: the information Frank disclosed in our counseling sessions suggested that he needed to review the events of his life, sort out his priorities, and establish a deeper spirituality—all tasks that could be aided by a supportive group. In one office visit, he told me about how his process of spiritual renewal began:

"When I reached the top professionally, I became a partner in my company. I had the latest Volvo 740 and a lot of people working for me, and I made my employees wash and wax my car. I felt on top of the world professionally, but personally I felt empty. For a while, I was involved in alco-hol. I was starting to toy with drugs, almost as though I were eighteen or twenty again," he admitted. "On the surface, I was the picture of a real family guy—a wife, two kids, a house, young, up-and-coming. But even though I was a Christian, I got involved in extramarital affairs. Then the business began to suffer. One day I came home from work and my wife had left me. She had taken the kids and everything in the house. It was the day before my birthday. She had unloaded a three-level, three-bedroom townhouse, and all the furnishings, in one day. She even dis-connected the light fixtures!"

Frank never took time to grieve the loss of his family, or his mother's death that same year. Nor, at first, did he own up to his responsibility in the marital breakup.

"I was crying out to God in desperation, but I wasn't crying out to him in repentance," he says.

The business continued to fail—or, as Frank says today, "I began to fail the business. Some of the basic things I had done, I stopped doing. I'm sure I was depressed during that period, but I didn't recognize it and I continued to find other diversions."

Frank set up a meeting with the company's accountant to discuss the financial problems resulting from the decline of the business. "Things were going progressively downhill. We were looking for solutions, and I suggested that maybe we could bring another partner into the business. The accountant, who by the way was not a Christian, just looked at me and said, 'I don't think you need a partner. I think you need a savior.'

"Of course, what my accountant meant is that the business couldn't be salvaged, that it was all over, beyond fixing. But I heard something dif-ferent in his words. I heard what God wanted me to hear—that I person-ally needed a Savior to lift me out of the mess I'd gotten myself into.

"After the meeting with the accountant, I hopped into the Volvo with the Corinthian-leather seats and the little bun-warmer underneath. It wasn't raining that night, but I'll tell you what—I needed windshield wipers to get me home. I drove forty-five minutes to my house with tears just pouring out in repentance to the Lord. God was speaking to me and telling me to come back to him."

In response to his sense of God's call, Frank gathered up his courage and joined a men's-prayer and Bible-study group. At first, he felt uncertain about the group; plagued by concerns that the other men would judge him, Frank revealed very little. Eventually, though, when another man confessed that he, too, was struggling with depression, Frank was able to open up. Today, the group provides spiritual companionship and mutual accountability. Frank takes comfort in a Bible verse that ordains such a relationship: "Bear one another's burdens, and in this way you will fulfill the law of Christ" (Galatians 6:2). After a lifetime of rejoicing in his self-sufficiency, Frank is slowly learning to depend on others and to listen to what they have to say to him.

Though his depression has remained under control for several years, Frank's life has remained a struggle. He remarried, but, despite his spiritual renewal and personal growth, he continues to have difficulties sustaining close relationships. Recently, his second wife asked for a separation—a move that Frank vigorously resisted. When his wife insisted, Frank acceded reluctantly. They have entered marriage counseling in the hopes of building a stronger relationship that will last.

The problems with his marriage have been difficult for Frank, but he has not become depressed again. Relieved of the bleak outlook and troubling physical problems that characterized his clinical depression, Frank is working on his marriage and grappling with difficult issues in his own personality.

"My life's not a 'happily-ever-after' story, not yet anyway," Frank said recently, "but one change that has really stuck has been a closer relationship with God. That's what the depression was for. See, I'm one of those guys that God uses a two-by-four on. The depression helped me grow spiritually and is still helping me grow."

✦

I can understand my patients' struggles with depression on a deeply personal level, because, as I said earlier, I myself have experienced this disorder. Early in medical school, as I struggled to digest mountains of facts and to keep up with the grueling pace of my training, I found myself sluggish and unable to concentrate on my work. I had always been a straight-A student; academic work was enjoyable and easy for me. But now I felt overwhelmed and was struggling even to pass the tests. I was running as hard as I could to stay in the same place. Humble pie was a new taste for me, and I didn't like it. Fortunately, my episodes of disabling depression were brief, lasting only a few weeks at a time (two weeks is the minimum time required for a diagnosis of clinical depression). But less intense symptoms of depression stayed with me for several months. Even though my depression abated and I successfully completed medical school, I can still remember that sense of heaviness and despair.

Moving on to my internship, I plunged into the best of times and the worst of times. It was exhilarating to know that patients depended on me, but the hundred-hour week took its toll. I was unable to maintain the exacting standards I set for myself. As one of only two brothers out of five to reach adulthood in good health, I felt that I needed to be a standard-bearer for my family; I put a great deal of pressure on myself to succeed. I love challenges, and in high school I had gone on the grueling wilderness-survival course, Outward Bound, whose motto I claimed as my own: "to serve, to strive, and not to yield." I believed in myself and felt that there was nothing I couldn't handle. I had heard the stories about how difficult internship could be, and I had observed its corrosive effect on other interns, but I would be different. I could make it without buckling; I *would* make it! I would "strive and not yield." I never imagined that I would have any difficulty fulfilling my responsibilities.

But in the middle of my first year of internship, my worst nightmare happened. I became quite depressed. I had to get off the battlefield. I took ten days of emergency leave. It was painful to realize that my colleagues had to pick up the slack as I struggled with my profound feelings of darkness and sadness. At first, I interpreted my depression as a defeat, a failure, and a lack of will, and I felt even more forlorn. But then something wonderful happened: gradually, over the course of a few months, I came to the conclusion that this was meant to be a transformative experience. In the past, I had relied completely on myself to meet life's challenges; though I was a religious person, I very seldom turned to God when times turned tough. The experience of depression showed me that my ability to help myself was limited. In times of despair, I could not motivate myself to get my work done, to overcome my sadness and confusion, or to change my outlook. I learned that I had to "let go and let God" help me deal with my feelings and problems, and at last I understood what St. Paul meant in his passage about "the thorn in the flesh":

. . . a thorn was given me in the flesh, a messenger of Satan to torment me, to keep me from being too elated. Three times I appealed to the Lord about this, that it would leave me, but he said to me, "My grace is sufficient for you, for power is made perfect in weakness." So, I will boast all the more gladly of my weaknesses, so that the power of Christ may dwell in me. Therefore I am content with weaknesses, insults, hardships, persecutions, and calamities for the sake of Christ; for whenever I am weak, then I am strong. [2 CORINTHIANS 12:7–10.]

Reframing this episode of depression as a "thorn in the flesh" and a reminder of the need for humility and self-acceptance was the beginning of the death knoll for some of my intense perfectionism. Fortunately, my mood gradually improved over the course of a month without any pharmacological assistance; I benefited greatly from counseling. Prayer, time, and time off helped me heal. Even when I resumed the intense schedule of internship, I could better cope; and the depressive symptoms have not returned.

The lessons I learned from my "defeat" have helped deepen my faith life and have prepared me for a life of helping others who struggle with depression and similar illnesses.

BEATING BIPOLAR DISORDER

One of the most severe forms of mood disorder is bipolar disorder, which is also known as manic-depressive illness. In this mental illness, the patient swings between periods of great energy and intensely "up" feelings—mania—and periods of deep depression. For my patient Claudia, age fifty-three, this illness has frequently been disabling, and she has probably had it since she was quite young. Her siblings show signs of it as well, which is to be expected, since there is a genetic component to the illness. But until Claudia was in her late forties, she did not know the name of her illness, nor did she receive treatment to make it better.

"I was sick my whole life," Claudia remembered. "I had depression. I had physical illnesses. Some years in school I would miss more days than I would actually make it, and as a result I was really having a hard time."

As an adult, Claudia found her depression manifested itself in fits of rage: "I had extreme, violent anger. I just couldn't seem to control it, and the violence would come on so fast I wouldn't even know it was coming. I lost a marriage that way. I had trouble with my children. Someone would say to me, 'Well, you should count to ten before you do anything when you're angry.' But I couldn't count to ten. I couldn't even think!"

Despite her debilitating anger, Claudia held responsible jobs. A Catholic with skills and training in institutional administration, she was placed in charge of all nonacademic programs for a large parochial school. In this and other positions, her rage would erupt. But then the manic side of her illness would resurface. While in the manic phase, Claudia would rebuild the bridges she had burned while depressed; she was also able to work twice as hard and twice as creatively as any of her colleagues. Her sporadic but exceptional effectiveness on the job helped mask her illness.

"I'm holding down a major job, doing fine, so how can I really be a wreck?" she would ask herself. Because her illness included many physical symptoms, like aches, pain, and fatigue, Claudia sought help from many doctors, but without good results. She became disgusted with the entire medical profession and avoided doctors as much as possible.

But while seeking therapy to help her cope with problems in her second marriage and other relationships, Claudia was referred to me for evaluation. At our first meeting, she angrily told me how she felt about doctors.

"I wasn't ready to trust you, no matter how nice you seemed," Claudia recalled several years later. "If you had looked at me cross-eyed I would have yelled at you, because I was just so defensive."

Fortunately, I didn't "look at her cross-eyed." Having enough psychiatric training to recognize that Claudia was projecting all her anger at doctors onto me, I reacted sympathetically, allowing her to vent her feelings. Slowly, Claudia and I established a rapport, and after examining her and talking with her at length, I gave her my diagnosis of bipolar disease and placed her on lithium, the treatment of choice for stabilizing this condition. Claudia continued therapy with the psychologist who had referred her to me. In addition, because Claudia told me she was a person of faith, I suggested that she pray for her healing and read a number of Bible verses. Today, Claudia feels like a different person.

"I have no more rages whatsoever," she told me during a recent office visit. "I can almost pray a lot of the anger and depression away. It's amazing how much I've changed."

Claudia feels pangs of regret when she thinks of all the years she was sick and did not know the nature of her illness. She looks at pictures of herself as a child and a younger woman, and she sees a terribly unhappy face looking back.

"I couldn't change what I didn't know existed, and that is sad," she said, reflecting on her years of suffering. "But because of my illness, I have a lot of compassion for hurting people."

Retired from her job as a school administrator, Claudia is now active in her church, teaching Bible-study classes and working with troubled individuals.

"One of the guys I'm helping now is a prisoner. Another fellow just came out of prison; he had been beating his wife and had raped her. That's awful, of course, but I can still talk to him," she said. "I've been through so much and done so many bad things myself, it's hard for me to be critical of anybody else, even this guy who did such terrible things."

Thanks to her active faith and her diligent use of medicines and therapy, Claudia has her illness under control. She dislikes some of the side effects of her medication, such as excessive thirst, diarrhea, and a prominent tremor. But she has come to understand that she must continue taking it. Like many others with bipolar disorder, she has occasionally stopped the medication, believing herself to be healed of the disorder. The eventual return of some of her symptoms leads her to resume medication, which she now accepts as inevitable, like a diabetic taking insulin. She is grateful that she can now give to others instead of screaming at them in blind fury.

"I've never known the happiness I have now, never before in my whole life," she said. "Maybe that's why it's so easy for me to laugh now. Before, I never knew how to laugh."

EASING ANXIETY

People with depression report feeling numb, emotionally paralyzed, sad, and physically slowed down. Anxiety, on the other hand, is often marked by a feeling of being speeded up, "wired." An everyday worry will turn into an enormous, urgent demand that constantly occupies the sufferer's mind. Physically, anxiety patients report racing and skipping heartbeats, a sensation of choking or being unable to get enough air, bowel disturbances, and weakness and trembling. When anxieties manifest themselves as phobias, patients will go to great lengths to avoid the factor that sets off the phobic episode or panic attack. Phobic patients come to fear not only the initially frightening event or situation, like flying in an airplane, traveling on a bridge or through a tunnel, or being near the edge of a tall building or cliff; they also fear the dramatic physical reactions of the phobia itself. Patients with phobias and panic attacks have what I call the "Franklin D. Roosevelt syndrome"—they have "nothing to fear but fear itself."

Just as my personal experience of depression helps me care for patients with this disease, firsthand experience with panic disorder gives me insight into this group of illnesses. I remember vividly my one and only panic attack; it came when I was facing an anatomy test in medical school. I felt inadequately prepared for the exam, and when the test was handed to me, I drew a complete blank. Suddenly a choking feeling developed in my throat, and I felt as if I could not control my vision, my mood, or my thinking. I left the room abruptly, heading to the restroom to collect myself. After about ten minutes, the panicky sensations passed, and I was able to complete the test successfully. But I will never forget the frightening feeling of being out of control that enveloped me that day—a feeling that millions of patients cope with regularly.

For most people with anxiety, prescription drugs, cognitive and behavioral psychotherapy—and church attendance, prayer, and Bible reading—can help control their symptoms. Researcher Harold Koenig assessed the relationship between religious involvement and anxiety disorders in 2,969 individuals in a 1993 study. Young and middle-aged individuals who attended church at least once a week were significantly less likely to have anxiety-related disorders than those who did not attend church regularly. Among younger subjects, devotional activities such as prayer and Bible study were found to be linked with lower incidence of agoraphobia and other forms of anxiety.

Anxiety can also manifest itself as tension in the body—tension severe enough to be paralyzing, especially when fear becomes extreme. Betty, a travel writer in her forties, was living with her husband, a military officer, in Japan when anxiety started causing real problems. Looking at this immaculately coiffed and elegantly dressed woman, I found it hard to envision her crumbling under the weight of anxiety, but her outer poise was not always matched by inner equilibrium.

"I had been subject to headaches that were tension-related, according to the neurologist I had consulted," she recalls. "They caused a great knot in the back of the head and horrible pain. I could barely move my head. I would have to take a prescription medication and also coffee, for the caffeine, and apply heat to the head. It would be several hours before I'd get relief."

Though she was a person of deep faith, Betty never considered praying for relief of the tension headaches and the anxiety, until one day a headache threatened an outing she had planned.

"I had a friend who was timid and nervous, and we were going to go to Seoul, Korea, together. This meant we had to drive from our base, near Tokyo, to the army air base. It was about an hour's drive through Japan, by ourselves, to where we were going to try to find a flight that would be available, so we could go to Korea for two or three days of shopping and exploring. Just thinking about this drive through Japan terrified me. The traffic is wild, you can't read any of the signs, *and* you drive on the other side of the road."

But Betty, an adventurous person, was willing to try. "I had driven with my husband up to this base, and I thought I could find it again by looking for little landmarks along the side of the road. The morning we were scheduled to leave, I was so nervous that, half an hour before I was supposed to pick up my friend, I had this horrible pain and a knot about the size of an orange in the back of my neck. If this kept up, I wouldn't be able to drive.

"I knew the responsibility for this trip was on me, because my friend was a total nervous wreck. The fact of being responsible for her was what was really getting to me. So I went to the bedroom in the back of our house and I knelt down by the side of the bed and asked God to help me. I asked for help with being responsible and wanting to get there safely.

"When I finished the prayer, I felt as if a finger had lightly touched the back of the neck, and I felt as if this ball of pain had literally crumbled, as if it were a ball of dry clay, and the pain disappeared. And I got us there in the car safely and we had a marvelous time."

Since her prayer that day, Betty's tension headaches have decreased in frequency and severity. "I used to get twelve to sixteen a year, and they were fierce. Now I'm down to two or three a year, and they're nothing like they were. I very rarely have to take the medication prescribed by the neurologist."

Was it prayer alone that reduced the frequency and severity of Betty's headaches? According to her, no other changes in lifestyle have occurred, and she has not switched medications. From the medical point of view, I believe that Betty may be invoking Remedy No. 1 of the faith factor, the Relaxation Response, when she prays, thus reducing muscle tension in her neck and relieving her headaches. The experience of finding relief through prayer may also have helped Betty avoid the feelings of anxiety that would make her tension headaches even more severe; now she believes there is a remedy that works in addition to medication, so she can reassure herself, thus avoiding greater tension.

✢

Insomnia often accompanies anxiety—not just an occasional restless night, but a persistent inability to get to sleep or to stay asleep. Many of my patients have successfully dealt with their anxiety through medication and also through prayer.

Brooke, a twenty-nine-year-old administrator at a nonprofit organization, found herself unable to sleep after an automobile accident took the lives of her father and brother-in-law and left Brooke responsible for caring for her mother and sister, who survived, severely injured. At the time of the accident, Brooke told me, she was anything but devout:

"I'd left the church because I was angry about sexism in the institution," she said, "and though I'd never renounced my belief in God, I had really drifted away from practicing my faith."

But in the aftermath of the accident, when Brooke could not sleep night after night, she found herself returning to the resources of religion almost instinctively.

"So many nights I'd find myself thinking about my father trapped in the wreckage of the car, or what was going to become of my mother and my sister, who were now disabled and widowed. Sleep would get further and further away," she said. "I'd then get even more worried because I couldn't sleep. It was as if I was hearing a constant chattering voice reciting all my worries to me as I lay there trying to sleep. My whole body was tense and I could not relax. How would I ever be able to deal with all these problems when I was physically and mentally exhausted, too? The next day, at work, I'd sit at my desk and stare into space. I could handle only the most boring, routine tasks. I began to worry that I'd lose my job on top of everything else."

One sleepless night, a familiar prayer came quietly into Brooke's mind.

"As a child in the Episcopal Church, I had learned to sing an ancient plainsong version of the Lord's Prayer. One night, without even thinking about it, I began to sing the Lord's Prayer to myself silently, over and over again. I would go over it in my mind, note by note, until finally I would fall asleep."

Despite long-term psychotherapy to help her deal with her grief, Brooke continued to struggle with insomnia and other forms of anxiety, as well as occasional bouts of depression. Even though she was experiencing a gradual renewal of her faith, there would be days when she couldn't get out of bed, or when hopelessness would seize her. When she became my patient, several years after the accident, I suggested that she try antidepressant medication as well as more prayer.

"You are a perfect candidate for prayer and Prozac," I told her. Brooke was ready for the prayer; she was a bit reluctant about the Prozac, but agreed to try it.

"Can we pray for the medicine?" I asked her. She agreed, and I prayed aloud, thanking God for the gift of medicines and asking God to make the medicine effective, to bless it, and to use it for Brooke's healing.

Brooke had a remarkable response. Her insomnia and the anxious internal chatter that broke her concentration have reappeared only when she stopped Prozac for several brief periods. She believes her recovery could not have been achieved without both faith and medicine.

"I had gone back to church, and I was trying to pray and read the Bible regularly, but the depression and anxiety really hampered the growth of my spiritual life," she said. "Once the medication kicked in, I was calm and stable enough to have a prayer discipline and to get involved with some projects at church. I was also much better able to handle taking care of my mother and my sister.

"Once I was back as a member of the flock, I got a lot of support from my friends at church and my priest. I prayed constantly for strength, while caring for my mother and my sister before they were able to care for them-selves again. I have attended many healing services and asked for prayer for healing of my depression, anxiety, and other problems," Brooke told me. "There haven't been any quick fixes in all of this, but I really have seen good come out of a great deal of suffering in my life, and today I feel as if I've been restored spiritually, almost as if I'm a new person."

In dealing with the many challenges facing her, Brooke has prayed sev-eral scripture verses regularly, but she does have one particular favorite:

"It's been tough for me to accept my limits, to understand that I can't make things all better for my family, and to accept the fact that I need medication for my anxiety and depression," she said recently. I told her that I, too, had struggled with perfectionism, and suggested that she pray the same verse that meant so much to me, where God says to Paul, "My grace is sufficient for you, for power is made perfect in weakness" (2 Corinthians 12:9).

Just as it did for me, this great scripture verse became an anchor of sta-bility for Brooke. "Every time I think I should be able to do more, be better, please everyone, I remember that verse," she said. "I hold on to it like a lifeline, because I really want to stay well." She still takes Prozac and will probably be on it indefinitely; when she has tried to stop taking it, her insomnia and anxiety symptoms return within several months, even though there are no major stress factors in her life at this time.

"I like sleeping at night," she said. "I think I'll stay with the prayer and the Prozac!"

✢

Fear truly rules the lives of some who suffer from anxiety. When he ini-tially came to see me, I noticed that David, a forty-five-year-old self-employed remodeling contractor, looked at first glance to be hale and hearty. A tall, muscular man with long brown hair and a beard, he reminded me of the "hippies" of the 1960s and 1970s. Indeed, as it turned out, David had been involved in that period's counterculture, but left it behind as he grew older and returned to the practice of the Jewish faith of his child-hood. David's faith had remained strong, but, despite his robust physical appearance, he had developed anxiety that grew continually worse, despite his best efforts to "talk myself out of it."

I asked David to tell me about the disease's progression.

"At first, it was just like my heart was racing and I was sweating, mostly when I had to drive over a bridge or through a tunnel," he said. "I know that's ridiculous, but that's what started the whole thing. Then it got so that I had diarrhea all the time—I still do. I've had several doctors check me out and there's no physical reason for it, but it's pretty uncontrollable, no matter what I do. So I installed a portable toilet in the back of my truck. That way I don't have to worry about finding a bathroom in a hurry."

David's fear of driving over bridges and through tunnels caused him to make enormous detours, sometimes taking him hundreds of miles out of his way. As a contractor, he works at sites throughout the Baltimore-Washington area, so the detours cost him valuable time—and money. Still, as the years went by, the fears grew worse.

"I don't even like to look at *pictures* of a bridge, Doctor!" David confessed ruefully. "Here I am, a grown man, and I get the shakes just thinking about them!"

I explained to David that anxiety disorders and phobias have nothing to do with a person's level of emotional or spiritual maturity. "This is a disease, David," I told him. "You didn't create it. It's not your fault. Millions of people suffer from phobias like yours, and I think I can help you overcome it."

I prescribed antianxiety medication for David, and asked him whether he had prayed for relief of his anxiety.

"I really haven't," he said. "I can't see bothering the Lord with my little problem."

"David, the scriptures tell us to trust in God to care for us and to take care of our needs," I said. On learning that David had not consulted his rabbi about his problems, I urged him to do so and suggested that he meditate on several passages from the Hebrew Bible, including:

For thus said the Lord God, the Holy One of Israel: In returning and rest you shall be saved; in quietness and in trust shall be your strength. [ISAIAH 30:15.]

I also showed David how to use deep-breathing and muscle-relaxation techniques whenever he felt the anxiety symptoms coming on, and recommended that he join a phobia-treatment group focusing on his particular disorder. Such groups use desensitization therapy—or carefully controlled, gradually increasing exposures to the situations that elicit the phobic reaction—to help people manage their phobias.

As I worked with David over the course of a year, he slowly began to gain control over his symptoms. Eventually, to his great relief, he was able to dismantle the portable toilet in the back of his truck. Then, at last, David experienced what was for him the ultimate triumph. I found out about it when I collected my messages from my secretary one day. There, on the pink slip of paper, was a simple message from David: "Made it across the Chesapeake Bay Bridge—no sweat! Thanks!"

Today, David can handle high bridges and long tunnels with little fear, thanks to a three-pronged approach to his anxiety disorder—medication, supportive group counseling, and a daily period of early-morning meditative prayer that helps him face the day in a calm and centered state of mind.

✢

Not long ago, people with illnesses like depression, bipolar disorder, and anxiety lived lives of despair and agony. Before the advent of effective drugs for these conditions, many patients were disabled by them, and some even committed suicide. Today, when doctors diagnose these illnesses properly, many treatment resources are available. Prescription medications now form the medical cornerstone for recovery from mental illness, but psychotherapy, support groups, and the resources of faith appear to help people change their thought patterns and make constructive changes in their lives. For many of my patients, suffering through depression or anxiety has actually brought them closer to God—perhaps not right away, but ultimately. Once out of the grip of these frightening illnesses, they find new meaning in their lives and often go forward with a desire to grow spiritually and to serve others. The illness can serve as a wake-up call for some to change destructive life patterns. People who have listened to the message and heeded its call have often done better.

Unfortunately, many individuals with depression and anxiety don't know they are ill, and resort to substance abuse to medicate themselves. Let us turn our attention now to addictions—to drugs, alcohol, tobacco, and other substances—the devastating disorders in which we appear to lose the God-given freedom to control our behavior.

CHAPTER 5

Healing Addictions:
Regaining Our Freedom

Nowhere in medicine has the faith factor proved more powerful than in the field of addiction recovery. Science has shown faith's resources to be critically important in preventing and treating many kinds of substance abuse and addictive behavior. In most clinical studies measuring the impact of spiritual beliefs and practices on the prevention and treatment of nicotine, drug, and alcohol addiction, religious involvement has been found to have a positive effect.

Studies have shown repeatedly that religiously observant people are less likely than others to abuse alcohol. This conclusion might not be surprising in view of the tenets of major religions and denominations that emphasize abstinence from any form of addictive drugs, such as Islam, the Church of the Latter-Day Saints, and the Seventh-Day Adventists. But the data indicate that the protective effect of religion against alcohol abuse holds true even among people who do drink. In a 1995 study, investigators measured signs of dependence on alcohol (blackouts, intense desire to drink, hand tremors, elevations in heart rate and blood pressure) and social consequences of drinking (arrests for drunk driving, problems at work or job loss, family problems, loss of friends) experienced by the subjects, as well as a number of other variables, including religious involvement. Over 40 percent of the drinkers ranked religion as "very important." These individuals were only half as likely to show three or more alcohol-dependence symptoms, and not quite half as likely to have experienced two or more social consequences of drinking, as the subjects who ranked religion as less important.

Though we know its devastating effects on the body, mind, and spirit, doctors are not immune to alcoholism. Fortunately, physicians, too, may find help in avoiding alcoholism through religious involvement. A 1990 study of graduates of the Johns Hopkins University Medical School found that 13 percent showed signs of alcohol abuse at some point in their careers. The strongest single predictor of alcohol abuse after medical school was a lack of religious affiliation. One interesting but unexplained additional finding of the study was a difference by religion: medical students who were Jewish by affiliation or ancestry were found to be less likely to abuse alcohol than their non-Jewish counterparts.

The antiaddictive effects of religion are particularly important during adolescence, when peer pressure and the need to separate from parents make young people particularly vulnerable to the use of alcohol, cigarettes, and illicit drugs. A significant body of research indicates that young people who are religiously involved have a much greater chance of avoiding substance-abuse problems and the delinquency that often accompanies them. The degree of parents' religious involvement also influences children's substance-abuse behaviors. A 1996 study of adolescents and their mothers found that the mother's religious involvement was the most significant predictor of reduced alcohol use among adolescents, and a 1985 study showed that family religiousness protected against alcohol and drug abuse among adolescents, with the father's belief in God being the most significant factor. In fact, the medical data now in hand suggest that any "war on drugs" or other substances may be a losing battle if faith is not part of the arsenal.

Scientists have also found that people who are addicted to drugs and alcohol are likely to be less spiritually or religiously active than their non-addicted peers. One study shows that this holds true even among a group of people at high risk for substance abuse—patients at mental-health centers. Researchers who analyzed factors influencing alcohol and drug abuse in 835 such patients found that those with a high level of religious involvement were half as likely to abuse alcohol and only one-third as likely to abuse drugs as their peers who had no significant religious involvement.

It is best, of course, to prevent addiction, using spiritual and other resources at our disposal. But when people *do* fall under the sway of an addictive substance, the resources of the faith factor offer help and hope for restoring wellness. To name one prominent example, programs like Alcoholics Anonymous have provided the best long-term answer for many addicted people. These Twelve Step programs are based on spiritual principles and lead to spiritual growth among participants.

While addressing the spiritual component of addictions is critically important, doctors must also consider addicted people's very real physical dependence on substances ranging from alcohol to nicotine to cocaine. For most people, recovery begins with a wrenching separation from the substance to which they are addicted, a period of "drying out" which may occur in an inpatient or outpatient setting. Drug addicts may need to be weaned slowly from their substance of choice to avoid provoking withdrawal symptoms of craving, anxiety, restlessness, headache, and bowel disturbances. Smokers benefit from nicotine-replacement therapy to help combat the insistent physical cravings for this tremendously addictive drug. Often, doctors find that addicted patients need treatment for mental illnesses like depression or bipolar disorder. Addictive behavior can arise out of an attempt to "self-medicate" emotional pain, so prescription medications and psychotherapy may be necessary to help prevent relapse.

But many people who are successful in kicking addictions cite the spiritual component of recovery as a major factor in regaining and maintaining their sobriety. In a 1991 study of alcoholics and drug addicts, researchers found that alcoholics who had achieved long-term sobriety (four to sixteen years) had developed spiritual practices in conjunction with their Alcoholics Anonymous participation; 100 percent said they meditated or had "quiet time" daily, 100 percent prayed regularly, and 97 percent read a meditation book daily.

The spiritual practices that helped these alcoholics achieve and maintain sobriety are not based on will power, or an attempt to resist temptation out of one's own strength, but on surrender to God, or to the less-defined "Higher Power" of the Twelve Step movement. As the first two of the Twelve Steps put it:

STEP ONE: We admitted we were powerless over alcohol—that our lives had become unmanageable.

STEP TWO: We came to believe that a Power greater than ourselves could restore us to sanity.

Admitting one's powerlessness over a substance runs counter to our cultural need to be "in control" and to overcome our problems through will power. But for many addicted people, coming to terms with their weakness is the only way to gain strength, and depending on the power of God is their only hope for maintaining sobriety. Their way of regaining control is to "let go and let God."

Let us examine the process of recovery from addiction as it is lived in people's lives, noting especially how recovery is frequently prompted by a profound spiritual change, such as a religious conversion, or how people experience spiritual growth through their attempts to deal with addiction. As psychiatrist Gerald May writes in *Addiction and Grace:*

> . . . any sincere battle with a particular addiction is likely to bring us to some kind of spiritual confrontation, and any sincere spiritual journey is certain to involve very practical struggles with addictions.

RELEASE FROM BONDAGE: QUANTUM RECOVERY

As alcoholism expert Dr. William R. Miller notes, many addicted people seem to undergo a sudden, profound transformation that starts their recovery. The value system of such "quantum changers" is often completely and quickly reversed, and they experience a deep awareness that the addictive behavior cannot continue. Sometimes they also feel as if their desire to drink or use drugs has been removed by a force outside themselves.

Medical science has no convincing explanation for such overnight transformations. Psychiatrists expect (and usually observe) gradual improvement, achieved by patients who work consciously on their problems. But the world's great religious traditions are full of stories of *metanoia,* a complete turning about that leads to a renewal of life. Here again, the resources of religion and spirituality can shed light on how people with addictions undergo sudden but profound change that frees them from emotional, physical, and spiritual bondage. Julia, an alcoholic who battled to quit drinking for years without success, experienced such a "quantum change," and credits her lasting recovery to God.

Julia grew up as the oldest daughter of a distinguished navy officer. At parties in their home and at the officers' club, "drinking was a part of our world." Still, Julia wasn't much of a drinker until after college, when she, now a young navy officer herself, met Dennis, the man she would marry.

From the start, Julia had unrealistic expectations about her relationship with Dennis and her stepchildren. "I was very impressionable, and I had a savior complex," she said. "All my life, I had wanted to be a hero like St. Joan of Arc. When Dennis came along, I saw my chance to do something heroic. He had full custody of his two children from a previous marriage. Their mother had mental problems. I was going to save this family and make everything all right." When Dennis and Julia married, she became "instant mother" to John, eight, and Chris, six.

Dennis and Julia's relationship was grounded in drinking together. "It was just what we did," she said. "We loved the taste of alcohol—Scotch, martinis, wine, all of it. Drinking seemed okay to me because I had grown up around a lot of social drinking, and my colleagues in the navy also drank together a lot."

Within just a few years of meeting Dennis, Julia was consuming half a quart of Scotch each evening, though she started to drink only after the workday was over. "My professional life was fine," she remembered, "but we'd come home from work and drink until we passed out or fell asleep, every night."

Though Julia's own life was spinning out of control, she accelerated her attempts to create a "perfect family" with her stepchildren. Incensed by the usual squabbles and ups-and-downs of family life, her emotions magnified by alcohol, Julia would fly into rages when things didn't go her way.

"Why can't we all pull together?" she would yell at the children and their father. "Why can't we help and love each other and not argue?"

Julia's efforts to create a model family caused resentment and rebellion in her stepchildren. The family situation was further from perfect than ever. Frustrated, Julia drank even more.

Then the navy sent Julia across the country to study for an advanced degree; because of Dennis's job, he stayed behind. Living alone, she drank even more. "I didn't have a car, but I'd ride my bike to the grocery store and buy booze, putting it in my knapsack on my back for the ride home. I started going around to different places so nobody would know how much I was buying."

Raised a Christian, Julia believed her drinking was interfering with her relationship with God. She resumed going to church occasionally, but this did not help her addiction. "I was afraid to stop," she recalled. "Just the thought of not being able to have a drink was enough to stop me from thinking about quitting."

Julia's career continued to thrive. Returning to the Washington area after completing her degree, she was assigned a high-profile post working with top navy brass. "I was just thirty, and the secretary of the navy was using stuff I had written when he reported to Congress and the president. It was a heady time, and I worked constantly—from eight A.M. to eight P.M., seven days a week. But our home life was a disaster."

Around this time, Julia became pregnant with the first of her two biological children. Pregnancy did not deter her from drinking or cigarette smoking, even though she knew better: "I remember knowing that drinking wasn't right, but I also remember that I thought beer was okay because it was loaded with vitamin B!" Jennifer and Harry were born one year apart, and soon Julia was assigned to a new duty station, in Florida. Dennis could not find a job there, so the family split up: Julia took her babies but left Dennis and her stepchildren in suburban Washington, D.C. It was in Florida that her drinking became a problem on the job.

"I would sometimes be late, or people could smell the booze," Julia said. "I didn't drink in the mornings, but every night I would drink a whole lot, and that was with having two small children with me. A friend told me I needed to stop drinking. I can remember really battling this, whether to stop drinking or not—fighting it out in my mind, sobbing about it. But I couldn't stop."

Today, Julia shudders, remembering how her drinking endangered her children. "I would come home, drink, and pass out. It was really by the grace of God that I did not cause or allow harm to happen to Jennifer or Harry. I was a drunken mother, I was incapable of taking care of them."

Throughout her drinking years, Julia never stopped believing that God existed, but she couldn't seem to reach him through the haze of alcohol. "For years I prayed the words of Jesus I remembered from church when I was a little girl: 'Come unto me, all ye that are heavy laden, and I will refresh you,' " she said. "I prayed, 'I am heavy laden, I need you, Lord.' But for a long time God could not answer, because I had made booze my God. I couldn't hear what God was saying to me."

At the end of her Florida assignment, Julia returned to the Washington area to face daily life with Dennis and her stepchildren. While she had been away, their home—an eighteenth-century farmhouse in the countryside near Washington—had deteriorated drastically. Dennis and the stepchildren were living in squalid conditions with infestations of ticks and mice. Dennis, too, was drinking heavily, and one day Julia came home to find him in bed with a prostitute. Her stepson John, now a teenager, became increasingly rebellious and violent. One evening, during an argument with his father, John picked up a baseball bat and started swinging. Julia jumped in to break up the fight, and John left in a rage.

The "perfect family" illusion had been destroyed, and Julia could not cope with the reality: a drunken, unfaithful husband; a violent, out-of-control stepson; a pest-infested, ramshackle, filthy house; responsibility for two toddlers; and a high-pressure job. Julia fell apart emotionally. Unable to make herself go to work, she called a navy friend and admitted she had a problem with alcohol. Her friend took her to the Bethesda Naval Hospital, where she was immediately admitted to a thirty-day inpatient alcohol-rehabilitation program and placed on antianxiety medications to ease withdrawal symptoms.

"In going into the program, you had to admit that your life was out of control and that you had no control over alcohol, and that you are helpless before God," Julia remembered. "I had to write an autobiography and go to Alcoholics Anonymous meetings. I remember I knew at my first meeting that *this* is how the Christian life was supposed to be lived. For the first time in my life, the whole thing clicked, though nobody ever said anything about Christ."

Julia's surrender to a Higher Power—for her, God in Jesus Christ—came when she admitted to her A.A. group that her drinking had led her to abuse and neglect her children. "That slayed me," she said. "That was a humbling experience."

One day, as she joined other rehab patients on a van going to an A.A. meeting, Julia heard God speak to her. "It was an inner voice, and he said that he was pleased with me, that I had done the right thing," she said. "I was totally flooded with peace. It was just like when God spoke to Jesus when he was baptized and said, 'You are my beloved Son and I am pleased with you.' That's what he said to me. Then I knew I didn't have to worry about anything—not about being separated from Dennis while I was in treatment, or my children, or my career."

It has been eleven years since Julia had a drink, even though Dennis continued drinking after she returned home. She believes that her desire for alcohol has been completely removed by God. "God knew how frail I was, and he gave me a special healing," she told me. "I never had to go through the one-day-at-a-time business; the desire to drink just left. God knows us inside out. I suspect he knew what my limits were." Though she enjoys a near-miraculous recovery from alcoholism, Julia has not found release from her addiction to tobacco; she continues to smoke two or more packs of cigarettes a day, despite repeated attempts to quit.

Still in thrall to alcohol, Dennis left the family several years ago and rarely visits Jennifer and Harry. The older children have grown up and moved out, and now Julia is in effect a single mother with two teenagers. To have more time with them through their growing-up years, she retired from the navy and works part-time. She is an active member of her church and enjoys gardening, hosting dinners for friends, and listening to music. Things are not always easy for Julia and her family. Money is tight, and Dennis's absence from the family creates a lingering sense of loss. But Julia is free of the bondage of alcohol, and her family life is peaceful, if not perfect. Jennifer and Harry are doing well in school, enjoying sports, and participating actively in church as members of the choir and youth group. Julia has time for the children and for the elderly members of her congregation who need rides to the doctor or the grocery store. Her days are ruled by her sense of God's call in her life, not by the pressure and prestige that marked her navy career. Most important, alcohol, the idol she once worshiped, has toppled, and in its place stands the God to whom she has dedicated her life.

CHANGE FOLLOWING CONVERSION: AMENDMENT OF LIFE

You might consider the "quantum changers," like Julia, to be the lucky ones. Their relief from addiction comes suddenly and, it seems, almost effortlessly, as their entire personalities undergo drastic change. For Julia and others like her, a deeper spiritual life came *after* the addiction was relieved. For other addicts, conversion comes first, and with it a sense of urgency about amending their lives to conform to new and higher standards of behavior. In the following story, we will see how a husband and wife worked to become free of their addiction to tobacco after their mid-life religious conversions. The need to restore their bodies as fit "temples of the Holy Spirit" gave them the courage to grapple with their addiction.

✢

Cigarette smoking is one of the most addictive and destructive behaviors known to human beings. Approximately forty-eight million American adults smoked in 1994, according to the Centers for Disease Control; public-health experts estimate that smoking costs our society around $50 billion each year in medical costs alone. The emotional cost of suffering and grief is immeasurable. Today's nicotine-replacement drugs, including chewing gum and nicotine patches, can help people overcome withdrawal symptoms that follow the attempt to quit smoking—irritability, restlessness, headaches, problems concentrating, sleep disturbance, increased hunger, etc. But in many cases, nicotine replacement alone is not enough. As with other addictions, spiritual means for coping with cravings can help break the dependency.

I urge my patients who smoke to quit, and, to help them, I often prescribe the patch. If they are people of faith, I will also "prescribe" prayer, religious involvement, and Bible verses to help them get through the first terrible days or weeks. My patients Becky and George took things a step further, developing their own method of aversion therapy to overcome their decades-long addiction to cigarettes. They created a series of disturbing mental images to focus on whenever they wanted to smoke. Though images of charred, shriveled lungs from autopsies of smokers had not deterred them, images of Christ suffering on the cross—out of love for them—did.

A tall, earthy Texas native with a ready sense of humor, Becky lives in a chaotic but happy household. "Four teenagers, a dog, a cat, two birds, three hamsters, and George and me in a three-bedroom townhouse. Picture it!" she said, laughing. Her husband, George, is quieter, but he is just as likely to crack a terrible pun as he is to communicate a profound spiritual insight. He let her tell me their story of recovery from nicotine addiction.

Becky started smoking at the age of thirteen, even though as a child she had proudly sworn never to do so. "I gave in to peer pressure when I went to junior high school," she recalled. "I began to smoke Kool cigarettes, so I'd be cool."

By the time she reached adulthood, Becky was a chain smoker, averaging three packs a day. While training for a career in medical technology, she witnessed her first autopsy—performed on the body of a smoker.

"The pathologist knew I was a smoker, so he pulled the lungs out and said, 'Look at this.' Normal lungs are very pink and white, and this guy's lungs looked like charcoal. It was disgusting. After that, I would try to quit for short periods of time, but I never could."

Becky met and married another medical technologist, George, who also smoked. Even when she tried to give up the smoking habit, she would relent after a few hours when George lit up. Other smokers—friends and family members—would try to derail her attempts to quit: "Come on, have a cigarette. You know you want one." And she would fail again.

During her four pregnancies, Becky found the inner strength to cut back drastically on her cigarette smoking. "From the time I found out I was pregnant till the child was born, I allowed myself one or two cigarettes a day," she said. "I was able to do that during pregnancy because it wasn't for me—you *have* to take care of that baby!"

Becky had been raised a churchgoer, but religion had become unimportant to her as she grew up. As she and George prepared to marry, they became furious when the minister who had counseled them was denied the opportunity to perform their marriage ceremony by his superiors because the minister himself was grappling with personal problems. After the wedding ceremony, George and Becky vowed not to darken the door of a church again.

But almost twenty years later, Becky had a sudden spiritual awakening. A friend challenged her to take her children to church. "He said, 'You were raised with the church, so at least you have a basis for faith. Your children don't have that, and it's not fair to them.' Then, the week before Christmas, my mother said, 'Why don't we go to church on Christmas

Eve as a family?' I said okay. The kids wanted to go, and George said he'd come, too, even though he was an agnostic. We went, and then, the next week, Mom suggested that we go to the regular Sunday service at a different church, nearer our home."

On the way to church that Sunday, Becky's mother said, "Oh, by the way, the pastor at this church is a woman." Becky was aghast: "I had a real problem with women pastors. I sat there in the pew listening to her sermon, and I thought, 'Well, you deliver it well enough, but what man wrote it for you?' "

On the way out of the church, as the pastor was greeting the congregation, Becky shook hands with her and had a surprising reaction. "I looked into her eyes, and I knew I was seeing the eyes of Christ," she remembered. "I said, 'I need to come and talk with you.' Kate said, 'Any time.' "

Over the next few months, Becky met with Kate frequently, talking about faith, life, and God. With Kate's encouragement, Becky attended a women's weekend retreat to learn more about the Christian life. It had a powerful effect.

"I knelt by my bed at the retreat house and I said to God, 'Here I am—take all of me.' And it was at that point that the transformation started."

Returning from the retreat, Becky knew her lifestyle needed to change. "I knew this holy temple shouldn't be contaminated with nicotine," she said. Soon George, too, had a remarkable conversion experience, and together they decided it was time to quit smoking. They turned to their God for help in a unique way.

"Being medical people, we went to the medical library and researched exactly what death by crucifixion is like, all the gory details," Becky recalled. "And then, when one of us would want a cigarette, the other would say, 'I wonder what it was like to have a nail driven into your wrist.' And that would keep us from smoking." The most powerful image for Becky made it impossible for her to pick up a cigarette: "I would think, how much love did it take to push up on a nail that was driven through your feet in order to fill your lungs with enough air to utter, 'Father, forgive them'? And how could I fill my lungs with smoke, then? It had never dawned on me before that Jesus suffocated. When I realized that, it seemed especially vulgar to be polluting our lungs."

For Becky and George, the image of Jesus on the cross and the prayer support of others made the impossible possible: "It's the only way we could have done it, because in actuality *we* were not doing it," Becky said. "We were truly and completely giving it to Christ and putting it on the cross with him. There were a lot of tears and a lot of prayers. Our kids prayed like crazy. They'd been asking us for years to quit."

Was their approach morbid? Maybe, but it worked for them, just as showing people photographs of cancerous lungs works for others. I encourage my patients to find the thoughts, images, and new habit patterns that will work for them as individuals. For some, the use of frightening or upsetting images can help in the battle against addiction. In Becky and George's case, the imagery was indeed disturbing, but it was also deeply meaningful for them—and it worked, even without nicotine-replacement therapy to ease the physical cravings. I would certainly not recommend a negative-imagery approach for everyone, but when patients develop their own recovery strategies, I endorse them, unless actual harm might result.

Four years after quitting smoking, Becky laughingly said, "Sometimes I'll think, 'When I'm one hundred years old, I'm going to the closest 7-Eleven store and buying a pack of Salem 100s.' But I know I can't. I won't contaminate my body that way. And I grieve for people who are addicted. I cannot comprehend how anyone has beat drugs or other addictions without God."

✢

Food is not an addictive substance in the same way nicotine, alcohol, and drugs can be, but people can relate to food in an addictive way, developing eating disorders like compulsive eating, bulimia, and anorexia. They frequently experience cravings and want to eat in order to soothe painful emotions. Eating disorders are usually linked with negative body image; patients who see themselves as "too fat" may develop anorexia in an attempt to starve themselves thin. My patient Celeste, age thirty-seven, came to me originally hoping to find the long-sought answer to her compulsive eating, overweight, and poor self-image. She had struggled with these problems all her life, but after she underwent a mid-life renewal of faith, it seemed especially urgent for Celeste to stop mistreating herself, physically and emotionally. Uprooting the habits of many years would prove very difficult.

Celeste starting overeating as a small child in rural Virginia. Years later, as an adult, she came to see the relationship between her emotions and her eating. "Whenever I am anxious or upset about anything, I'll want to reach for food, especially sweets," she told me. "And I just keep gaining weight. I've tried everything—drugs, therapy, hypnotism, every diet you can imagine. I even went to an expensive 'fat farm' for a month. I'll lose the weight, then gain it back—plus more."

Like many patients who struggle with compulsive eating and the overweight that often results, Celeste saw herself as "fat and ugly." On her first visit to my office, she told me that she was frightened of doctors—and of me.

"All my life, doctors have ridiculed me, shamed me, and made me feel that I was worthless because I couldn't lose the weight," she said. "I had to force myself to make an appointment with you. I haven't seen a doctor for at least five years."

I asked Celeste to tell me about her childhood and the circumstances of her present life. She grew up in a poor family, and, though usually loving, her parents conveyed their anxieties about money and health problems to young Celeste.

"I always felt Daddy was going to die while he was away at work," she remembered. "These thoughts preoccupied me, and I got every childhood illness that came along as well as other illnesses that the pediatrician could find no physical cause for."

Celeste also felt like a misfit at school, where her exceptional intellectual abilities set her apart from her classmates. "I was the kid who always got straight A's—*and* I was fat, and my clothes were different because Mom made them at home so we could save money," she told me. "The result was that I had no friends and was ostracized systematically by everyone except for a couple of teachers."

Celeste found solace in music—she was a piano prodigy—as well as reading, writing poetry, and spending hours alone in the woods. Food, too, was an important comforter.

"We had little in the way of material things," she remembered. "I had a piano because one of Daddy's great-aunts gave us a beat-up, ancient upright when she moved to a retirement home. But we always ate well, even when we couldn't pay our electric bill, because Daddy planted a vegetable garden and raised chickens, ducks, and rabbits."

As Celeste's weight increased, her pediatrician prescribed severe diets. The little girl who had turned to food for comfort was distraught.

"Then I seemed even weirder to the kids at school. I went to the lunchroom with my Metrecal [a canned diet drink] or my tiny little half-sandwich and an apple," she told me. "All the other kids were eating ice cream, but not me. I felt that I was being punished. So I rebelled by eating whenever my mother's back was turned at home. I'd fail on the diet and feel even worse about myself."

The pediatrician then prescribed amphetamines—diet pills—for the eight-year-old.

"I'd take the pills in the morning, then by lunchtime I felt like I was zooming around the room. I hated that 'speedy' feeling. My blood pressure went up, and the doctor took me off the diet pills. I hadn't lost any weight—I had failed again."

As Celeste grew up, she learned how to make friends and became a gregarious, outgoing, and high-achieving student, but the eating problem—and the weight—persisted.

"I look back at the pictures of me as a teenager, and I remember how awful I felt about myself," she said. "I thought I was absolutely enormous—but I wasn't. In reality, I was a big girl, but I was very pretty. But no one could convince me of that fact. Perversely, I would eat to make myself feel better." Celeste and her parents were faithful churchgoers, but faith didn't seem to help Celeste cope. She felt like a misfit at church, too, and wondered if God could really love a fat girl like her.

Celeste received a number of scholarship offers from universities around the country, and chose one at a distance from her overprotective parents. "I got away, and I cut loose," she told me. "I promptly started sleeping with a number of different guys. It was all about proving that I was attractive even though I was fat." She continued dieting, losing as many as fifty pounds, only to gain back that much and more.

As she sat in my office on that first appointment, Celeste confessed that, though she was now happily married, had a profound spiritual life, had established a successful business by the time she was thirty-two, and though she had many friends, she still felt terrible about herself.

"The only weight-loss technique I haven't tried is stomach-stapling or jaw-wiring," she said. "Yet I'm bigger today than I've ever been. I look in the mirror and I say, 'Yuck.' I push myself to enjoy my life anyway, but those bad feelings are always there."

As our interview drew to a close, I asked Celeste if she would feel comfortable proceeding with a physical examination that day. Tentatively, she said yes. When I met her in the examining room, I took her hand.

"Celeste, I am sorry that anyone, including doctors, ever made you feel bad about your body," I told her. "You are a child of God, and you are precious in his sight just as you are."

Tears filled Celeste's eyes and she nodded. "I know that's how I'm supposed to feel," she whispered. "That's how I *want* to feel."

Several years have passed since I first saw Celeste in my office. I have advised her to pray before eating and to read the Bible instead of reaching for food. Together we have prayed for her release from the bondage of compulsive eating. I have referred her to a therapist who specializes in eating disorders and prescribed antidepressant medication for her long-term, low-level depression. Her recovery from the compulsive-eating cycle has been slow, but, with much prayer and long-term therapy, she is making progress.

"I can't diet, because dieting starts the cycle of deprivation and bingeing that has gotten me where I am today," she told me recently. "Instead, I'm learning to eat in response to actual physical hunger. All my life, I've eaten because I was angry or anxious or sad—regardless of whether I was hungry or full. Now I'm learning to stop before eating and really ask myself if it's food that I need or something else, like a hug, or a talk with a caring friend, or some quiet time with God."

Self-acceptance has been an important component in Celeste's healing.

"I realized finally that all those inner voices that told me I was ugly and awful had nothing to do with God," she said. "God would never abuse me like that! *I* was abusing me, repeating the taunts and jeers of children on the playground. I internalized the prejudice against fat that's so rampant in our society, and I punished myself. Slowly, with a lot of prayer and the acceptance of my church community, I have come to understand that being fat does not mean being unacceptable or ugly. I'd like to lose weight, but even if I'm never thin, I am okay. I'm God's beloved child, as you told me several years ago."

"That's right, Celeste," I said. "Fortunately, salvation is not dependent on our Body Mass Index!" I encouraged her to continue with her therapy and to learn how to live in a healthy way regardless of her weight. Today, Celeste exercises regularly, strives to eat healthfully, and nurtures her spiritual life faithfully, attending church at least once a week and participating in a small group that meets for prayer and fellowship weekly, as well as taking daily time for individual prayer.

From the world's viewpoint, she has not succeeded, because she has not become slender. But her internal transformation is real, and by drawing on the resources of faith, Celeste is forging a new path, breaking a lifelong cycle of compulsive eating and self-hatred.

✦

While Celeste struggled with eating and weight, her husband, Tom, a publishing executive, suffered from a long-standing addiction to marijuana. Like Celeste, Tom was able to function reasonably well in the world despite his addictive behavior, but the misery underlying his addiction could not be resolved until he stopped smoking marijuana and began to deal with profound emotional and spiritual issues. For Tom, stopping was impossible until his conversion to Christianity, which followed Celeste's renewal of faith.

Tom started smoking "dope" in high school, like many of his generation. Because he was raised in a nonreligious family, he did not enjoy the protective effect of the faith factor against teenage drug use. I have seen many patients who, without the mooring provided by religion during the rocky teenage years, succumbed to drug abuse. This certainly was the case with Tom, who was thirty-eight when he first came to see me.

Tom's mother, an alcoholic, died suddenly of a cerebral aneurysm when he was thirteen. His parents had been separated at the time of her death; Tom went to live with his father, who soon remarried. Tom and his new stepmother did not get along, and his father retreated emotionally, beginning to drink heavily himself.

"I was in so much pain," Tom told me. "It was hell on earth for me. There was a lot of unresolved grief, and I felt really uncertain about where I fit in my family and whether I was wanted." Though Tom attended a prestigious church-based private school, neither he nor his parents believed actively in God; there were no faith resources to help Tom through these terrible years.

Tom started using marijuana during high school. "It was partly peer pressure," he remembered, "but I also wanted to do it. I had a lot of feelings that I didn't want to look at. I was part of a rebellious crowd—we were members of Students for a Democratic Society, we protested the Vietnam War, and we were generally disaffected with the life of Washington's rich and powerful, who surrounded us."

His marijuana habit accelerated at the intensely competitive college he attended. "I got heavily into smoking dope, especially on weekends. By the summer after my first year of college, I smoked four or five times a week, and I was smoking cigarettes, too. I stayed away from alcohol—I didn't want to be an alcoholic like my mother."

A serious and committed student of ancient languages and philosophy, Tom didn't think the marijuana smoking interfered with his academic work. "I still managed to be a really good student, but I know in retrospect that I wasn't really giving it what it deserved." By his third year of college, Tom was "stoned" almost all the time. "I felt I couldn't go on without it, that I absolutely needed it. Morally, I felt as though I wasn't hurting anybody but myself. I had this notion that being stoned helped me deal with people and kept me in touch with what was going on around me."

Tom graduated from college, married Celeste, and started working. His father was diagnosed with cancer and died soon after Tom's graduation, compounding his grief and melancholy. His marijuana use continued, though for several years he did not smoke during the day. But at his second job, as a research assistant for a large consulting firm, Tom met young drug users who smoked marijuana *and* used cocaine and other drugs on the job. His own drug use accelerated, though he stayed mostly with marijuana.

"Smoking dope let me go blotto," he said. "It allowed me not to face the pain of not knowing what I wanted to do with my life, and of not being able to deal with all my grief."

A career change helped Tom cut back on his drug use. "I started a new job in a new field when I was about thirty-two. "There was a lot to learn, and it really engaged me. Nobody was using marijuana at this new office, but I quickly found out who sold it and who could get it for me. It was still really important that I have a supply for nights and weekends."

During these years, as Celeste experienced a renewal of her childhood faith, she urged Tom to examine his beliefs and to seek God, as well as to enter psychotherapy, which he did. "Coming to faith was slow," he said. "I had to come to a place where I could trust people, first of all, before I could trust God. I trusted the strength of my relationship with Celeste, and that's what got me through. Watching her was inspirational. I thought, 'Well, she's not a nutcase, so this faith thing must be real.' At the same time, the dope was beginning to pale for me. It just wasn't delivering the results it once had. Sometimes it was just as painful as it was fun."

After several years of watching Celeste's faith life develop, and of seeking his own spiritual path and reading a number of Jewish and Christian spiritual classics, Tom went on a silent retreat at a Trappist monastery. Still searching for faith, he attended the monastic services, but did not feel as if he fit in. One day, as he was walking to the refectory for dinner, an old priest, also a retreatant at the monastery, broke the silence and spoke to Tom, gently asking why he was on retreat.

Tom found himself telling the priest about his search for faith, his confusion, and his longing to find God and to be found by God. After listening carefully to Tom's story, the priest offered to help him make the next step.

"I could counsel you and baptize you while we're on retreat here," he said, "if you feel you are ready for that."

"My grandmother had me baptized when I was a little boy, Father, but I have never received communion," Tom said, feeling a mixture of excitement and fear. The priest explained there were a number of steps Tom would need to take before receiving communion in the Roman Catholic Church.

"I'm available to talk with you, Tom, when we get back to the city," the priest said. The two men entered the refectory for dinner. They did not speak again, because Tom, upset and confused, fled the monastery that evening, before he could be asked to say grace at one of the common meals. Heading home, he tried to sort out his feelings. Eventually he began to attend Episcopal church services with Celeste. He did not partake of the sacrament of communion, administered weekly at their church; he felt unready and "not good enough."

Then some friends invited Tom and Celeste to a house-blessing ceremony. With the other guests, they followed the priest from room to room, praying for the house's occupants and their life in the new home. The ceremony concluded with the guests and priest gathering in a circle in the living room, celebrating communion and passing the bread and wine to each other.

"Here I was, standing in a circle of people, totally unable to escape without making a scene," Tom remembered. "I had to make a decision, fast. I decided to stay in the circle."

With his first communion, Tom began to see himself as a "real" Christian and to take an active part in the life of the church, but he continued smoking marijuana for several months.

"It still didn't come down to a choice between dope and God for me, not at that point," he said. "I could feel the tide changing, but I still had an ear open for any marijuana source that might open up. The only person I could find who would sell me dope insisted that I have it delivered to the office. That's when I woke up. Just exactly how much was I willing to risk? I thought it didn't make sense for me to throw my career away just because I needed a high. And the faith was really making a big difference in my life. I had an underpinning, I had a place to take my pain. I was getting solace from the community and the church."

Now Tom appeals to God whenever he has the urge to find a marijuana source. "That's been a successful formula for me. I realized that dope wouldn't do anything for me any more, but I still needed God's help to resist temptation. When I have difficult feelings now, I talk to God about it, about what's going on in me, and what's wrong, and what needs fixing, and I feel that I get God's reassurance that everything's okay. I prayed to be released from this addiction and to find meaning elsewhere. I never heard bells or had visions, but I think God did answer my prayer."

Carrying a burden of guilt about his years of drug use, Tom needed to find forgiveness. "I often feel like I've wasted a certain amount of my life, and that's hard for me," he said. "I have to work pretty hard not to blame myself a lot for smoking dope for all those years. I do believe God forgives me. In some ways, God's forgiveness seems to diminish the importance of the whole thing and take the sting out of the issue for me."

Today, Tom finds his "highs" in other places: "I find joy in very simple things now—a good meal, just sitting around with Celeste, a pretty day.

I feel as though I really have reconnected to life and can enjoy things again."

In the course of searching for faith, Tom read St. Augustine's *Confessions,* and there he found the book's opening phrase that aptly summarized his own experience: "Our hearts are restless until they rest in Thee."

"That's been a very important sentence in my life," he said. "In fact, *The Confessions* was probably the most important book leading to my conversion. My heart was restless, and I was flailing around. Now I'm not flailing. In some ways I'm still struggling. I don't always feel that God is close to me. But generally I feel so much more rooted than I ever was before.

"I don't think I'm ever going to go back to marijuana," he said. "I don't have any desire for it anymore. After years of craving it daily, that's fascinating to me! It's like, 'I did that years ago, and I don't want to do it any more.' I feel, if I went back, God would forgive me. It's not like God is saying, 'Don't you dare do this!' On the contrary! It's knowing that I'm forgiven by God that helps me make a free choice."

Tom's experience of God is quiet and ordinary, yet completely revolutionary. "That simple-grace thing, that's it for me," he said. "It's not some big light flash. It is just very simple. And very quietly right."

RECOVERY THROUGH SPIRITUAL COMMUNITY

Many addicts need a great deal of support and structure in order to overcome their addiction. The twelve-step programs—Alcoholics Anonymous and others—provide a therapeutic community for recovery. Within the Twelve Step programs, many people who have been alienated from the religions of their childhood can find a renewed spirituality. They also find a network of caring people who share their commitment to sobriety.

In a sense, an A.A. group is like a church or temple, and a meeting has some of the components of a religious service: set rituals, including prayers; a meeting of established duration; specific ways of relating to others that are carefully defined; and even a shared scripture—*The Big Book,* or *Alcoholics Anonymous.* Members share common wisdom, including slogans like "One day at a time," "Easy does it," and "Let go and let God." Outside the meetings, Twelve Step group members support one another as sponsors and friends. In effect, these programs operationalize a number of important spiritual principles which we have defined in chapter 2 as elements of the faith factor, including social support, shared beliefs, transcendence, confession and forgiveness, and meaning.

Researchers R. E. Hopson and B. Beaird-Spiller have defined four major ways in which A.A. helps participants achieve and maintain sobriety. First, they say, it *encourages the expression of feelings,* helping alcoholics vent the troubling emotions that can lead to drinking. Second, it *facilitates acknowledgment of participants' lack of control* over life circumstances, leading to the "let go and let God" position that brings equanimity. A related effect, *relieving the participant from self-effort,* also sets the stage for peacefulness and tranquillity as the alcoholic no longer struggles to control what he or she has come to understand is essentially uncontrollable—the desire for alcohol. And, fourth, they say that A.A. provides *structure and accountability* to help the alcoholic build a new life that is not centered around drinking.

From the experiential point of view, my patients who are members of Twelve Step groups tell me the most important benefit of membership is a sense of being connected and at home among people who understand their experience.

✢

Louisa, age forty-six, a business consultant, has found peace and recovery from alcoholism through her membership in Alcoholics Anonymous. Her relationship with alcohol is long-standing:

"There's a family picture of me as a baby holding a bottle of Miller beer," she told me. "I was still in diapers!" Louisa's father drank beer steadily; to entice her to sit with him in the evenings, he offered her sips of it.

Louisa was repeatedly sexually abused by another male relative when she was a child. As it so frequently does, the abuse led to low self-esteem and self-destructive behavior, including sexual promiscuity. To ease the emotional pain she felt, and because drinking was the chosen activity for popular teenagers in her small town, Louisa started drinking regularly from the "booze cupboard" in her home when she was about thirteen.

"I never had any feelings of self-worth," she told me. "I was always willing to spread my legs, open my shirt, let someone beat me up, work overtime and not get paid for it—just give and give and give, and I thought that would get me loving returns."

Louisa met her first husband "in a bar—where else?" They married when she was only twenty-one. Both drank and used illegal drugs throughout their years together. For a while, they grew marijuana in the Florida Everglades, selling it to support their drug habits.

Louisa told me about the tempestuous nature of this marriage: "We would get into fistfights, then afterwards we'd sit and look at each other's bruises. We'd compare wounds, say we were sorry, and get on with the day. We would drink, take drugs, and act out."

Finally, Louisa left the marriage. Soon she was dating again, and met the man who would become her second husband, Richard. Soon, the pair, both heavy drinkers, were living together; when Louisa became pregnant with their daughter, Emma, they married.

"I abstained from drinking during the pregnancy," she remembered. "But after she was born, everybody told me beer helps you relax, so I started drinking again."

Louisa and Richard established a business together. She described a typical day: "We'd get up at noon, and I would roll a joint and put my makeup on as I smoked it. We'd eat, go to the office, conduct a little business, then go to a restaurant and drink all afternoon. Then we'd go back to the office, work for a few more hours, leave, and drink all night. Emma was with the babysitter all this time."

Louisa reluctantly agreed to join her husband in "swinging"—meeting other couples for partner-swapping and group sex. "I was not an eager participant, but if I had enough marijuana, coke, and alcohol, I could join in," she remembered. "I was doing an awful lot of stuff I didn't like, and I was really hating myself."

By combining cocaine and alcohol, Richard "got really whacked out and ended up in rehab." Louisa rejoiced: "Our lives are going to be fine now!" After a thirty-day rehabilitation program, Richard started attending A.A. meetings, and Louisa went to Al-Anon, a Twelve Step program for the loved ones of alcoholics. Richard's drinking was the problem, not her own, Louisa thought, but at the A.A. meetings she attended with him, reality started breaking through.

"I marveled at how much I understood, at how much I knew where these people were coming from," she told me. "Richard didn't. After

126

three years, he was drinking again. I had stopped drinking 'for Richard's sake,' but when he did that, I bought a gallon of wine and drank the whole thing as I drove to see a friend who was in the program."

Her friend, Steve, looked at Louisa and said: "One of these days, you're going to realize that you need to go to this program for yourself." Louisa knew Steve was right. She started attending A.A. for herself as well as Al-Anon, and began to "work the program" rather than simply attending occasional meetings. "Working the program," a term frequently heard in the Twelve Step movement, included attending daily meetings for the first several months, then several times a week; studying and applying each of the Twelve Steps to one's own life; and finding a sponsor, an A.A. member who had achieved long-term sobriety and who could mentor the person in the recovery process.

"Working the program" worked for Louisa. But after about five years of sobriety, she rebelled. "I told my sponsor, 'I didn't get sober to spend my life in A.A. I got sober to get back in the mainstream of life.' " Louisa stopped going to meetings. Neither she nor Richard was drinking, so life seemed all right for the moment.

Then financial disaster struck. "We had to reorganize our business and file for bankruptcy," Louisa said. "We had nothing. We had used every penny for drinking and drugging. We owed a lot of money in taxes, and bankruptcy did not resolve that. My husband said he'd handle it, and I believed him."

Soon Louisa started having terrifying nightmares—nightmares so bad she would stay awake to avoid them. A huge rolling black cloud seemed ready to come and smother her at any moment. To stay awake at night and avoid the nightmares, she started eating constantly. Her weight ballooned up to 230 pounds. Seeking help for her compulsive eating, Louisa made an appointment with an eating-disorders therapist, who, after learning about Louisa's sleeping problem, promptly referred her to me.

After an extensive interview and physical examination, I determine that Louisa was severely depressed and potentially suicidal. I recommended immediate hospitalization.

"You need to be pulled out of the mainstream for a while and go into the hospital for a month or so," I explained to Louisa.

"That's a cute idea," she said defiantly. "I have a business to run and a little girl to raise. What's Plan B?"

I discussed hospitalization further with Louisa, but she was unwilling to consider the option. Reluctantly, I presented Plan B: "If you really will not go into the hospital, I would like to prescribe an antidepressant medication for you and to see you on a regular basis. I'd also like to refer you to a therapist," I said. I asked Louisa about her faith life; she told me that A.A. had led her back to the faith of her childhood, Roman Catholicism, and that she was active at church, but that nothing seemed to help her deal with the nightmares and anxiety. I urged her to schedule a follow-up appointment soon, and to call me immediately if she continued to be unable to sleep.

"That night, I slept well for the first time in months," she told me. "After a couple of good nights' sleep, I decided all my problems had arisen from being tired—there wasn't anything else going on. I started going to meetings again. I got another sponsor, a lady who loved me until I could love myself. This lady would put her arms around me and say, 'I'm really sorry you're hurting.' She insisted that I attend daily meetings and share with others about all my problems, including the hate mail I was getting twice a week from the IRS."

To no one's surprise but Louisa's, Richard was not helping pay off the significant tax debt the couple had accumulated. He had taken over a business in a city about a four-hour drive away, and when Louisa went to visit him, she discovered he was having an affair. At the same time, Louisa's beloved mother was dying. It was an unimaginably difficult year.

"I demanded that God send me somebody who could get me off the hook," she remembered. "I turned to an accountant, a friend in A.A., and asked him to review our situation. I was sure he'd find a loophole, but he looked up from the piles of papers at me and said, 'Louisa, you're in trouble. You owe the government over two hundred thousand dollars, and there's no way out of it except to pay it.'"

Louisa remembered the moment clearly: "I said, 'Excuse me.' I went out to my car and cried for a minute, blew my nose, came back into the house, and said, 'What do I do from here?' It was time to stop blaming Richard for this and to get on with my life."

Louisa started paying the debt, but now she needed to face reality about her marriage. "One Sunday, after Mass, I sat in church praying to God, 'What do I do?' I heard God say, 'What makes you think you were ever supposed to marry this man in the first place?' I finally realized I needed to let go of this marriage—that, if I wouldn't open up my fist and let go of it, God couldn't put anything good in my hand."

Louisa started divorce proceedings, and she started to get better. Then the next crisis hit.

"I was getting healthy, so our daughter, Emma, who was twelve, could finally let her guard down. She attempted suicide. She had just about had it with me and her father."

Emma went into therapy and joined Alateen, a program for the teenage relatives of alcoholics. "She's an amazing girl," her mother proudly says. The pain of her past remains; her father rarely contacts her. But she has become a leader in Alateen and, at sixteen, is doing well.

"Emma and her dad don't have a relationship, and she thought it was because she had done something wrong or been a bad daughter," Louisa said. "Getting her to understand that it isn't her fault took a lot of work. Last Christmas her father sent her a last-minute Federal Express package with a little necklace and a twenty-dollar bill in it. She looked at me and said, 'I suppose I should have gotten him something for Christmas.' I said, 'Do you want to?' 'Not really,' she said. I told her she wasn't obligated to give him anything, and she accepted and understood that."

As a divorced woman, Louisa has had to grapple with the issue of sexuality. "I had always thought God wanted me to find the right man and get married," she told me. "Now I think maybe I'm supposed to be celibate. But at first I couldn't imagine it! I wanted so badly to be touched and held by a man. One day I was praying in church after Mass, holding myself and crying. I said to God, 'I wish you could put your arms around me and hold me. I can't stand this another day!' A few minutes later, a woman came up behind me and put her arms around me. She said, 'I don't know what's wrong, but I'm praying for you.' Where did this woman come from? There I was, asking to be held, and somebody holds me! I looked for a rational explanation for this, but I couldn't find one."

Louisa began to seek God's presence more and more frequently, believing that her relationship with him was the underpinning of her sobriety and of a healthy life.

"I realized, if I didn't start getting some of this God business in my life, even with ten or eleven years of sobriety, I was risking drinking again," she said. Today, she continues to work as a consultant; her business has been successful, and over a period of years she has managed to retire most of her debt to the IRS. Once that debt is retired, Louisa plans to spend more time in the activities that nourish her soul, like coordinating an annual women's retreat at a local retreat house. Every day, Louisa says the rosary and reads the Bible and A.A. literature, as well as listening to religious tapes in the car. She spends a lot of time with Emma and teaches dancing on the side. Because she knows now that A.A. is her lifeline to sobriety and health, she attends several meetings a week, talks to her sponsors daily, and serves as sponsor to four women. Louisa's life is full and busy, but she is adamant about finding quiet time.

"God rested on the seventh day—why? Because we need it! When I get destructive thoughts in my head, it's guaranteed that I haven't taken the time for quiet. I'd better find time to be still, so I can sort out what's going on in my life.

"In all those years of drinking and drugging and partying, I was looking for love from outside myself," she continued. "The Bible says, 'Love your neighbor *as* yourself,' but I didn't love myself. I thought I could get the love I needed by pleasing people, but the love has to come from inside. Elijah experienced God as the still small voice, the whisper. That's how God speaks to me. He leans over and whispers. When I'm too busy with my day, I don't hear him. And then I get into trouble."

Louisa will soon celebrate her twelfth anniversary of sobriety. As she has done for the past several years, Emma will attend the A.A. meeting celebrating this anniversary, and she will give her mother the "chip," or commemorative token, awarded by A.A. to mark such milestones.

✢

In 1986, a study appeared in *The Lancet,* a British medical journal, documenting the rise of a new illegal drug epidemic in the Bahamas: the use of freebase or "crack" cocaine. Soon afterward, I met one of the authors of the study, Dr. David Allen, who, after recognizing the epidemic, had begun to develop a treatment program. He invited me to look at his program, and I agreed to join him in a new research venture. We traveled back to the Bahamas and interviewed a number of recovering crack-cocaine addicts who had started successful recoveries in a Christian psychiatric-rehabilitation facility called The Haven. We wanted to learn about the men's psychological and religious histories, to determine any factors they might have in common which would predispose them to crack addiction; and we wanted to learn how these former addicts had successfully kicked the crack habit—one of the most potent addictions known, and one of the hardest to break.

After interviewing a dozen crack-cocaine addicts, Dr. Allen and I knew that these men were living, not one *day* at a time, as recovering alcoholics do, but one *minute* at a time. We found, too, that The Haven's residents had experienced a deep conversion to the Christian faith in conjunction with their recovery; we heard again and again from the men that they were able to overcome their longings for crack only by appealing to the Spirit of Christ.

Before becoming addicted to crack, most of the men had experienced emotional difficulties and disruptions in their lives, including:

- poor relationships with their fathers, who were likely to have been alcohol abusers, and/or who had abandoned the family
- close relationships with their mothers—sometimes unhealthfully close, with the mother overprotecting the son or enabling him in his self-destructive behavior
- familiarity with drug abuse through other family members, often a sibling
- poor performance in school, poor self-esteem, and heightened vulnerability to peer pressure

Most of the men had started their drug abuse with marijuana; it made them feel "mellow, relaxed, happy." But crack cocaine went far beyond marijuana's relatively mild effects. It gave them a "rush" or a "lift," accompanied by feelings of omniscience and omnipotence. While high on crack, the men felt in control of their lives, peaceful, and even ecstatic; once hooked by this extraordinary feeling, they found themselves striving constantly to experience it again through repeated crack use. Small wonder that the men, many of whom were unemployed and who had poor relationships with spouses and family members, wanted to maintain the crack high. Small wonder, too, that breaking this seductive addiction often required a powerful spiritual experience within the structure of a carefully designed program like The Haven's, where the men participated in precisely scheduled household chores, Bible study, group meetings, worship, and job training or remedial education.

Interestingly, the study's subjects told us that it was not the experience of conversion *per se* that helped them overcome addiction. They did not depend on the emotional "high" of a "zap" conversion in their daily struggle against crack. Rather, it was the structured, disciplined aspects of their spirituality—daily Bible study, prayer, and fellowship—that gave them the strength they needed. This echoes the lessons learned by many in Twelve Step programs: it is not the *concept* of religious belief, but the *living out* of such beliefs, the steady and regular application of them in day-to-day life, that makes the difference. This highly structured approach to faith may appear to be just another addiction replacing the dependence on crack, but, given the destructive nature of cocaine addiction to body, mind, and spirit, a disciplined life of faith, however rigorous, seems a better choice.

✣

The experiences of addiction chronicled here run the gamut—from alcohol to marijuana to tobacco, from food abuse to crack-cocaine use. The individuals profiled come from different religious and ethnic backgrounds and different walks of life. Some required medical intervention (including a thirty-day hospital program for Julia) and counseling to aid in their recovery process; some did not. But they have one thing in common: through hard experience, they have learned that, for them, a highly developed spiritual life is the *only* way to stay free of the bondage of addiction. This does not mean that they never have cravings or weak moments, or that all the problems of their lives have been solved. Indeed, recovery is precarious for many people, which is why frequent contact with spiritual resources like Twelve Step groups is so important; only with constant reinforcement and support can they continue their sobriety.

In the Gospel of John, Jesus says to his disciples, "You will know the truth, and the truth will make you free" (John 8:32). For the individuals whose stories are told here, the truth of a living relationship with a Higher Power helped bring about a freedom that can seldom be attained any other way—freedom to live fully, without the crippling effects of addiction.

Liberated from slavery to a substance or behavior, Julia, Becky and George, Celeste, Tom, and Louisa can work on building healthy, positive lives. According to current research, they are likely to find in these new faith-based lives a better ability to cope with difficulty and a greater sense of satisfaction and meaning than they have ever before known. They will, in other words, experience an improved *quality of life*—yet another profound benefit available to those of us who are willing to tap into the faith factor.

CHAPTER 6

The Quality of Life:
Living Abundantly

Is there a guaranteed way to inoculate people against life's stressful events, or to transform an unhappy existence into a purposeful, joy-filled life? As much as I would like to say "yes," I cannot: no matter how blessed we may be by the good things in life, we will all face loss—failure in our work or finances, strain in important relationships, grief when a loved one dies, and, in many cases, some loss of our own capabilities as we age. Throughout the millennia, wise people in every discipline—medicine and other sciences, religion, politics, art—have sought a vaccine against pain and a panacea to end all misery. In fact, the quest for relief from suffering has characterized the human experience.

Modern medical research suggests that we may find relief—not a vaccine or a panacea, but real help nonetheless—from another great human quest: the search for ultimate meaning that so often leads to faith in a Divine Being. As we enter into a relationship with "the God of our understanding" (to borrow a phrase from the Twelve Step movement), and as we grow spiritually as individuals and as members of a community of faith, we begin to enjoy an unparalleled array of benefits that equip us for handling life's difficulties, provide us with a sense of meaning and purpose, and enable us to create and sustain positive, satisfying relationships with others.

Whereas contemporary culture has often portrayed religious people as repressed, sour-faced prudes or wild-eyed fanatics, scientists are finding the opposite is more likely to be true: people of faith are happier—more excited about life, more fulfilled as human beings. A study published in 1988 followed 1,650 individuals, looking for the effects of religious involvement on their well-being. This study was remarkable because of its length: the subjects were followed for *forty years*, a period far exceeding that of most studies. The adult respondents were asked about their religious beliefs and practices, and asked to rate their overall life satisfaction, as well as their satisfaction with marriage, work, and community. Respondents who attended church regularly reported a significantly higher degree of overall life satisfaction, and those who reported strong religious beliefs were more likely to have happy marriages. Even after researchers applied controls to the data to account for the influences of gender and income, church attendance and personal religious belief were still powerful factors in determining the happiness of these individuals.

A 1984 study of fifteen hundred Americans also examined the relationship between religious activity and well-being. Participants were asked to rate their happiness, excitement about life, satisfaction with various aspects of their lives (family, friendship, community, hobbies), and physical health. The study found that happiness, excitement, and satisfaction were linked with both frequency of church attendance and strength of religious preference, the two measures of religious involvement used in the study. Among the African-Americans surveyed in the study, the link between well-being and religious involvement was even stronger than among whites.

Looking at the relationship between church attendance and well-being in another American ethnic population, researchers Jeffrey Levin and K. S. Markides surveyed 750 Mexican-Americans in San Antonio. Participants filled out questionnaires that asked about frequency of church attendance as well as health, age, education, marital status, and life satisfaction. Frequent church attenders, especially women, reported higher life satisfaction than those who attended church less often or not at all. This finding—that women benefit even more from the faith factor in terms of life satisfaction and well-being—has been echoed in a number of studies. One study focused on younger married women caring for at least one child under five at home; the most religious among the sample of 188 women enjoyed the highest degree of life satisfaction and well-being.

The faith factor's effects on well-being and life satisfaction become even more dramatic among older individuals. A Canadian study of eighty-five individuals, aged sixty-five to eighty-eight, found that participants became more religious as they grew older, and that religiosity was linked to happiness and personal adjustment. A 1982 study of 719 married or widowed women between sixty and seventy-five years of age measured demographic characteristics, religiosity, health, and fertility history, so that the impact of childlessness on older women could be assessed. The researchers found that religious involvement was the most reliable predictor of contentment among the women; for widows, whether childless or not, religion was linked to general well-being. And in a large national survey of 1,493 individuals aged sixty-five and over, researcher L. Y. Steinitz discovered that church attendance was positively associated with happiness, health, and excitement among women and whites. Among African-Americans in the study, those who had confidence in organized religion reported that they gained higher levels of satisfaction from their families than others, and the respondents who believed in life after death had a greater sense of excitement in life.

For younger people, too, religious involvement, quality of life, and improved health outcomes appear to be connected. Researchers examined this link in 299 students at the University of Western Ontario, looking not only at feelings of well-being, but also at physical-health complaints among the students. The students affiliated with a campus faith group reported that they enjoyed better moods, higher satisfaction, and less stress than their nonaffiliated counterparts; the faith-group members also enjoyed better health, with fewer emergency-room, physician, clinic, and dental visits than the nonmembers.

DEEPER THAN SURFACE LEVEL:
THE CONNECTION BETWEEN FAITH AND WELL-BEING

Many of the studies mentioned above used frequency of church attendance to measure religious involvement, but personal religiosity—private prayer, meditation, and the sense of intimacy with God—is also an important indicator. Just as people with intrinsic, or inwardly authentic, religiosity seem to enjoy more benefits of the faith factor than the extrinsically religious, it may well be that certain types of personal piety lead to greater degrees of happiness and contentment. In studying well-being among religious people, sociologist Margaret Poloma has defined four types of prayer:

1. *Colloquial:* talking to God informally, as if you were talking to your best friend. The relationship with God is marked by a sense of easy intimacy.

2. *Petitional:* asking God for things for yourself and for others; focusing prayer on what God can provide.

3. *Ritual:* using formal prayers or rites, like a rosary or prayers in a prayer book. The relationship with God is more formal.

4. *Meditative:* focusing the mind on an aspect of God for a period of time; calming the conscious mind and dismissing extraneous thoughts. Also known as *contemplative* prayer, this form of prayer is similar to the meditative activity that evokes the Relaxation Response detailed in chapter 2.

Dr. Poloma measured well-being in 560 survey respondents in Summit County, Ohio, also assessing the type or types of prayer each person used most often. In addition, she asked respondents about their frequency of church attendance, church membership, and feelings of closeness to God. The respondents who most often used colloquial, or informal, prayer reported a higher degree of happiness; those who favored meditative prayer were more likely to experience religious satisfaction and existential well-being, or satisfaction with the meaning and purpose of their lives. Individuals who used only petitionary and formal, ritualistic prayer reported *less* happiness and lower levels of life satisfaction.

These findings point to the importance to well-being of one's perceived *relationship with God* as expressed in prayer. If we think of God only as a great divine switchboard, answering or denying our requests, or if we feel we can relate to God only through prayer formulas devised for us by others, we are less likely to enjoy great feelings of happiness through our faith. If, on the other hand, we conceive of God as a friend we can talk to any time, about anything, or if we meditate on the nature of God and his goodness, we are likely to find a deep sense of satisfaction and even joy in our prayer and in our lives.

We see similar findings in a study by researcher C. G. Ellison, who assessed the faith/well-being link among 1,481 respondents from a national sample. As with most of the well-being studies, Ellison found that happiness and life satisfaction were linked with church attendance, but he also discovered a strong link between satisfaction and a sense of intimacy with God. Going to church or synagogue just to "go through the motions," or to conform with social standards, yields fewer benefits than worship attendance combined with a strong sense of personal devotion to God.

Since the nature of our relationship with God depends upon our image of him, people who view God primarily as a loving Being will tend to report a closer relationship to him and thus to enjoy greater contentment. In a 1990 German study of 115 women and 91 men, researchers assessed participants' images of God as well as levels of life satisfaction, loneliness, and neuroticism. Contrary to the popular myth that religious people are more neurotic than the nonreligious, the study found that the more religiously active individuals were *less* neurotic. Patients who saw God as primarily loving and helpful reported less loneliness and greater life satisfaction. Conversely, those who viewed God as wrathful were lonelier and less satisfied.

A REASON FOR LIVING

In chapter 2, we defined *meaning* as one of the components of the faith factor. Without a sense of purpose, human beings suffer psychologically and spiritually. In order to thrive, we need to know that we are important to someone or something. For many people of faith, religion provides a sense of meaning, a reason to live, or a meaningful interpretation for difficult events. Often, people will find their sense of purpose in helping others, especially others who have been through travails similar to their own. We see this in the case of the recovering alcoholic who follows the Twelfth Step of the Twelve Step movement by rendering service to fellow alcoholics; for the founders of Alcoholics Anonymous, service to others was a vital part of the prescription for recovery. My patients continually report the great satisfaction they find in reaching out to others, whether their service is to fellow recovering addicts, homeless people, newly arrived immigrants, sick people, or others.

Even people who are sick and disabled can gain a sense of purpose by finding ways to help others. My patient Melanie, age thirty-nine, suffers from severe chronic fatigue syndrome (CFS). Once the owner of a thriving retail business, Melanie cannot work; on a good day, she manages to drive to the grocery store or take her dog for a quarter-mile walk. The symptoms of this mysterious illness—extraordinary fatigue, muscle aches, fever and chills, depression, inability to concentrate, among others—have forced this formerly dynamic young woman to move at a snail's pace.

"Sometimes it's all I can do just to get out of bed," she told me on a routine office visit. "Yesterday I managed to wash my hair after getting up in the morning—but then I had to take a nap."

Melanie told me that she was grieving—not only for her formerly active professional life, but for her extensive church activities, now curtailed by CFS.

"I used to run the homeless program at church," she told me. "I taught Sunday School and sang in the choir, too. This was in addition to working seventy-hour weeks. But now I can't do anything. My concentration is so bad I can't even read the Bible as much as I want to!"

"I know that you'd like to be more active, Melanie," I told her. "And I hope that the medical treatment you'll be receiving will help you feel better. But until that happens, I have a suggestion for you. I can think of a tremendously important ministry that you can do, even when you're lying in bed."

"What's that?" she said. "I hope you don't mean making phone calls, because that wears me out, too."

"No phone calls," I replied. "You can pray, for yourself and for other people, even when you're at your worst physically." I told Melanie about the scientific data showing that prayer can have a positive effect on health and well-being, as discussed in this book. "Could you pray for people who are sick, or lonely, or under a great deal of stress?" I asked. "You may really be making a difference, even if you're forced to stay in bed all day!"

"Yes, I can certainly do that," she said. "I could make up a prayer list and keep it beside the bed. Then, when I'm unable to do anything else, I can pray for these people."

On her next visit, Melanie told me her prayer ministry was giving her a sense of fulfillment even on her worst days. She was particularly pleased that a few of the people she had been praying for called her to say that her prayers for them had been answered. We cannot know if, in fact, Melanie's prayers brought about these results, but it is clear that having a prayer ministry gives her a sense of purpose and satisfaction that was lacking in her life because of her disabling illness.

Of course, it is not only religious people like Melanie who participate in service to others, but religious involvement does encourage the altruistic behavior that gives people a sense of purpose. A study of students at Wilfred Laurier University in Ontario found that students with an intrinsic religious orientation were more likely to volunteer for both religious and nonreligious charitable organizations than were students with an extrinsic religious orientation. In a fascinating study of 663 male respondents in a city hit by a tornado, researchers assessed religious involvement as well as measures of helping behavior. Respondents were asked how often they helped motorists with car trouble, donated money to charitable causes, and took food to bereaved families in nonemergency settings; they were also asked about their helping activities during the post-tornado emergency, such as donating money to relief agencies, providing needed goods for tornado victims, and performing disaster-relief services that were not connected to their employment. Frequency of church attendance and personal religiosity were strongly correlated with helping behaviors, both routinely and in the emergency caused by the tornado.

Though the "look out for Number One" mentality has infiltrated our popular culture, the most satisfied people are those who have a sense of purpose, and that almost always includes helping others, whether the "others" are family, friends, or strangers. All the great religious traditions promote the importance of reaching out to people in need; most religious congregations undertake in charitable activities like feeding the hungry and ministering to the sick. It is not surprising, then, that the faith factor bolsters our sense of well-being and life satisfaction, because religious involvement so consistently points us in the direction of doing good for others—which is also good for us.

The absence of a sense of purpose can result in a feeling that one's life has been wasted. This can be devastating emotionally, particularly as life's end draws near. Recently I saw a new patient who was one of the saddest people I have ever met. Ellen, a woman in her sixties, has lung cancer. Her oncologist is treating her with chemotherapy and radiation, but she needed care for her symptoms of abdominal discomfort and vomiting. As one might expect in such a sick patient, Ellen's whole demeanor was listless and sad.

"How are you handling your illness, Ellen?" I asked her.

"The cancer doctor says it's terminal," she told me matter-of-factly. "So I've been thinking about my life, and I have to tell you, it adds up to zero. There's been no point in my life."

"Tell me about your life," I said.

Continuing in a monotone, Ellen reviewed her life for me, first saying she had never been married and had no children, which she regretted.

"I haven't even had any real friends," she said. "My jobs have been just jobs—nothing special. There's been no point in my life, no purpose in anything that's happened."

Because Ellen's cancer had been diagnosed as terminal, I thought it important to ask about her spiritual life.

"Are you a person of faith, Ellen?" I asked.

"Not really," she said. "I grew up Roman Catholic and I changed over to the Lutheran Church when I got older, but none of it really has made any difference to me. I don't go to church anymore, haven't gone for years."

I asked Ellen about her views on life after death.

"It's just rest," she said. "I don't believe we'll be happy or active in heaven. We'll just rest."

It was the matter-of-fact tone in her voice, this banality of meaninglessness, that distressed me so much in listening to her. After talking with her at length and examining her, I pondered whether giving her an antidepressant medication was appropriate, but decided that she did not meet the criteria for depression; she simply had found no purpose in her life and was facing a bleak ending, without even a hope for relief in the afterlife.

Ellen had tried religion but, for reasons she could not explain, it did not answer her needs. Of course, social support and purpose in life can be found outside of religion, but Ellen did not find them. I cannot pretend to know why her life lacked purpose, or why her religious involvement did not go deeper than occasional attendance at church, but I hope that, as our relationship develops, I will come to understand her better, and perhaps to help her find hope, even in the dying process.

All of us, of course, are dying; each day is another step in the relentless march to death. Yet those with a strong religious commitment are more likely, in Jesus's words, "to have life, and have it abundantly" (John 10:10). Seizing a purpose in life will lead to greater zest for living, more contentment, and, according to the research data, better physical and mental health.

COPING

As we have seen in previous chapters, the faith factor's measurable effects on physical and mental health have been documented by many scientific studies. Being religiously involved actually reduces incidence of illness, assists significantly in recovery, and in some cases appears to prolong life. Of course, no one—no matter how holy—can count on an existence free of illness and suffering, but people of faith have been found to meet these challenges with greater resiliency than do their nonbelieving counterparts. Let us examine together how the faith factor strengthens people to meet some of life's greatest crises—serious illness, disability, caregiving for a sick or disabled loved one, and bereavement.

Serious Illness and Disability

When I tap on a patient's elbow or knee, I expect to see, in a neurologically healthy person, an involuntary reflex as the arm or leg responds to the stimulus. When they were little, my children enjoyed this reflex so much that they would ask me to tap on their knees or elbows "just for fun!" According to common wisdom as well as a number of clinical studies, there is a "religious reflex" in those who are tapped by the hammer of sickness. Many people reach instinctively toward God when illness befalls them. According to a study of 114 adolescents in Children's Hospital National Medical Center in Washington, D.C., even teenagers pray when they are sick, and the sicker they are, the more emphasis they place on their religious experiences. In another study, a research team led by

Theresa Saudia, an Air Force nurse, found that 97 percent of patients awaiting coronary-artery bypass surgery rated prayer as "very helpful" in dealing with illness and upcoming surgery.

The tendency to pray when confronted with illness becomes even more pronounced among the elderly. In a study of eighty women aged sixty-five and over, researchers found that their single most frequently used coping response in medical illness was prayer. The respondents were asked, "Who assisted you when faced with these stressful medical problems?" Their most common response, given by 85 percent of the participants, was "God." In comparison, only 60 percent named a friend, 57 percent named a family member, and 28 percent named a minister.

A 1990 study by L. B. Bearon and Harold Koenig echoed these findings. The investigators interviewed forty men and women aged sixty-five to seventy-four in Durham, North Carolina, asking about their physical symptoms and whether they had prayed about the symptoms. Fifty-three percent of the subjects said they had prayed about their illness; if the symptoms had been discussed with a physician, 63 percent of the patients prayed about them. In addition, 78 percent said they believed health to be a blessing from God.

We know that people young and old turn to religious resources to help them cope with illness. But what is it specifically about religion that helps people? According to a 1990 study of 586 patients from Midwestern churches by Kenneth Pargament and his colleagues, the following elements of religious coping are the most helpful:

• *Belief in a just, loving God.* Again we see the importance of one's image of God: individuals who see God more as a judging, punitive Being will find less comfort in religion during times of stress.

• *The experience of God as a supportive partner in the coping process.* If God is loving and caring, then it follows that we can experience him as a true helper, someone who is always there for us in times of need. Compare this to a theology that sees God as a "divine watchmaker," one who made the universe and now allows it to run without his help or interference; there is little solace in such a concept.

• *Involvement in ritual.* As I discussed in chapter 2, ritual, a component of the faith factor, has distinct soothing and calming effects. The

Pargament study shows that individuals who take part in worship services and special rituals like healing services appear to benefit more from their faith when coping with stress.

• *The search for spiritual and personal support from religion.* This study seems to indicate that, if we undertake a search for support from religion, and expect to find what we need there, then we are indeed more likely to have that search positively fulfilled.

By activating these mechanisms of religious coping, people who pray, and especially people who pray in their churches and synagogues, face illness with more resilience, succumbing less frequently to the feelings of passivity, depression, and despair that frequently accompany sickness. Even in situations calling for high-tech medical interventions like heart transplantation and hemodialysis, faith can play a crucial role. In a study mentioned in chapter 1, researcher M. E. O'Brien examined the role of religious faith in the lives of patients undergoing long-term hemodialysis, a time-consuming medical procedure required several times a week for individuals whose kidneys have failed. The study assessed feelings of powerlessness among the patients, one of the most common emotions experienced by those undergoing long-term hemodialysis, who may come to feel that the dialysis machine controls their lives. Their schedules are seriously disrupted by the need for sessions that take up as much as half a day. Social isolation and withdrawal often follows. In response to the powerlessness they feel, some dialysis patients will relinquish the degree of control they *do* have in their lives. Frequently this leads to depression; for some, it leads to lessened compliance with their life-saving medical regimen.

But among the more religious patients in the study, a pattern of greater adjustment emerged. The patients who attended worship services weekly maintained the highest levels of social interaction, as well as the greatest compliance with their demanding medical regimen. Those who indicated that their religion was "always important" to them reported the lowest degree of powerlessness, social isolation, and alienation. For 27 percent of the patients, religion increased in importance over the course of their illness; they did not "give up on God" when they got sick, but, rather, found greater meaning and support in their spiritual lives than they had experienced previously.

Researchers examining the role of religion in the long-term health and well-being of forty heart-transplant patients found similar results. The patients were interviewed three times—two months, seven months, and twelve months after their heart transplants. Those who expressed strong religious beliefs in the initial interview were most likely to experience better physical functioning, fewer health worries, and less difficulty following their demanding medical regimen than those who were less religious. The patients who attended religious services frequently were less anxious than those who did not.

As mentioned in chapter 1, researchers found similar benefits of faith in a study of patients with spinal-cord injuries. Among the hundred paraplegics and quadriplegics studied, those who were more religious reported a greater sense of well-being. Other factors were also important, including higher incomes and levels of social support. Many of the respondents told the researchers that they had found a positive purpose in their injury and disability—a true example of making lemonade when life hands you lemons.

For elderly women recovering from broken hips, the faith factor boosted recovery from surgery. Researchers used a three-item scale called the Index of Religiousness to measure the patients' religious involvement; this scale includes questions about frequency of attendance at religious services, how religious the subject believes himself or herself to be, and how much strength and comfort he or she derives from God or faith. The women who scored high on the scale were able to walk farther at the time of discharge than those whose scores were lower, and those who attended church more frequently were less likely to become depressed, regardless of how severely ill they might be.

The faith factor's effectiveness in helping people cope with illness is not surprising, given that serious illness really presents a spiritual crisis, a crisis of meaning. As long as we are well, we can remain relatively independent, and we can gain feelings of self-worth and purpose from our work in the world, from our role in the family, and from our hobbies and volunteer activities. Once serious illness strikes, some or all of these sources of satisfaction may be blocked. We can no longer derive our self-esteem from our accomplishments; we may no longer even be able to care for our own bodies. For most people, serious illness provokes a re-evaluation of life's meaning and purpose. For many, it causes a radical reversal of lifestyle. My patient Loretta and her husband, Clarence, began such a radical reversal when Loretta became seriously ill for the first time in her life. Clarence called an ambulance, and their journey through life-threatening illness began.

Loretta and Clarence, both in their late fifties at the time her illness was discovered, are African-Americans living in the Anacostia section of Washington. The proud parents of five children and grandparents of ten, they have worked hard throughout their thirty-year marriage to maintain their modest home, raise their children well, and serve their Lord. Before they were married, Loretta asked Clarence to attend church with her; from that time on, the couple shared a deep faith and commitment to their Pentecostal church. In 1975, Clarence, a security guard at the headquarters of a large national association, perceived a call to become a pastor. He kept his regular job, but at night and on the weekends, Clarence preached, called on the sick, administered a small church, and attended to the many other duties of a pastor to his flock, with little, if any, pay. Loretta took care of the household and the children, becoming very involved as a volunteer in their schools; to pick up some extra income, she ran a babysitting service as well.

"I got my satisfaction from helping others," Loretta told me. "I always said, 'If I can help somebody along the way, then my living won't be in vain.' "

When I became their internist recently, Clarence and Loretta told me the story of her illness, which came on suddenly four years ago.

"Loretta had a terrible headache and she was really confused that day. Then, all of a sudden, she passed out. I called 911, and an ambulance came. They took her to D.C. General Hospital," Clarence recalled. Later, he would learn that Loretta's heart had stopped twice while she was in the emergency room. "They checked her and found that her condition was really serious. She had a brain tumor that was the size of an egg. The doctor told me it was a touch-and-go situation. They couldn't do the operation there, so they took her to Howard University Hospital."

Speaking hoarsely because of the tracheotomy tube installed in her windpipe to aid her breathing, Loretta told me her memories of those first few hours of her illness: "I heard my husband and my children in the hall of the hospital crying, and I said to myself, 'Oh God, what can I tell them? What can I say to them?' I didn't realize how bad I was. When they came in to see me, I told them, 'Don't worry about me. I'm in God's hands.' That's all I could think of to say."

Clarence called on the members of his church to pray for Loretta. "The 'saints' were praying, and they went on a fast, praying that she would recover." Every church member undertook a two- or three-day complete fast on behalf of Loretta. As Clarence explained it, "The church goes on a fast to look for God to do a healing. According to the Bible, he hears the prayers of the righteous. The fast moves God, when a child of God is really in a bad predicament. He knows the heart of his children, and the prayers of the righteous will move him."

Clarence and Loretta believe that the church members' prayers were answered, resulting in a recovery that surprised Loretta's physicians.

"The doctor came out of the operating room and he said, 'All went well,' " Clarence told me. "He was just amazed at how she pulled through that surgery. It could have easily gone the other way, he said. He told me they had taken out as much of the tumor as they could."

But Loretta's ordeal was far from over. She was transferred to another hospital for long-term physical therapy. Clarence wept as he watched nurses and attendants move Loretta.

"At first, they had to hoist her in a sling to get her in and out of bed," he told me. "She was just a lifeless body hanging in the air. I'd look at her and I just couldn't hold the tears back. She was like a baby who had just been born."

After the brain surgery, Loretta could not talk or read for a time, but, to her doctors' amazement, she was soon able to speak, though her diction was slurred. She remembered and spoke aloud the names of her husband and children.

"Then I remembered my phone number," she said, smiling, "and I called my husband at home on a Saturday, the day we worship. I said, 'Hi, Dad!' But he didn't think it was me! He couldn't believe it! I said, 'Are you going to church today?' He said, 'Yes,' and I told him to put in a good word for me."

Today, she is confined to a wheelchair and has some paralysis on her left side. The tracheotomy tube makes speech difficult for her, but, despite this obstacle, she is an animated, outgoing woman with a wonderful sense of humor. At a recent office visit, I asked her if she had struggled with depression during the course of her recovery.

"Yes, I have," she said, "but after you carry that burden for a while, you realize there's nothing you can do about it. Either you've got to hold on to it or let it go. So I let it go. I have my good days and my bad, and I decided to dwell on the good things and forget about the bad, since I can't do anything about the negative things in my life."

"What do you think about when you dwell on the good things?" I asked, wanting to hear more of this radiant woman's approach to life.

"I think of the goodness of Jesus, and all that he's done for me," she said. "I think about what they did to Jesus, how they nailed him to the cross. I think about the hardships that he went through. Then I say to myself, 'Well, if he can go through it, so can I.'"

"Amen," said her husband. "The Lord has been good to us. He's been faithful! The doctors just can't understand how well she's done. They'll look at her and say, 'Loretta, you're a miracle!'"

But neither Loretta nor Clarence denies that they have suffered substantially. Loretta longs to be able to walk again, and she misses singing in their joy-filled, celebratory worship services:

"I used to love to sing," she told me with a tinge of sadness. "But now I sound just like a frog! I think it's because of the 'trach.'"

"Yes, it probably is," I told her, "and if the trach tube can be removed someday, perhaps you will be able to sing again."

"Do you think my brain will learn to cooperate with my body again?" she asked me. "You know, sometimes I know what I want to say, but the words come out wrong. I might say, 'Please bring me the towel from over there,' when I really mean, 'Please bring me my comb from upstairs.' That's very frustrating."

"Only God knows the answer to that question, Loretta," I said. The amount of damage her brain received from the tumor and subsequent surgery made it impossible to predict the degree of her recovery, but for such faithful people, there is always hope.

After adjusting Loretta's medications for hypertension and for post-surgical epilepsy, I regularly pray with Loretta and Clarence during our office visits. Their enthusiasm for God moves and inspires me deeply. Our visits help me as much as I help them.

"Doctor, you're our prayer partner!" Clarence said recently. I can't think of a greater honor than to share in the spiritual journey of these courageous people of faith.

In the months following Loretta's surgery, Clarence had to cope with new duties and burdens he had never expected to carry. In addition to worrying about Loretta and praying for her, he could no longer take refuge within the smoothly operating household she had run; he could not look forward to her supportive companionship at home or at church. He was deprived of the many gifts Loretta had given him, *and* was required to take on new responsibilities in caring for her.

"For all those months, I would go to work, then go directly to the hospital," he told me. "I would sit at her bedside all evening, then try to creep away when she was sleeping. But she would wake up and beg me not to leave. Then I also had to talk with the doctors and sign papers and talk to the insurance company—and that's a lot of work. When it snowed and driving was too dangerous, I would have to ride buses and the subway and walk long distances at night, just to get home in time to fall into bed."

Like many caregivers, Clarence found his new role overwhelming. Under the stress of his routine, his appetite dwindled and he lost a great deal of weight that he didn't need to lose. But as Loretta's condition began to improve, Clarence, too, began to feel better, and he received another boost to his health and good spirits when he decided to retire after thirty-two years as a security guard. Now Clarence has more time for his unpaid pastoral duties and for caring for Loretta, who needs help with most of the simple tasks of living—even getting in and out of bed.

Though Clarence never complains, I was worried about the stress caregiving placed on his body, mind, and spirit. Once, when he visited me alone, I asked him, "How are you holding up?"

"I couldn't make it without the Lord," he replied. "I'm just so glad she pulled through! Now, I won't pretend that things have turned out the way we'd planned. But God has other plans for us. He still gives me a lot of joy."

Looking at Clarence, who is in excellent health and looks much younger than his sixty-three years, I cannot help thinking that his profound faith, as well as his deep love for Loretta, have allowed him to meet the demands of her illness with unexpected resilience. According to scientific studies of caregivers like Clarence, this is not an uncommon phenomenon. A 1994 study examined the role of religious and nonreligious coping among parents of young children with chronic illnesses—juvenile diabetes, juvenile rheumatoid arthritis, cystic fibrosis, epilepsy, and spina

149

bifida. The researchers found that parents' age, marital status, educational level, child's age, and length of child's illness had no significant effect on the parents' coping ability. What *did* make a difference was their ability to derive comfort and strength from religion. Those who were consistent "religious copers" also used nonreligious coping mechanisms to good effect for dealing with financial, family, and social problems. These findings indicate that religiosity in times of crisis may strengthen people's ability to handle problems of every kind, at a time when they most need such heightened ability.

People caring for patients with Alzheimer's disease face a particularly difficult task: these patients lose most, if not all, ability to care for themselves, experiencing the dementia that erases memory and even personality. A study of caregivers of Alzheimer's and cancer patients found that those with a strong religious faith coped more effectively with their caregiving roles, whether or not they attended worship services regularly. Since many caregivers cannot leave their charges long enough to attend worship, perhaps they adapt to their circumstances by finding new modes of spiritual fulfillment within the tremendous constraints of their daily routines.

My patient Priscilla was a person of faith when caring for a sick loved one became a part of her life, but she found she needed to develop a deeper and more authentic relationship with God in order to cope with the challenges of her situation. Priscilla's seventeen-year-old son, Phil, was nearly killed in an automobile accident; doctors told Priscilla not to expect his survival, because his head injuries were so severe. But Phil survived, though in a coma. After several weeks had passed, Priscilla asked Phil's doctors if he might wake up someday.

"We don't want to encourage any false hope," the doctors said. "He'll probably be in a vegetative state. You might want to look into the possibility of long-term nursing care for Phil."

"What will happen to him then?" Priscilla asked.

"Eventually, he will die of pneumonia," she was told.

Priscilla never gave up hope, however, and turned to her faith for help. "I closed up my ears and kept on going. I read the Bible and prayed constantly," she told me. "I just about wore my Bible out! I'd sit in Phil's room reading the Bible to him, playing Christian music, or just holding his hand and praying. I fully expected him to come out of the coma one day."

And, one day, he did. Priscilla arrived for her regular daily visit to find Phil's doctor and a speech therapist talking intently outside Phil's room.

"Tell me what's going on," she demanded.

"He woke up," the doctor said.

"He couldn't verbalize anything, but his mouth was forming a word," the speech therapist said. "The word was 'alleluia.'"

Priscilla went into Phil's room, not knowing what to expect. "He looked at me and formed the words, 'I love you, Mom,' with his lips, and he went back to sleep," she told me. "It's one of the miracles in my life."

But the family's struggle was just beginning. Phil would require twenty-six separate surgeries, as well as intensive rehabilitation therapy, over the course of the next few years. Priscilla reacted to her son's condition by learning everything she could about brain injury and recovery; soon, she became intensely involved in helping other families of brain-injured individuals.

"After Phil was injured, I jumped into the role of activist for people with brain injuries. My husband and I ran an advocacy group from an office here in our home, speaking, putting on conferences, and helping other families. We educated people, and we made a lot of things happen," she told me. "At the same time, we were one hundred percent responsible for Phil's ongoing care, and visited him daily. My heart and my mind were with Phil all the time. Even when I attended my daughters' graduations and weddings, I would be in tears because I knew I would probably never see my son experience those things."

Though Priscilla was eager to keep going full speed ahead on all fronts, her body had other ideas. When she first came to see me, she had a number of frightening symptoms.

"My husband and I went to our beach house a few weeks ago. We needed to get away," she told me, briefly explaining the situation with Phil. "But when we got there, I started shaking. I had terrible pains in my stomach and my head, and my whole body ached. I couldn't think. I tried to make lunch and I couldn't do it. I have no energy. This has been going on for weeks now, and it's not getting any better. I've been to five doctors, and they all say I'm fine, but I know I'm not."

I interviewed Priscilla in depth, discerning as much as possible about her emotional, spiritual, and physical states, then performed a physical examination. Meeting her back in my office, I said, "You're totally wiped out, even burned out, but I think I can help you." Knowing that Priscilla was a practicing Christian, I drew her attention to Jesus's parable about the vine and the branch:

> "I am the vine, you are the branches. Those who abide in me and I in them bear much fruit, because apart from me you can do nothing. Whoever does not abide in me is thrown away like a branch and withers; such branches are gathered, thrown into the fire, and burned. If you abide in me, and my words abide in you, ask for whatever you wish, and it will be done for you." [JOHN 15:5–7.]

"Priscilla, you're like the branch that is withering and falling into the fire," I said gently. "You need to get back in touch with the vine, to get the spiritual nurturing you need, in addition to medicine and some counseling to help you deal with the losses and stress you've been experiencing." I talked with Priscilla about the antidepressant medication I wanted to prescribe, referred her to a Christian counselor, and suggested that she become involved with a prayer group in her church if possible. I also suggested a scripture verse for her use in private prayer:

> Humble yourselves therefore under the mighty hand of God, so that he may exalt you in due time. Cast all your anxiety on him, because he cares for you. [1 PETER 5:6–7.]

At her next office visit, about one month later, Priscilla told me she was feeling better, and over the course of the following year, she came to understand her life in a new way. Though she had been a committed Christian for twenty years, something was missing in her faith life. That "something" was revealed by the stress of caring for Phil after his accident.

"Most of my life, I've been a person who likes to be in control. I liked to control my life and everyone and everything around me," she told me. "I'm a perfectionist, and I want things to happen *now*. I got so intense in working with my son. I got angry with people and cynical and tired of hearing the same things, with nothing good happening for brain-injured people. When I look back on that time, I can see that I was really relying on my own power rather than using God's power."

Priscilla developed depression and chronic fatigue as a result not only of Phil's injury, but also of her "in-control" lifestyle. It was time to "let go and let God," but this didn't come easily.

"Getting out of the driver's seat and letting the Lord control my life, that's very difficult for me," she said. But Priscilla came to understand that she had expected far too much of herself as a caregiver, a mother and wife, and an activist for brain-injured people. She started to say "no" to new projects and activities, limiting her advocacy work sharply and focusing instead on caring for herself as well as for Phil.

"I needed time off, time for prayer and quiet," she said. "I needed to take care of my body, too—better nutrition, exercise, sleep. I'm going to my aerobics class regularly now. For years, I'd go once or twice, then an important meeting would come up, and I'd stop going for months at a time. I'm really trying to keep myself healthy."

Today, Phil lives in a group home with other young men with disabilities and holds down a job. As his mother says, "He has come a long way, but everything is still so difficult for him. Still, his attitude and his faith are amazing. People send him notes about how he has touched their lives with his beautiful faith and his cheery outlook on life."

With the relief of her major caregiving responsibilities, along with medical treatment and lifestyle changes, Priscilla's depression and chronic fatigue lifted, although she continues to require ongoing medications for other medical problems, including asthma and hypertension. Her faith, she tells me, is deeper than ever before, and she is grateful that God sustained her and her family throughout their long ordeal.

BEREAVEMENT

Like Priscilla, Anne was experiencing many troubling symptoms when she was first referred to me, including fatigue, fever, aches and pains, and nausea. Neither her general practitioner nor a psychiatrist had been able to name her illness.

"I feel like I'm in a black hole and I'm never going to return," she told me tearfully. "I've got motion sickness, so I can't go anywhere by car or plane. If this keeps up, I will lose my job." Forty-two-year-old Anne worked in television production; her schedule was hectic and demanding.

Because Anne's symptoms led me to consider the diagnoses of depression and panic disorder, I asked her about her emotional and spiritual health. "Have you experienced any particular stress in the last year or so?" I asked.

"My daughter-in-law, Gloria," she said, then started to sob. After a few moments, she went on: "She died six months ago."

"Tell me more about it, Anne," I said quietly.

"She was just twenty-one, and she was pregnant," Anne told me. "She was terribly sick, and they found liver cancer." Gloria's baby boy was born prematurely and had a stroke during the birthing process, which caused some mental retardation. Gloria died soon after her son was born.

"I just can't help thinking, 'God, why did this happen? What else could happen next? How do you expect us to go on from here?' And I just don't know the answers." Anne explained that she was not a churchgoer, though she did believe in God. As a child, she had attended church, but when she married Walter, who was Jewish, both had left organized religion behind. "I'm more spiritual than religious, I guess," she explained.

I went on to examine Anne and to run some tests. I recommended bereavement therapy (psychotherapy focused on supporting those who are grieving and helping them to move through the stages of bereavement) and prescribed an antidepressant drug. Then I suggested that she and her husband turn to the Bible—particularly to the Psalms—to find comfort in their grief.

"Perhaps this reading would draw you and your husband together spiritually as well," I said.

"It's worth a try," Anne said.

"And I hope you'll keep praying," I continued. "Even when you ask God questions that are full of anger, that's a form of honest prayer. Just keep those lines of communication open, if you can."

Anne followed all of my advice, and over the course of the next year, she got much better. The depression and chronic fatigue symptoms abated, and her emotional distress, though not completely relieved, was eased.

"My husband and I are learning to live with Gloria's death," she told me. "We're coming to accept it, even though we may never really understand why it happened. But with all this praying I'm doing, I'm beginning to think I might understand, someday."

Anne understands firsthand how both medical and spiritual resources can help one bear the burden of bereavement. Her story is echoed in a number of scientific studies that show the power of the faith factor in coping with bereavement, including a study assessing the value of spiritual support in helping bereaved parents cope. The eighty-one participants were drawn from the membership of a support group for bereaved parents, Compassionate Friends. University of Maryland psychologist Kenneth Maton found that people who reported that religious belief was an essential component of their coping repertoire were significantly less depressed than the other group members. The study also confirmed the value of peer-support groups, but found that parents who used *both* spiritual and peer-group support had the lowest incidence of depression.

Losing a spouse is another of life's great storms in which religious belief can serve as an anchor. A study of one hundred recently widowed women between the ages of sixty-five and eighty-five showed that those with stronger religious beliefs coped better with the loss of their husbands; they experienced fewer emotional and physical problems than the widows with lower levels of religious commitment. And in a study of epidemiological data gathered in Washington County, Maryland between 1963 and 1975, researchers found that widows and widowers had higher mortality rates than nonwidowed people, but widows and widowers who attended church frequently had lower mortality rates than their non-church-attending counterparts. This finding points to the possible importance of church attendance to the health of individuals in an at-risk group. Researchers have found that losing a spouse can cause the immune system to function less well; religious involvement may help counter this effect. Unfortunately, widowed individuals are less likely than married people to attend worship services regularly.

Church attendance alone may not be the best health booster for widowed people. A study of 139 widows and widowers measured their depression levels and assessed their religious orientation as either intrinsic or extrinsic. The intrinsic/extrinsic distinction, which I have discussed previously, once again proved important: patients who had an extrinsic religious orientation experienced more grief and depression than those with an intrinsic orientation. Considering these data, I advise my bereaved patients to take care of themselves physically, to take medication for depression or anxiety if it becomes necessary, to attend worship services, and to develop their spiritual lives in a personally authentic manner.

✣

The data on the faith factor point strongly to the effectiveness of religious involvement in nurturing our well-being and in strengthening our ability to cope. In any life crisis, the studies say, people who can turn to spiritual sources of support cope more effectively than those without a spiritual anchor. Of course, you do not have to undergo a life crisis in order to experience the faith factor's life-enhancing properties; religious involvement improves the quality of life in everyday, ordinary ways as well, bolstering marriages, strengthening families, and providing a sense of purpose and meaning in life.

However, the advantages of belief can perhaps be seen most clearly in people who are facing life's challenges. Let us turn now to the ultimate challenge we shall each face—the loss of our own lives—and examine how the faith factor can assist us in making this greatest of all transitions.

CHAPTER 7

Faith and Mortality: Transforming Death

Because my wife, Demetra, is an accountant, I am especially aware of the certainty of taxes. Yet, although the arm of the IRS may be long, death is our most feared and relentless pursuer. Medicine and religious commitment can often help forestall death, but neither has found a way to overcome our ultimate fate as human beings: the certainty that our physical bodies *will* die. The truth expressed by the Psalmist centuries ago holds true today:

> As for mortals, their days are like grass;
> they flourish like a flower of the field;
> for the wind passes over it, and it is gone,
> and its place knows it no more.
> [PSALM 103:15–16.]

Even though most religious traditions offer the hope of an afterlife, we must still grapple with the reality that the life we live now will not last forever. Given this reality, people hope for two things: delaying death's inevitability as long as possible and, when at last we can delay it no longer, minimizing the emotional and physical pain of the dying process. In both of these efforts, the faith factor has been found to offer help and hope, in the experience of dying people and also in the scientific literature.

157

DELAYING DEATH

Is it possible to cheat death? Ultimately, of course, the answer is "no," but a solid and growing body of scientific evidence indicates that we can delay premature death in many cases through authentic religious involvement. In a carefully designed and executed study published in 1997, researchers W. J. Strawbridge, et al. followed 6,928 persons in Alameda County, California, over the course of twenty-eight years, tracking their mortality rates and frequency of attendance at religious services. During the unusually long period of the study, the subjects were physically examined at regular intervals. The study was also unusual in that it carefully considered and compared a large number of factors that might affect longevity—demographic factors (age, gender, education), health status, and social support. The study found that people who attend religious services frequently (once a week or more) had mortality rates 36 percent lower than those subjects who attended services less frequently. Even when the researchers "controlled for" (or made statistical adjustments to take into account), factors such as age, gender, ethnicity, education, health status, and degree of social support, these results held firm. Women benefited from frequent worship attendance even more than men.

The Strawbridge study reaffirms the findings of a 1979 survey of residents of the same community—Alameda County, California. In the earlier study, researchers L. F. Berkman and S. L. Syme found lower mortality rates among men aged thirty to sixty-nine who were married, had frequent contacts with friends and relatives, and were church members. For women of the same ages, lower mortality rates applied among those who had frequent contacts with friends and relatives, were church members, and belonged to one or more groups, like clubs or associations. This study found that social isolation and absence of church membership raised mortality rates significantly, even when the study data were adjusted to account for factors like physical inactivity, smoking, alcohol consumption, obesity, and lack of preventive health care.

In another noteworthy study, researchers U. Goldbourt, S. Yaari, and J. H. Medalie examined the factors leading to mortality caused by coronary heart disease among 10,059 Israeli men. Like the Strawbridge study, this study offers the advantage of following a large group of people over a long period of time—in this case, twenty-three years. The following table demonstrates their conclusive findings that mortality rates from coronary heart disease and from all causes were lowest among the most Orthodox Jews and highest among those who defined themselves as "secular."

	Deaths Per 10,000 Person Years	
	Most Orthodox Subjects	*Secular Subjects*
Deaths from coronary heart disease	38	61
Deaths from all causes	135	168

The most Orthodox, or religiously observant, Jews among the subjects experienced a dramatically lessened risk of dying from coronary heart disease, compared to the nonbelievers. To determine whether this effect could be explained by differences in the ages of the two cohorts, the researchers controlled for age, a standard statistical practice in mortality studies; the results indicating the importance of religious observance to longevity remained the same. Another study of Israelis shows that members of religious kibbutzim live longer than members of nonreligious kibbutzim. Over a fifteen-year period, 192 people in the secular kibbutzim died (8 percent of total residents), as compared with only 69 (4 percent) among the residents of religious kibbutzim, a startling 50-percent reduction in mortality. This study truly compares "apples and apples," not "apples and oranges," because residents of kibbutzim, whether religious or secular, are remarkably similar in terms of demographic factors apart from religious beliefs and practices. Both groups benefit from strong social support, but it is clear that those who also take part in frequent religious observance as part of the community enjoy enhanced health benefits.

It has been shown that social support is stronger among religious communities. For example, a 1994 study of 2,956 individuals in North Carolina found that frequent church attenders enjoyed more relationships with people outside their families and more frequent social contacts, both in person and by telephone, than others did.

Researchers have found a similar effect of the faith factor among African-Americans, one of the most religious groups in the United States. In a 1992 study of 473 African-Americans aged seventy and over, individuals who did not attend church services regularly were twice as likely to die during the four-year study period as those who did.

Religious involvement also helped decrease mortality rates in older individuals facing a very stressful event—being forced to move from their homes. Among 225 such elderly persons in New Haven and West Haven, Connecticut, religious people were twice as likely to survive the two-year follow-up period than the nonreligious, even though no association was found between religiousness and health habits. The religious elderly were also found to be psychologically healthier than their nonreligious peers. And in a 1981 study, religious individuals among the elderly residents of Veterans Administration nursing homes were found to survive longer than nonreligious residents.

However, the level of religious involvement in a community does not always predict greater longevity. When religious doctrine advocates the avoidance of traditional medical care, mortality rates can be higher, not lower, than among the general population. As mentioned in chapter 2, a study of pregnant women among the Faith Assembly communities of Indiana (who do not use obstetric care) found a maternal mortality rate *almost a hundred times higher* than in the general population, and the Faith Assembly's infant-mortality rate was almost three times higher. Childhood illnesses, like polio, appear much more commonly among groups who eschew vaccination. But when religious practice does not preclude medical care, mortality rates have been found consistently lower among people with a high degree of religious involvement.

Why do religiously committed people live longer? We know that better health practices account for part of the answer. Among Seventh-Day Adventists, Mormons, and other believers whose faith dictates abstinence from substances like tobacco and alcohol, lower rates of cancer and coronary heart disease can be easily understood and even anticipated, as mentioned in chapter 1. Even in a broader slice of the population, including members of less strict sects, the health practices of religiously active people have been found better than those without religious commitment. For example, the Strawbridge study mentioned above found that frequent church attenders were more likely to stop smoking and to increase their level of exercise. But temperance is not the only component of the faith factor that accounts for longer life among religious people; its other elements also contribute to greater longevity.

If you want to live longer, then, contemporary science tells us that attending worship services frequently (i.e., once a week or more) may help. But even among less frequent attenders—individuals who attend once a month or more—mortality rates appear to be lower than among people who attend rarely or not at all. The survival benefit of private religiosity (for example, watching religious programs on television) is less clear. Worship-service attendance, as mentioned earlier, is the benchmark used for religiosity in most of the mortality studies quoted demonstrating enhanced survival. From a scientific point of view, then, I feel secure in urging patients to attend the worship services of their choice at least once a week, for their health's sake. But because so many studies have indicated the greater value to health of intrinsic religiosity, as opposed to an extrinsic religious orientation (see chapter 2 for a detailed discussion), I also encourage my patients to develop an authentic, personal spirituality that includes but goes beyond weekly worship, to seek closeness to God in a manner that honors their individual pursuit of meaning, purpose, connection, and truth.

FACING DEATH WITH EQUANIMITY

As we saw in chapter 6, people of faith report a higher quality of life and greater sense of meaning than nonbelievers; they also draw heavily on the resources of faith to see them through difficult situations like illness and bereavement. Unless we meet death unexpectedly, we will all contend with the dying process, perhaps the most significant crisis any of us will face. Scientific research has established that, though religious and nonreligious people alike will search for meaning and comfort in the experience of terminal illness, people of faith are more likely to have this search fulfilled.

Religiously involved people suffer less from fear of death, or death anxiety, than do nonreligious people, according to a number of studies. A 1983 study of 1,428 Americans found that death anxiety was expressed by 13 percent of individuals who stated that they had no religious preference, versus only 5 percent of individuals who did have a preference, whether it was Protestant, Roman Catholic, Jewish, or another faith. In this study, the relationship between religious preference and death anxiety was even more pronounced in younger people. But older individuals, who are likely to be more aware of death's nearness than their younger counterparts, also benefit greatly from faith when grappling with death anxiety. A study examining attitudes about death among 260 older subjects found that highly religious people had the least fear of death and the strongest belief in an afterlife.

Middle-aged male respondents to a 1984 survey provided an interesting finding for researcher A. M. Downey. Those who were moderately religious experienced greater death anxiety than either those who were highly religious or those who were nonreligious. This curvilinear relationship between religious commitment and death anxiety points to the importance of intrinsic religiosity in evoking the benefits of the faith factor; lukewarm, going-through-the-motions, extrinsic religious commitment does not yield the same result.

The relationship between religious commitment and death anxiety is seen even more clearly when studies involve patients with terminal illness—people who are actively grappling with imminent death and who are likely to be experiencing physical suffering. Surprisingly, patients with life-threatening illness have been found to exhibit high levels of spiritual well-being. In other words, even seriously ill individuals can feel spiritually healthy, and can enjoy a comforting sense of the reality of God in a time of illness.

In a 1992 study assessing the spiritual health of patients with lung cancer, the patients scored very high in their response to a thirty-one-item Spiritual Health Inventory that elicited their agreement or disagreement with statements like "I believe God can help me." All the patients appeared to have high levels of spiritual health, but those reporting the greatest sense of spiritual well-being were older patients, and those experiencing greater physical well-being. It is safe to assume that all the patients in this study were in some degree of pain or discomfort, because lung cancer is not usually diagnosed until symptoms like coughing, shortness of breath, and weakness have appeared. We might hypothesize from this finding that the patients who experienced more intense pain found it harder to find relief in their spirituality, but the study did not directly address that question. Certainly up-to-date methods of pain control are an essential aspect of the care of the terminally ill. Proper pain control may itself provide an opportunity for the patient to nourish and employ more freely his or her spiritual resources.

In a study of twenty terminally ill patients, researchers D. K. Smith, A. M. Nehmkis, and R. A. Charter found that those who attended church had markedly lower death anxiety, and that, the higher the patients' own rating of their religious commitment, the greater their courage and hope for the afterlife. The more religious patients were also less likely to feel indifferent about death; it is probable that they took the transition from this life to the next more seriously and worked harder to come to a sense of resolution about their lives, so that they could face death as the important event it is for spiritually oriented people. In a 1978 study of terminally ill patients whose life expectancy could be measured in weeks, investigators found the lowest levels of conscious fear of death in patients who rated their religious beliefs as strong. Other factors related to lower levels of death anxiety in these patients included absence of pain and the patient's previous experience of having lost a loved one. Interestingly, these patients feared death less than patients in good health with whom they were compared.

Some religious people seem not to fear death, but to welcome it. I will never forget one patient of mine, a seventy-nine-year-old woman named Miriam, a practicing Orthodox Jew who had severe rheumatoid arthritis. Degeneration of her spine at the neck vertebrae caused her neck to teeter unsteadily. The circulation of blood to her feet was so poor that she was in imminent danger of developing gangrene of one foot. Without an operation, I told Miriam, gangrene would eventually take over her body, and she would die. But she had decided not to have the operation.

One day Miriam came to see me, traveling in a wheelchair with her maid and companion, Dora. In maneuvering Miriam's wheelchair into my office, Dora accidentally bumped Miriam's leg against the doorway, and Miriam winced in pain. She looked even more frail and pained than when I had seen her last.

"What's been going on, Miriam?" I asked, taking her hand.

"Well, Doctor, I'm still having a lot of pain," she said. "And you know about my leg—about the gangrene."

"Yes, I do know about it, Miriam. As I told you the last time I saw you, I strongly recommend that you proceed with surgery right away, so we can prevent this gangrene."

"I want to wait till the spring," Miriam said softly. I heard a little catch in her voice as she said "the spring."

No matter how many times I had stated my case for the operation, Miriam had stood firm, and as her doctor, I was bound to respect her wishes. "Tell me about the spring," I said, leaning forward expectantly.

She paused, then told me that she had experienced a vision. She saw herself standing in the front of her temple. A ceremony was taking place; all her friends and family were there. Her rabbi was saying solemnly, "Miriam, you will no longer be known by this name." Dressed in a beautiful white gown, Miriam walked out of the temple and down some stairs. There she met a handsome young man, who greeted her warmly. Taking her by the hand, he led her into a lush garden full of spring flowers; the sun shone gently on them, and Miriam was filled with joy.

"The whole world will be changed in the spring," she said, and paused again, her eyes filling with tears. "Thank you, Doctor! Thank you! You have always been my favorite doctor. You listen to me!"

My eyes glistened, too, and our glances met in an embrace. "Thank you, Miriam! You have told me of God!"

CARDINAL BERNARDIN'S "GIFT OF PEACE"

Though Miriam was a Jewish laywoman and Joseph Bernardin a cardinal of the Roman Catholic Church, they shared an important bond: both would find great meaning in the process of dying. When Cardinal Bernardin, archbishop of Chicago, learned he had pancreatic cancer, he decided to be completely honest with the public about his illness, instructing his doctor and his aide to hold a press conference at once. After surgery, radiation, and chemotherapy, the cardinal enjoyed relatively good health for fifteen months before learning that the cancer had spread to his liver. At that point, his oncologist informed him that the cancer was inoperable, and that he would probably live a year at the most. Within just a few days, Cardinal Bernardin called a second news conference. In his book, *The Gift of Peace,* the cardinal recounted his words to the media:

The room was so crowded with reporters and TV cameras that it was difficult to move. I shared the news about the latest diagnosis and the estimate that my life expectancy was one year or less. "I have been assured that I still have some quality time left," I said. "My prayer is that I will use whatever time is left in a positive way, that is, in a way that will be of benefit to the priests and people I have been called to serve, as well as to my own spiritual well-being."

Cardinal Bernardin proceeded to live his dying publicly and courageously, so that others might learn from it. He reached out to his fellow sufferers wherever he went. When hospital officials suggested he enter the oncology clinic from a rear door so as not to be overwhelmed by other cancer patients asking for prayers and comfort, the cardinal insisted, "I am a priest first, a patient second." He continued to minister to his fellow cancer patients until the very end of his life, finding great meaning and satisfaction in the person-to-person ministry he had had little time for as spiritual leader and administrator of the enormous Archdiocese of Chicago.

By necessity, the cardinal wrote, he found his own faith deepening as death neared. When he was lonely, he would think of Jesus in the garden of Gethsemane the night before his crucifixion; he would identify with his Lord's experience of desolation. For many years, he had started every day with one hour of prayer; now prayer became even more important to him. Pain and discomfort interfered with his praying, and he hastened to tell his friends and his flock, "Pray while you're well, because when you're sick you might not be able to pray!" As his illness progressed, the cardinal learned to let go of the ministries that had been so important to him. Knowing that death was coming, he put his house in order, making arrangements for a smooth transition in the archdiocese, finalizing his will, and saying goodbye to friends and family.

Thirteen days before his death in November 1996, Cardinal Bernardin completed his book manuscript. In part, he wrote:

As I write these final words, my heart is filled with joy. I am at peace. . . . I will soon experience new life in a different way. Although I do not know what to expect in the afterlife, I do know that just as God has called me to serve him to the best of my ability throughout my life on earth, he is now calling me home.

Cardinal Bernardin had received the precious gift of God's peace, a gift he wanted to share with others through his public dying and the book he left behind. He gave us a model for finding meaning in dying. In so doing, he became a vivid, living example of one aspect of the Roman Catholic Church's argument against assisted suicide and euthanasia: we are to live each day God gives us, serving God and accepting his will for us, learning to trust him more and more, rather than taking our fates into our own hands.

As a doctor, I am grateful to this great man of faith for his courageous example. Cardinal Bernardin showed us how the act of dying can bring grace, spiritual growth, and transformation. It is a lesson we urgently need to heed in a time of tumult over how our society views and regulates death.

ASSISTED SUICIDE: A DOCTOR'S LAMENT

How did we come to a place where doctors, the guardians of health and life, are being asked to help patients commit suicide? In a sense, scientific progress has brought about a new kind of adversity. Whereas most patients used to die quickly of infections like pneumonia, now we can often forestall death with powerful antibiotics. The sick are less likely to die of acute infections, leaving them more subject to the lingering effects and slow deterioration of chronic illnesses like prostate cancer, Alzheimer's, and Parkinson's disease. The increased likelihood of facing a prolonged dying process has spawned the cry for a "medical" end to suffering through assisted suicide.

But for doctors even to entertain the idea of euthanasia or assisting patients to commit suicide is an enormous turnabout and tragedy for medicine as a healing profession, a strange by-product of our progress. To accede to the growing demand for instant, controlled death goes completely against the very nature of our profession, overturning a specific proscription of the Hippocratic Oath and thousands of years of medical history. Rather than assisting in suicide, doctors can offer the suffering person many palliative resources, including the resources of religion and spirituality. I would much rather that a doctor inject the comfort and wisdom of Holy Scripture into someone's veins than inject potassium chloride. I would far prefer that a doctor encourage a patient in pain to breathe in the life and peace of the Holy Spirit than the carbon monoxide of euthanasia advocate Dr. Jack Kevorkian's death machine.

In the call for physician-assisted suicide, we can see the extent of our culture's dependence on the success of medical technology—and our spiritual impoverishment as a people. When disease presents challenges contemporary science cannot easily meet, many Americans look for a quick way out. Even though men and women throughout human history have faced suffering with courage and expected to find redemptive meaning in their pain, many individuals today feel justified in demanding access to a pain-free, sanitary, state-approved method for killing themselves. Interestingly, religious patients and doctors are less likely than nonreligious patients and doctors to endorse the idea or to request participation in assisted suicide.

For me, the mere existence of physician-assisted suicide points to our failure as a culture to grasp the profound spiritual opportunity presented by illness. But it also indicates that many people do not trust their doctors to help them cope with lingering physical and spiritual pain. In the cries of those who long for an easy way out, we hear a cry for medicine and doctors to show their heart and soul. Cardinal Bernardin could face death courageously because of his remarkable character and great spiritual depth, but he also had the advantages of excellent medical care from compassionate doctors and the comfort of a caring and supportive community. Perhaps the terminally ill patients who yearn for assisted suicide would feel differently if they could depend on similar resources.

The grace and transformation possible in the dying process, so beautifully demonstrated in Cardinal Bernardin's story, has been shown to us repeatedly by many of the individuals who have faced the most terrifying epidemic of our era, AIDS.

Though coronary heart disease and cancer continue to be the leading causes of death in the United States, the AIDS epidemic has compelled the attention of the media and the general public, in part because of the tragic drama of so many younger people facing death through this terrible disease. Patients with AIDS often find their illness and dying process complicated by the stigma attached to the disease, a stigma caused in part by the fact that the disease first surfaced in this country among homosexuals. In Orthodox Judaism and Christianity, the active practice of homosexuality is forbidden by scripture and tradition; this may have caused some religious groups to shun people with AIDS, regardless of their sexual orientation. Fortunately, many other congregations and religious organizations offer staunch support for those on the journey through this difficult illness, making the process much easier to bear for patients and their loved ones. To illustrate the faith factor at work in the lives of people with AIDS, I would like to share two stories with you.

✢

Martin is a forty-three-year-old musician and retired nursing-home recreation therapist who developed AIDS. Fortunately, neither his wife, Alice, nor his fourteen-year-old son, Joshua, has contracted the virus. Martin tested positive for HIV in 1989, after a six-month bout with bronchitis that just would not go away. He received the diagnosis of AIDS when his T-cell count dropped almost to zero and a bronchial infection brought him close to death. With the help of aggressive antibiotic therapy, Martin pulled through, slowly regaining strength. Today, several years later, his T-cell count is actually higher than it was at the time he tested positive, and he has few health problems except for fatigue, which was severe enough to cause him to retire from his job. Like many people with AIDS, Martin is taking three antiviral medications to stave off deadly infection.

Currently, dealing with extreme but unpredictable exhaustion is Martin's worst physical problem. "There are some days when I can do whatever I want, and there are other days when by two in the afternoon I'm done for the day," he said. Martin has taken up "house-husband" duties so that Alice can pursue a graduate degree while working full-time.

Their household is remarkably peaceful and even happy now, but this was not always the case. For years, Martin struggled with the emotional aftershocks of childhood sexual abuse. He was repeatedly molested by a step-grandparent, and though he did not consciously remember the abuse until shortly after he tested positive for HIV, it left deep and aching marks and laid the psychological foundation for compulsive sexual behavior in later life. Martin acquired the virus that causes AIDS through such extramarital sexual activity. For many years, his faith life did not go deep enough to bring healing to his painful memories, experiences, and behavior patterns.

"I've been a churchgoing person all my life, and, being a church musician, I've always enjoyed that work and had a sense of ministry in it," he said. "But in many other ways, my spiritual life was a mess. After six years of heavy-duty therapy, Twelve Step meetings of various kinds, and pastoral counseling, I've learned that the childhood sexual-abuse stuff was a big factor in why things were so messed up."

Before undertaking his journey of healing, Martin experienced a constant sense of alienation, from himself, from others, and from God. "There wasn't any sense of spiritual groundedness," he explained. "Fortunately, I got a therapist who was comfortable with talk of spiritual issues, and that was a wonderful thing."

Having suffered from a sense of being dissociated from his physical self as a result of the childhood sexual abuse, Martin needed healing experiences that would bridge the apparent gap between mind and body that has formed the basis for much of Western culture. "When I first went into therapy, and my T-cells were great, the HIV went on the back burner and the sexual abuse went on the front burner," he recalled. "I had periods where I did not feel connected to my physical body. Sometimes I would actually have difficulty moving physically, or I might lose the ability to speak for an hour, because my tongue wouldn't move. A part of the healing work was getting comfortable with being a physical person, and part of that came through learning better ways to take care of myself physically—eating and sleeping more appropriately."

But as he remembered the torture of his childhood experiences, Martin needed spiritual counseling as well. He began to see a minister at his church regularly.

"We had a lot of discussions about evil in the world, and how can God allow these things to happen to little children?" he said. "I don't know the answers to those questions, and I know I never will, but there was a period of time when I had to ask them. The minister told me, 'Get angry at God. Yell and scream at God. He's a big guy, he can take it!' And I did—in a slow, measured fashion, because anger is something that has always terrified me."

Martin's emotional healing of childhood trauma continued when he decided to share his history, as well as his HIV status, with his church community. It was time, he decided, to bring these dark places to light:

"I had all these secrets. It came to a point when I felt like I had to tell somebody other than Alice and my therapist. I had to connect it into church, somehow. I selected someone at church who seemed real safe. I shared my story, telling him about the sexual abuse and the HIV and so forth. And he didn't judge me, he was just there—accepting and supportive."

His friend's acceptance gave Martin the courage to approach his minister for pastoral counseling and spiritual direction. "She, too, accepted me. She told me, 'It's my job to beat you over the head with the love of God until you get the picture,' and she has done that."

Martin and Alice decided to tell more friends at church about his HIV infection. The reactions they received surprised them—pleasantly.

"Everywhere we went, people said, 'We're sorry. What can we do? We're praying for you. Come to dinner!'" Martin remembered. The church community's love and acceptance have given the entire family a sense of peace and assurance about the future:

"We haven't needed a whole lot from people yet, in terms of hands-on help, but we will," Martin said, "and it's wonderful to know that, when that time comes, two phone calls is all it's going to take. We would not have had the security of knowing this if we had not been willing to take the risk of being open. Our son, Joshua, shares that, too. He has grown up in this church, and he knows that we are accepted and loved by these people."

Through coping with his illness, Martin has found real peace with himself: "For years, I was always saying to myself, 'If people knew *this* about me, they'd reject me.' But now people know those things and they love me anyway. The love of God is great stuff, but I learned about what it is to be loved by God because all these people around me loved me. That's why now I feel like I'm able to handle anything that comes along."

Given the hope provided by new medical treatments like the protease-inhibitor drugs, Martin, like many people with AIDS, is asking himself, "What now?" A few years ago, his life seemed short, likely to end in a week or a month; today, he realizes that he may have a number of years left, and he is searching for the most meaningful way to live the time that remains.

On many Sundays, Martin substitutes as an organist and choir director at a variety of churches. When he's not playing, he enjoys worshiping as "just a parishioner in the pew" at his own church, where he takes part in healing-prayer services on a regular basis. He doesn't expect to be healed of AIDS, but he is certain he has experienced other kinds of healing through spiritual means. In a number of guided-imagery prayer sessions, he found a metaphor for his spiritual journey.

170

"One of the recurring images was a jewel—faceted, red, slightly magenta in color, a little smaller than a golf ball. It glowed, as if light was coming from inside it. In the meditations, I kept walking through forests searching for this precious jewel. Eventually I found it and took it with me. That jewel is about preciousness, which is something I never believed—that I was precious, to God or to anyone. And now I know that indeed I am, to God and to other people. The jewel image is also about finding my heart that was locked away inside a fortress, inside a deep woods, and claiming it as my own now."

Martin recalled another important image from these prayer sessions: "In one of the prayer times, Jesus appeared, and we were standing by a well. The well was full of tears, and I was supposed to take a ladle and to drink from it," he explained. "I didn't want any part of it! And Jesus was there saying, 'It'll be okay. I'm here.' So I did. And as soon as it touched my lips, I began to weep profusely, and caught all my own tears in my hand. Jesus was still standing right there, and my tears turned into diamonds, as a sign of how precious those are, too."

Though his faith has brought him great comfort through community support and a deeply felt sense of God's love, Martin does not think much about an afterlife. "I have never had a sense of the future, except in terms of anticipating something awful," he said. "The future is something I cannot conceive of, except as some sort of nebulous dread, or waiting for the other shoe to drop, though that fearfulness is infinitesimal now compared to the way it used to dominate my life.

"My journey in the Christian faith really hasn't been about preparing for the next life. If all that good stuff happens, fine. I'm trying to get through *this* life, and to me faith isn't about planning for then, as much as getting through now.

"If now spills over into everlasting bliss, cool," Martin said, laughing. "I'll take bliss any way I can get it!"

✣

Unlike Martin, my patient Serena counted heavily on the assurances of heaven provided to her by her strong Christian faith. A young African-American woman, Serena contracted HIV from her husband, who was an intravenous-drug user. When I met her in a room at Georgetown Hospital, she was in the late stages of AIDS and very sick with tuberculosis, coughing incessantly. She had lived for four years with *no* T-cells, and she had suffered through a number of serious infections, but her faith radiated throughout the special isolation room to which she was confined.

"Hallelujah!" she said repeatedly. "Praise the Lord!" Her musical voice sounded clearly through the mask she wore to prevent the spread of tuberculosis as she testified to her love of God; no mask could hide her insistent smile. It seemed that Serena's faith brought her more than just relief from anxiety, and she faced death with an unquenchable joy.

One day, I visited Serena, joining her father (who is a minister) and a family friend at her bedside.

"Let's all pray together," I suggested, and we joined hands around the bed. Serena's father began our prayer time, praying for Serena's release from the "demon of AIDS," and all of us confessed our sins and thanked and petitioned God together. Serena died a few days later, having lived much longer than expected, based on her devastating illness.

With another doctor from Georgetown, I attended Serena's funeral. Both of us were asked to speak at this wonderful "Victory Celebration" of Serena's life, and though we were the only two white people in the crowded church, I felt immediately at home worshiping God with these fellow Christians. Together in the midst of death's finality we sang a wonderful song—"I've got a feeling, things are gonna be all right"—and despite the grief Serena's family and friends were suffering, there was a real sense of rejoicing and homecoming for this great woman of faith. The bishop of the church district led the service, allowing Serena's father the opportunity to grieve rather than have the responsibility of leading worship. But he couldn't help himself. After another stirring song, he arose and told the stilled congregation, "Many of you have offered your condolences to my wife and me regarding the loss of our daughter. My wife and I thank you from the bottom of our hearts. But my dictionary says that, when people are lost, we have no idea where they are. My daughter is *not* lost. I know *exactly* where my daughter is—she is on her knees worshiping before the King of Kings and the Lord of Lords, praising and glorifying him! Glory!"

Shortly thereafter, the family motioned to me to speak. Picking up where Serena's father had left off, I asked the congregation to imagine where Serena was at that moment, in the throne room of heaven. Drawing on passages from the Book of Revelation, chapters 4 and 5, I described

St. John's vision of heaven, with a great throne surrounded by twenty-four thrones with a rainbow above it and a sea of glass before it, with thousands upon thousands of angels in joyous assembly singing, "Holy, holy, holy is the Lord God Almighty," and holding bowls of incense before the throne, which are the prayers of the saints. Truly, we sent up a bowlful of fragrant prayers that day!

Though missing Serena's earthly presence, I said, we could rejoice together in faith, knowing that she had, indeed, won the victory of eternal life.

✢

In the Book of Ecclesiastes, Solomon reminds us, "For everything, there is a season" (Ecclesiastes 3:1). There is a time to fight death, a time to heed poet Dylan Thomas's charge, "Do not go gentle into that good night." There is also a time to let go, a time to mourn. For everyone, death is a loss; even people like Serena, who have a clear and certain view of the next life, must confront the reality that *this* life, and all we hold dear in it, will one day be no more. As we cope with the inevitable loss of our lives on earth, we are more likely to make this ultimate transition with less pain and distress if we are people of faith.

A few weeks before his painful death from leukemia, my grandfather, a Baptist minister and missionary, preached his final sermon. His topic was dying and the afterlife. While serving as an orderly in France during World War I, in times of great despair over the brutal savagery of war, he would often imagine joyfully the scene at the end of the war, when at long last he would arrive in Washington's Union Station and find his train, the Dixie Flyer, to take him home to the red hills of Georgia. He'd see himself boarding that train with great eagerness, looking forward with blissful anticipation to that moment at the end of the line when he would first see his father again and run, like a little boy, into his outstretched arms. He concluded his last sermon by saying:

"When I think about where I'm headed now, I think again of the Dixie Flyer, for I believe the journey will be the same. There will be a long train ride—a bit bumpy and uncomfortable in places, perhaps—and that is the process of dying. But then—ah, then!—I will at last come to the end of the line. There on the platform will be my Father, my Heavenly Father. He will come running to me and he will open his arms to greet me and to place a crown on my head. And he will say the words I've longed to hear all my life: 'Welcome home, my beloved son.' And at last I will be home. Home with my Father, forever and ever."

I pray that, when the time comes for me, I will be able to meet death with my grandfather's assurance and faith.

✢

As we have seen in the preceding chapters, having an authentic faith improves the odds of our having better physical and mental health, and we increase our chances of meeting life's vicissitudes with courage, resilience, and peace. Developing authentic faith requires seeking God and nurturing the life of the spirit in a personally meaningful, God-honoring way. In the chapters to come, I will discuss some basic principles of living a spiritually rich life. Regardless of your faith tradition, and even if you would say you have *no* faith tradition of any kind at this time, I believe these principles of the spiritual life will help you explore how you can receive the health-giving and joy-filled potential of the faith factor by seeking, and finding, the source of health and joy.

PART II

―――――――――――― ✠ ――――――――――――

Spirituality

CHAPTER 8

⟡

Developing a Spiritual Program:
Seeking God in Your Life

Better physical and mental health, a longer and more satisfying life, a greater sense of purpose and fulfillment, a happier marriage, more courage and strength in times of difficulty—who *wouldn't* want to take full advantage of the faith factor's benefits? I hope that the preceding chapters have inspired you to consider the magnitude of these benefits, and to consider how *you* might respond to the wealth of data that show the connection between faith and health. Your response will depend largely on where you are in your spiritual life at this moment. If you are already a religious person, you may want to examine ways of deepening your faith. If you consider yourself spiritual but have no link to a church or synagogue, you may wish to re-examine your views about religious commitment and consider establishing a relationship with a faith tradition and community. If you do not consider yourself religious or spiritual, but are intrigued by the faith factor's potential, I hope you will think about developing a spiritual life that is authentic, meaningful, and healthy for you. The key component in this quest is the desire for a greater knowledge of the Divine, the thirst for a relationship with God, even if you feel you do not yet know who he is.

If you sense such a desire, I recommend that you consider beginning a *spiritual program,* a course of action designed to help you explore your faith and cultivate your spirituality. Your spiritual program will be yours

177

alone, because each person has a unique background, individual experiences, and particular needs, but it will also resonate with aspects of others' experience as spiritual seekers. In the three chapters following this one, I will discuss in depth what I consider to be the basic components of a spiritual program—prayer, scripture study, and participation in a spiritual community. But first we must examine our assumptions about what constitutes faith, religion, and spirituality.

There are thousands of ways to approach this topic. For millennia, great thinkers and spiritual leaders have developed entire theologies based on seemingly simple questions like "What is faith?" I do not presume to follow in their footsteps by presenting a comprehensive theology of my own. Rather, as a physician and research scientist, I can explain how religiosity has influenced the patients I care for, how it is measured by clinical researchers, and, given their definitions and assumptions, how we can hope to align ourselves with the people of faith who have benefited from religious involvement.

The scientists who have produced and reviewed the faith-factor data are not theologians and cannot take the place of spiritual leaders. But so that you can understand how your spiritual program might better tap into the faith factor's resources, let us look at the nature of faith. Then we will look at how researchers have defined it, and examine their findings about how various aspects of religiosity affect health and well-being.

WHAT IS FAITH?

First, let us consider faith, or belief, from a medical, nonreligious point of view. As I discussed at length in chapter 2, Dr. Herbert Benson has established the medical importance of our beliefs, stating in his book, *Timeless Healing,* "Our brains are wired for beliefs and expectancies. When activated, the body can respond as it would if the belief were a reality, producing deafness or thirst, health or illness." You have probably experienced this phenomenon while watching a movie. For example, though we know that an Alfred Hitchcock thriller like *Psycho* is "just a movie," we react to events like the stabbing in the shower as if they were happening to us. Our eyes and ears are flooded by sensory data that command our autonomic nervous systems to react in fear. Our bodies respond accordingly: hearts race, breathing becomes rapid and shallow, we begin to perspire.

Dr. Benson and other researchers have accumulated overwhelming evidence that our beliefs can affect our health. If we believe a certain pill will make us better, chances are good that it will, regardless of its ingredients. This is the "placebo effect," which formed the basis for much of medical practice until the twentieth century. In times when doctors knew nothing about bacteria and viruses, when their pharmacopeia was limited to a few herbs, and when surgery was more likely to kill than to cure, the effectiveness of many medical treatments depended upon the patients' expectations of positive benefits.

We know now, for example, that the eighteenth-century practice of bloodletting (removing blood in times of illness) did not help make people better because of its inherent physiologic effects. From the modern, scientific point of view, bloodletting should have made most patients sicker, in the same way that someone who begins to hemorrhage profusely can develop shock and ultimately die if the bleeding is not stopped. But patients often *did* get better after bloodletting, because they *believed* in its efficacy. Then, as now, the imprimatur of medical authority carried great weight. Famous physicians like Benjamin Rush, one of the signers of the Declaration of Independence, advocated bloodletting. Rush's authority as a medical leader certified the expectations of positive benefit that made bloodletting a frequently effective treatment.

Medical history is replete with examples of treatments that, like bloodletting, once appeared effective yet were proved later to have no actual curative powers greater than those achievable by the use of inert placebos. Some of these treatments sound barbaric to contemporary ears. Even as recently as my father's era of medicine, for example, doctors actually administered live hookworms to patients with the disease polycythemia, in which the body manufactures an excessive number of red blood cells. (In fact, polycythemia is one of the few diseases where bloodletting actually is effective!)

One interesting example of the power of belief in medicine was documented when researchers gave a pregnant woman the drug ipecac, which is customarily used to induce vomiting in people who have swallowed poisonous substances. In this study, the woman was told that ipecac was intended to *reduce* vomiting from morning sickness—exactly the opposite of the drug's actual pharmacological qualities. The patient's vomiting was reduced; the researchers' claims were supported. The woman's belief about the drug overrode its well-established pharmacologic effect.

Just as this patient's beliefs literally reversed ipecac's usual effects on the body, doctors know that the sizes, shapes, colors, and names of pills can influence their effectiveness. For example, to even the most casual observer of medical advertisements, it appears that pills must have the letter "z" or "x" in their names to be successful. In recent years we have witnessed a proliferation of such names in new medications like Prozac, Paxil, Xanax, Zantac, Zestril, and Zoloft.

The placebo effect also influences the outcome of surgery. Until the late 1950s, a surgical procedure called the internal mammary artery bypass was a common treatment for heart disease. However, using a research technique that today's ethics committees would not allow, researchers set up a "sham-surgery" experiment to test the effectiveness of this procedure. One group of patients received the internal mammary artery bypass surgery. Patients in another group were simply cut open and stitched closed again, without surgery being performed. Both groups had the same degree of relief of symptoms immediately after surgery, and, in fact, patients receiving the sham surgery were more likely to have at least a 50-percent reduction in their angina pectoris (heart pain) one year later when compared with the group that received surgery. The results of this experiment soon banished the internal mammary artery bypass procedure to the graveyard of outmoded techniques.

How many of our surgical procedures today might also be based on the placebo effect? Since we now consider it unethical to do sham-surgery experiments, we may never know. But we *do* know that surgery's effectiveness must be influenced, to some degree, by patients' expectations, especially because surgery is such a powerful intervention and symbolic act. It evokes spiritual images, including the administration of anesthesia ("putting people to sleep," the cultural and Biblical metaphor for death), having patients "wake up" in the recovery room (as if they were being resurrected from the dead), and granting mythical power to the surgeon, who is given the unique, astounding privilege of entering and leaving other people's bodies. Such profound images abound particularly in cardiac surgery. In coronary artery bypass surgery, for example, the patient's heart is literally stopped (for centuries a medical criterion of death) and the patient's circulation maintained through mechanical means for the duration of the surgery, after which the heart is restarted and circulation restored.

What we believe about our doctors and our medical treatments will markedly affect our illnesses and our recoveries. Such belief is an important form of faith, but it does not address our larger questions—the meaning of life, the purpose of existence, the nature of a relationship with the One who created us. People grapple with these questions largely through spirituality and religion, which, as the faith-factor data show us, can also significantly affect physical and mental health.

RELIGIOUS FAITH:
"THE ASSURANCE OF THINGS HOPED FOR"

"Secular faith," like our faith in medicines and medical procedures, profoundly affects other areas of our lives as well. Without faith, explorers and immigrants would have stopped far short of the New World of America, preferring safety at home to the promise of a better life. Without faith, early American pioneers would have stopped at the Blue Ridge Mountains, deterred by rugged terrain; only their belief in what lay beyond the mountains kept them going. In our own era, the space explorations of the 1950s and 1960s demanded faith, for, even if scientists could make some assumptions about the nature of space travel, they could not know with certainty what lay ahead for the astronauts. Imagine the faith required of Neil Armstrong to make his "one small step for man, one giant leap for mankind"!

But though this kind of faith has advanced the cause of humanity, and though it forms the basis for many accomplishments in life, it is overshadowed by the transcendent scope of religious faith. Even the excitement of discovering a new world cannot assure that human life has ultimate meaning. Even the greatest of human accomplishments do not defeat or delay the grave. For most of us, religious faith seems to offer the best access to the supreme meaning that gives purpose to our lives on earth and hope for a life in the world to come.

The Bible says that faith is "being sure of what we hope for, being certain of what we do not see" (Hebrews 11:1, NIV). By definition, faith is

181

not based on visible proof but, rather, on trusting the invisible. We act out that trust by making a commitment, stepping out in a direction. This action was characterized by Pascal as a "wager" and by Kierkegaard as a "leap." Cinematically, it was captured beautifully in *Indiana Jones and the Last Crusade,* where Indiana Jones, facing an abyss between himself and the Holy Grail, steps out in faith, and a bridge suddenly appears underneath his feet.

Our spiritual searching will ultimately lead us to a similar leaping-off point. How that leap is made—at what point in our lives, under what circumstances, and with what belief system as our safety net—will be determined by many factors unique to each person's personality, experience, and religious tradition. The choices we make may well have an impact on the faith factor's potency in our lives. Faith appears to be beneficial to health and well-being, but its efficacy in this regard will be determined in part by how we live out our faith commitments.

SPIRITUALITY OR RELIGION?

If your goal is to improve your health and well-being by activating the faith factor in your life, it's important to understand the similarities and differences between spirituality and religion. These are important distinctions in our era, when many people who are disillusioned by religious institutions or dogma have chosen to create a highly personal form of belief, often a smorgasbord of religious elements from various traditions which they define as their spirituality. Among believing people, some identify themselves as spiritual, some as religious; many are both. Because these distinctions have significance in the research on the faith factor's medical effects, scholars have worked hard to define the differences and the similarities between religion and spirituality. The concepts I share here are one effort to synthesize this work.

We might define religion as an organized system of beliefs, practices, and symbols designed to bring about closeness with God, and spirituality as a quest for answers to ultimate questions about life and meaning, which may or may not lead to the development of specific rituals and practices or the formation of community or religious doctrine. In short, spirituality poses questions; religion composes answers.

Concepts of spirituality and religion have much in common. Both address a "search for the sacred" and fundamental, eternal issues—issues about meaning, the use of our time, the nature of our relationships and our community with one another. Both acknowledge the transcendent, that which is outside of ourselves, and both offer methods for coping with suffering, meaninglessness, loss, and issues of guilt and shame. But whereas religion and spirituality often overlap, their differences are significant. Please note that these distinctions are tentative and not absolute, a series of proposed continuums.

Religion	*Spirituality*
More focused on establishing community.	More focused on individual growth.
More objective and measurable to the outside observer.	Less objective and measurable to the outside observer.
More formal in worship.	Less formal in worship.
More behavior-based, focused on outward practices.	More emotion-based, focused on inner experience.
More authoritarian, with patterns of prescribed and proscribed behavior.	Less authoritarian, with few prescriptions or proscriptions.
More particularizing, distinguishing one group from another.	More universalizing, discouraging separateness from others.
More orthodox and systematic in doctrine.	Less orthodox and systematic in doctrine.

For Jews and Christians, certain fundamental beliefs about the nature of God and human beings differentiate religious commitment from the kind of individualistic, nontraditional approach that some identify as "spiritual but not religious." For example, religion from the Judeo-Christian perspective implies belief in a Being greater than ourselves; this differs markedly from the idea of a divine potential of each human being, which, according to some philosophies, can be "actualized" through spiritual practices. Nor does Judeo-Christian tradition promote a view of God as merely a source of cosmic energy, which exists in and around all things and beings. The results of most of the studies we have looked at have evaluated the effect of religiosity of a traditional monotheistic (and largely Judeo-Christian) nature, in which:

• God is seen as a personal Being to whom we can relate as persons. We can, in various ways, listen to and speak with this God, who is portrayed in Judaism and Christianity as "Father," "Lord," and "King."

• Though we are made in the image of God, he is transcendent—far greater in every way than we can imagine, omniscient and omnipotent. Therefore, God is worthy of our praise, worship, and obedience. As C. S. Lewis writes in *Mere Christianity,*

> In God you come up against something which is immeasurably superior to yourself. Unless you know God as that—and therefore, know yourself as nothing in comparison—you do not know God at all.

• God is omnipresent, always with us, and actively involved in our lives as a loving parent with his children. We are to ask God to supply our needs, to thank him, and to trust him as the ultimate protector and provider.

• There is a moral code to be obeyed; the Ten Commandments of the Hebrew Bible form the cornerstone of this code. God has ordained rules and boundaries to guide the ways we live. These ways are certainly open to differing interpretations, but people of the great traditions all seek to know God's will and, insofar as they are able, to live by it.

• Though he seeks us continually and yearns for us to turn to him in loving obedience, God has given us free will, the ability to choose his ways (to obey) or to depart from them (to disobey). We are not automatons, or pawns being manipulated by some celestial puppeteer; God does act in our lives, but we can choose to follow him or to reject him.

These Judeo-Christian precepts form a particular religious structure that is distinctly different from a more generic, open-ended, and individualistic spirituality. This difference is important to note, because researchers have measured subjects' religious involvement or religiosity, rather than spirituality, in almost all the faith-factor studies. As mentioned earlier, religious involvement is much easier to measure than spirituality. For example, from the researcher's point of view, looking at the frequency of church attendance among patients is a simple, valid, and easily measurable variable that can be used to compare patients' religiosity. There is no such variable to apply among people who are spiritual but not religious. Their beliefs and practices tend to be idiosyncratic and to elude standardized measurement. For example, rather than going to church on Sunday morning, a person defining herself as spiritual might choose to meditate while walking on a beach, a solitary activity that could be construed as either spiritual or nonspiritual. Only the walker herself knows the intentions of her heart; the mere fact of her being present on the beach signals nothing about her intent. An observer could not be certain whether or not her Sunday-morning walk is a spiritual exercise. On the other hand, an observer who noticed a woman attending Friday-evening synagogue services faithfully every week could assume with some degree of certainty that she had religious purposes in mind. Though the woman going to synagogue may or may not be deeply religious, and though both women may have very similar spiritual outlooks and experiences, only one provides an easily measured, observable gesture of her religious intent.

As we have noted throughout this book, an overview of the research studies tracking the faith factor shows that religious involvement is good for your health. It does *not* show that spirituality without religious involvement provides the same benefits. This may be because the difficulty of measuring spirituality has led researchers to measure primarily religious activity, rather than personal spiritual practices. If spirituality could be measured more accurately, perhaps scientists would find that it offers health benefits similar to religious involvement. We will not know whether this is the case until the appropriate studies are designed and executed.

What's the best possible way to approach the religion/spirituality mix? Some scientific studies indicate that people who are spiritual within the framework of religiosity—those whose religious involvement is accompanied by an inwardly experienced and highly personal awareness of God—derive the greatest benefit from the faith factor. For example, in the study of patients undergoing open-heart surgery conducted by Thomas Oxman, M.D., which is described in more detail in chapter 1, regular churchgoers were three times more likely to survive the surgery than non–church attenders. But within the pool of churchgoers, thirty-seven of the patients described themselves as obtaining significant "strength and comfort" from religious practices, and all of these patients survived the six-month period. This indicates that a person's internal experience of relating to God is a valuable asset to health, beyond the benefits of worship attendance alone.

This result is perfectly compatible with the Biblical approach to living our faith. God asks us to undertake certain practices in order to be holy, but he asks for much more: He wants our whole hearts, our whole beings. In answer to the question "Which commandment is the first of all?" (Mark 12:28), Jesus summarizes Jewish teaching by saying:

> "The first is, 'Hear, O Israel: the Lord our God, the Lord is one; you shall love the Lord your God with all your heart, and with all your soul, and with all your mind, and with all your strength.' " [MARK 12:29–30.]

In the Judeo-Christian tradition, we can best aspire to answer this call by attempting to be both religious *and* spiritual. Attending worship services is a fundamental step in this quest, and, according to the faith-factor data, it is central to reaping the health benefits of religion.

WORSHIP-SERVICE ATTENDANCE: THE ONE KEY VARIABLE

As noted by epidemiologist Jeffrey Levin, frequency of worship-service attendance is the bellwether religious variable, the one that has been shown most often to have a pronounced impact on the health of patients in the studies. Why should this be so? Why can't we benefit equally from praying at home, or from worshiping God privately in the beauty of nature, the "church of the open skies"? Does it matter whether we worship in a pew or on a putting green on weekend mornings? I believe that frequent church attendance is a particularly valuable aid to health because when individuals participate in worship services they are exposed to every one of the faith factor's components, previously discussed in chapter 2:

Remedy No. 1: Equanimity—Overcoming the Wear and Tear of Life

Most worship services engender some of the faith factor's stress-buffering effect by providing time for silent prayer or meditation, which in turn may elicit the health-boosting Relaxation Response. Even if there is no opportunity for silent meditation in the worship service, stress is relieved as people take time out from the busyness of their frantic schedules and reconnect to their ultimate sense of meaning within a community setting (see Remedies 6 and 9, below). In my wife's Greek Orthodox tradition, attending the Divine Liturgy is literally considered "heaven on earth"—you are participating in the Sacred Mysteries, worshiping while surrounded by invisible angels and the "communion of saints," including the spirits of departed loved ones. The broader view of life provided by such a respite from daily stress helps us put our problems and worries into proper perspective.

Remedy No. 2: Temperance— *Honoring the Body as a Temple of the Spirit*

Church or synagogue services may include scriptural messages focusing on the importance of taking care of the body, thus shoring up our resolve to avoid unhealthful habits like smoking and to nurture healthy behaviors like exercise. We react to a positive form of peer pressure, refraining from habits like smoking, when we are in church. It seems, too, that the act of worship itself encourages us to focus on our bodies as temples of the Spirit. We dress up, or at the very least make sure we are neat, clean, and presentable, fit to come into the presence of the Lord. Many worshipers will don their "Sunday best" for church. In past years, when bathing was a weekly, rather than daily, occurrence, family members took their baths on Saturday night, so as to be clean for church on Sunday morning. By preparing our bodies in these ways, we honor God, and we remember that worship services are not the *only* time when our physical beings are profoundly connected to the Holy One. Thus, worship reinforces the need to care for ourselves lovingly and responsibly.

Remedy No. 3: Beauty— *Appreciating Art and Nature*

Entering a church or temple, we often find beauty in many forms. For example, in the great cathedrals of Europe, like Chartres or Notre Dame, one is overwhelmed by the majestic spires and arches, intricate stained-glass designs, and soaring worship spaces. We may be equally moved by the beauty of a rustic chapel or an outdoor worship space at a retreat center.

When worship includes music, as it frequently does, we encounter beauty aurally, too. Sacred music uses beauty in audible form to communicate God's splendor to us. The smell of incense or altar flowers, the poetry of liturgy, the taste of communion wine, the appearance of wall hangings, statues, and paintings stimulate each one of our sense organs, and may also evoke the deep sense of peace and meaning that comes from this contemplative appreciation of beauty in all its forms.

Remedy No. 4: Adoration—
Worshiping with Our Whole Beings

When we pray aloud, sing, chant, genuflect, kneel, stand, lift our arms in praise, or dance as part of our worship, we find inner harmony in worshiping God with our souls *and* bodies, a unifying experience that is as good for us as it feels. This effect holds true for quieter gestures, too; many people who pray contemplatively will use a prayer bench to support them in a semikneeling position for an hour or more. Simply turning the palms upward during prayer symbolizes our willingness to receive what God wants to say to us and give us through our communication with him.

Remedy No. 5: Renewal—
Confessing and Starting Over

In the three great Western religious traditions, confessing our sins to God, repenting, asking forgiveness, and receiving assurance of forgiveness form part of many liturgies. Unburdening ourselves of guilt, to God and to another, leads to intimacy with God and helps maintain community. After we confess our sins, we receive a "clean slate" and can leave worship with fewer burdens than we brought when we came in. We can let go of the burden of sin and start afresh, receiving a balm for the soul—and the body!

Remedy No. 6: Community—
Bearing One Another's Burdens

Community grows in the context of people gathering for worship on a regular basis. Coming together in worship is a strong foundation upon which supportive social networks can be built. The relationship between believers is symbolized in some Christian churches by the "passing of the

Peace" before Holy Communion. In this practice, the minister or priest turns to the congregation and says something like, "The peace of the Lord be always with you"; the congregation responds, "And also with you." Then the congregants turn to one another, to clasp hands or embrace and to wish one another peace. This ancient practice, restored to the eucharistic liturgy in recent decades, is an acting out of our connectedness to one another.

If we are connected, we will help each other in times of trouble. A simple and familiar example of such support is the common response when a family in the congregation loses a loved one—congregants bring food to the bereaved family's home and offer other practical and spiritual help. To know we are not alone in facing life's hardships gives us tremendous emotional support, which, in turn, is beneficial for our health.

Remedy No. 7: Unity—
Gaining Strength Through Shared Beliefs

Worship is a community's expression of the beliefs it holds sacred. We may feel isolated and unsupported in our religious beliefs during most of the week, but when we gather to worship, we find we are not alone, and we glean strength from the power of shared beliefs. This is particularly important in our era, with its growing isolation and fragmentation. Our culture, with its emphasis on "rugged individualism," has long held up heroes like those portrayed by John Wayne as the ideal. Though our ability to go it alone and to forge our own paths is important, we also need— even crave—connectedness with our fellow beings in terms of our most deeply held convictions.

Such connectedness does not always come easily, especially for men. Perhaps this is why the Promise Keepers movement has swept the nation in recent years. This ecumenical Christian program invites men of all denominations to come together in football stadiums and arenas for several days of prayer, worship, and small-group sharing. Over two million men have gathered for Promise Keepers weekends since the ministry's founding in 1991.

Programs like Promise Keepers can provide an additional (and intense) dose of unity, but many believers will experience this bracing remedy routinely in weekly worship, where focus on the transcendent helps us rise above differences between individuals.

Remedy No. 8: Ritual—
Taking Comfort in Familiar Activities

Ritual finds an ideal home in worship services, where ways of communicating with God are codified in various actions, postures, gestures, words, and songs. In rituals, we create patterns that are deeply ingrained in our minds; there is comfort in repeating the familiar, reassuring expressions of our faith. When a temple service opens with the Shema ("Hear, O Israel, the Lord our God, the Lord is One"), Jews who have heard this prayer every week of their lives find its repetition to be grounding and centering for worship. When a Catholic priest blesses the congregation and worshipers make the sign of the cross, as they have done thousands of times before, they literally embody the blessing and experience the peace it gives all the more deeply; its habitual nature makes the blessing *more,* not less, meaningful. Group recitation of prayer or creeds builds unity in the midst of ritual, combining the benefits of Remedies 7 and 8.

Remedy No. 9: Meaning—
Finding a Purpose in Life

Attendance at worship, where the story of our faith is regularly presented to us, shores up our spiritual sense of meaning and purpose. The stories of the heroes and heroines of faith become our stories. Our lives, in turn, become connected to the deepest meanings and mysteries of our faith. As we repeatedly celebrate the central significance of our existence through liturgy, we strengthen our convictions about our reasons for being. In worship, we are reminded of our highest ideals, such as love for God and love for humanity. We come to know ourselves as part of something much bigger than just ourselves, and therefore we know that our lives and actions have significance.

Remedy No. 10: Trust—
"Letting Go and Letting God"

By reminding us that God is all-powerful and loving, worship reinforces our ability to trust God and to relax our grip on the reins of our lives. It offers us the opportunity to pray for ourselves and to lift up our concerns for others, asking God to bless those we love and to help those who suffer. When I am worried about a particular situation, I look forward to weekly worship, because there I will have a formal opportunity to present the problem to God in the presence of others who share my beliefs and who worship alongside me. In some instances we may choose to inform fellow worshipers of our needs and ask them to pray for us as well. We can truly leave worship feeling that we have laid our burdens down, and that God will act for the good to help us resolve or deal with the problems in our lives.

Remedy No. 11: Transcendence— Connecting with Ultimate Hope

Again, through our liturgies we are reminded of the nature of God and strengthened in our connection to hope. As we take part in worship, the very act of praising God—and thus reflecting on his all-glorious nature— can help us rise above the grinding daily concerns that can keep us in the grasp of stress. When you come into a beautiful, sacred place and are surrounded by the sound of singing and prayers, when scripture is read aloud and an encouraging message is preached, you can be uplifted, as you remember and act out the truth of God's glory and his love for each of us. We connect with the past—the "communion of saints," the martyrs who gave their lives for the faith, our ancestors and loved ones who kept faith alive throughout the generations. We also connect with the future, to a day when "mourning and crying and pain will be no more" (Revelation 21:1–4).

Remedy No. 12: Love— Caring and Being Cared For

Love of God, love for our neighbors, and love for ourselves are central foci for worship in the Judeo-Christian tradition. When the Bible is read aloud in worship, we are likely to hear about some aspect of love; many great scriptural passages are flooded with images of love. When we pray, we express our love for God, acknowledge his love for us, and remember his charge to love others. And when we greet our fellow worshipers, we experience love in the context of religious community.

✢

Every one of the faith-factor remedies can also be experienced outside of worship, but it is rare to encounter them all in one place and in a relatively short period of time. Frequent church attendance delivers a highly concentrated, regular dose of these remedies. In fact, I can think of no other event, practice, or circumstance that can match church attendance in its efficiency as a "method of delivery" for the faith factor. No wonder, then, that frequency of church attendance has been found time and again to be such an important determinant in prevention of disease, recovery from illness, achievement of well-being, coping with stress, and prolonging of life.

EXTRINSIC VERSUS INTRINSIC: THE IMPORTANCE OF REALLY MEANING IT

Just showing up in church week after week seems to provide some health benefits, but a number of studies have pointed out the additional potency of an intrinsic faith orientation. How can you discern whether your orientation is extrinsic or intrinsic? In all probability, you already know your true motivations for participation in religious activities. If you feel you are simply "going through the motions," you may have an extrinsic orientation to faith. (It may also be true that you are going through what the saints and mystics call a "dry" period in your spiritual life, when signs of God's presence are rare or completely absent.) Extrinsic religiosity can result from lack of exposure to a more authentic form of spirituality, or it can be a result of an unwillingness (conscious or unconscious) to become more intimate with God. A desire for more satisfaction and meaning from spiritual activities will usually lead the seeker away from an extrinsic orientation and toward a closer relationship with God. In both the Hebrew Bible and the Christian New Testament, we are assured that God is yearning for a closer relationship with us, and that he will meet us if we seek him sincerely. God's promise to us is simply this: if we look for him, he will let us find him. There is, then, every reason to believe that an extrinsic religious orientation can be changed to an intrinsic one. Following the spiritual program outlined here will help extrinsics develop a deeper spirituality.

What if your spirituality is intrinsic in nature, but you still feel something is missing? I would like to discuss two different ways in which this dilemma might manifest itself.

"I'm Very Spiritual, But Church Is Not for Me"

I have spoken to many patients, particularly very idealistic and sensitive individuals, who say something like this: "I'm very spiritual, but I can't stand organized religion. Churches [or temples or mosques] are full of hypocrites; the people there are not really interested in God at all, but in their own selfish agendas. There's no way I could be a part of that."

I am always sad when I hear this, particularly because I know there is some truth in this statement. Yes, religious communities *do* harbor some hypocritical people. Yes, religious people *have* committed atrocities in the name of their creed. Yes, some clergy and other church leaders *have* abused their offices. To deeply faithful people, these realities are tragic. What could be worse than to hurt other human beings in the name of our loving God?

But just as it is untrue to deny the wrongdoing perpetrated by religious communities, it is also false to say that *all* of organized religion is worthless because of such wrongdoing. Even if you have been deeply hurt at the hands of organized religion, and I know many people who have been, the church where you experienced pain is not the only church available to you. I would urge anyone who feels he or she has been victimized by religious leaders or a religious community to seek healing. A part of that healing, I believe, should come from the church itself—perhaps a different congregation, denomination, or branch of the church, but definitely from within organized religion, under whose aegis the harm was done.

If your dislike of worship services stems more from a sense of boredom or apathy than from pain over past hurts, I would encourage you to try new churches or synagogues until you find one where you are being truly nurtured spiritually. A huge variety in terms of liturgical styles, congregational focus, clergy talents, and theological emphasis awaits you. Do not give up easily in your search for the right place, and remember that you may not discover the treasures of a given congregation until you have taken the risk of being a part of its life for some months.

If you do already consider yourself a spiritual person, there are treasures, including greatly enhanced benefits of the faith factor, waiting for you when you connect with the right congregation of worshipers.

"I'm Not Satisfied with My Church: I Want Something More"

In all likelihood, a person who makes this statement is poised on the threshold of further spiritual growth. The longing for *more* in the spiritual life usually signifies a greater desire for intimacy with God. This is good, of course, but the ways we can respond to such an urge differ, and offer different results.

Sometimes people will find themselves growing "stale" spiritually, and will conclude that they need to change churches or synagogues. This may in fact be the case, but the decision should not be made hastily. Rather, we should pray, talk with a pastor or spiritual director, and wait to see if the dryness we feel may actually be rooted in our interior life, and not in the life of the congregation. Making such a decision requires spiritual maturity, discernment, and assistance from our spiritual brothers and sisters. If we accede to the urge to "church-hop" too readily, we will never build a stable life within the community, and this will hamper our spiritual growth instead of aiding it.

✣

Wherever you may be today on your quest, I believe that you may find new spiritual riches by looking earnestly and honestly for God's presence and activity in your life, asking for guidance from representatives of your religious tradition, and listening for "the still, small voice within" that will guide you in the right path.

SOME PATTERNS OF SPIRITUAL GROWTH

In the stories of my patients recounted in this book, we have seen how a number of people grew spiritually when illness, addiction, or loss brought them face to face with a need to go deeper in their spiritual lives. In most cases, they did not consciously approach their quest as a deliberate spiritual program, but we can learn about some of the steps involved in deepening our relationship to God by looking at their experiences.

As the stories demonstrate, each individual's path to a more intimate relationship with God will be different. It is important to realize, too, that their stories do not end here. All of the patients we have met will continue their spiritual development throughout their lives. They, and we, can nurture that development by deciding upon the right steps to take at any given time. The possibilities are many, but I encourage my patients to focus on the three areas I will discuss in the following three chapters—prayer, scripture study, and participation in a religious community.

I have been privileged to witness actual conversions, like Tom's (chapter 5), in a number of my patients. Like other developments in the spiritual life, conversions can take many forms. Some people feel haunted, or even hunted, by God for years before they allow him to enter their lives. God seems to seek us out, yearning for us to respond to him in love, with our whole hearts. Conversion starts this intimate relationship with God, and it can come in many forms. It can happen gradually, as it did with Tom, requiring years of emotional and spiritual growth before faith can take root. Sometimes religious conversion means an abrupt turn away from an old way of life, and toward a life centered on God. Stories of conversion are as unique as fingerprints. But the common element to all these stories is that the individuals who underwent dramatic conversion were looking for God, or at least looking for ultimate meaning.

One notable fourth-century Christian had such an abrupt conversion. The young man who would become St. Anthony of Egypt, founder of a great monastery in the desert and father of the monastic tradition, was a churchgoer but apparently more of an "extrinsic" than an "intrinsic" person of faith. But one day in church, Anthony heard the story of the rich young man who asks Jesus how he can inherit eternal life. After learning that the rich young man was already following the commandments, Jesus said: "You lack one thing: go, sell what you own, and give the money to the poor, and you will have treasure in heaven; then come, follow me" (Mark 10:21).

Millions of people have heard this Gospel lesson read in church, yet few are moved, as Anthony was, actually to obey Jesus's words. He sold his goods and, with the exception of a provision for his sister, gave everything to the poor. Taking up a life of asceticism and complete devotion to God,

Anthony eventually felt led to go into the desert alone. He attracted a band of followers for whom he served as a spiritual guide. Anthony never intended to start a movement of any kind, but his life laid the foundation for the monasticism that would enrich Christianity in the centuries to come.

Sixteen hundred years later, such conversions continue to occur. My patient George, whom I told you about in chapter 5, became a Christian after his wife, Becky, had renewed her childhood faith. George was even more reluctant than Becky to give organized religion a second chance, and he dismissed most spirituality as "nice but not relevant to my life." But Becky's dramatic return to faith forced George to look once again at his relationship with God—"if there *is* a God," as he said at the time.

Becky and George talked for hours about God, George trying to understand what had happened to his wife of twenty years after her recommitment to God took place.

"What happened to you? You're totally changed," he asked, puzzled. "I don't understand how one weekend retreat could make this kind of a difference!"

Though Becky tried her best to explain what had happened, George could not grasp it. For some time, he remained skeptical and a little hostile.

"I almost felt like I was competing with God for my wife's attention," he said. "It scared me to think that I was losing her to him! She told me she still loved me, but I knew things were different—she was radiant, and it wasn't because of me."

One night, as he worked the four-to-twelve shift at the hospital laboratory, George was particularly troubled by all of this. Taking a cigarette break, he walked outside to the hospital courtyard. It was getting late, and this semirural hospital was quiet; no patients were coming or going, and George was the only person around. Preoccupied, he gazed absently at the hospital's entrance doors, which opened and closed automatically when triggered by an approaching person, and he prayed a strange but honest prayer:

"Okay, God, if there *is* a God. If you're really there, you've got to give me a sign."

As George stood puffing on his cigarette, the sign came: the hospital doors slid open, though there was no one around to trigger the electronic eye. Even today, three years later, George gets tears in his eyes when he talks about this experience.

"There's no way that door would have opened on its own," he said. "I'd never seen that happen before, and I've never seen it happen since. I *knew* God was responding to my demand for a sign. I started praying right then and there!"

Since there were no other eyewitnesses to this event, we cannot determine if there are alternative explanations to account for the door's mysterious opening. But whatever the cause, no one who knows George can deny the importance this "sign" has held for him. He began to attend church regularly with Becky and their children. He, too, sought counseling from their minister, and went on a weekend retreat like the one that had made such an enormous difference in Becky's faith life. Today, George has joined Becky in ministry; together they lead the youth group in their church. He also helps coordinate retreat weekends, transporting and delivering crates of hymn books, prayer books, and other supplies to retreat facilities throughout the state.

"My entire life has changed a hundred percent since those doors opened," George said. "I *know* God is real, and that he loves me. I have a joy and peace I never had before. The only way I can say 'thank you' is to do whatever I can to serve him."

Whether it is gradual, like Tom's, or it starts with a bang, as it did with George, conversion is a process that continues throughout our lives. As I have learned, our relationship with God will not remain the same; like any important relationship, it will change and grow over time. Wherever you are spiritually today, I hope that your ongoing process of spiritual growth will be helped by this book. In the next three chapters, I will discuss three essential components of a spiritual program designed to support your faith development and help you enjoy more of the faith factor's benefits. We will start with prayer, the mundane yet mystical activity in which we communicate with God.

CHAPTER 9

✠

Prayer:
Conversation with God

Bright Tibetan Buddhist prayer flags flutter in the wind. Votive candles burn and flicker on an iron rack in an ancient Greek Orthodox cathedral. Hasidic Jews pray earnestly, rocking back and forth, at the Wailing Wall in Jerusalem. Five times a day, Muslims around the world answer the call to prayer, facing toward Mecca, their spiritual home. And in countless homes, faithful people pray together before meals in a custom we have come to call "saying grace."

Indeed, prayer in all its forms is a way of articulating grace in our lives, the God-given grace that merits acknowledgment and thanksgiving. But, most simply defined, prayer is our vehicle for communication with God. Theologian Peter Kreeft has called prayer "the great conversation," and indeed it is, for human beings, the transcendent form of communication.

For most people, prayer seems to come naturally. A poll commissioned by *Newsweek* in 1996 found that 54 percent of Americans pray daily, with 29 percent reporting that they pray more than once a day. Even people who aren't sure they believe in God will find themselves praying "just in case," or simply crying out "Oh, God!" in times of distress. We pray in our cars and in the shower, at the doctor's office and in the still of the night when we can't sleep. Unhampered by intellectual doubts, many small children will pray spontaneously, needing little in the way of explanation in order to talk to God.

As we have seen in the preceding chapters, prayer can have a significant impact on health. Basically, this effect has been studied in two ways:

1. *Measuring the effect of intercessory prayer—prayer undertaken on behalf of others.*

2. *Measuring the physical and mental health, well-being, and coping levels of individuals who themselves pray regularly.*

Before addressing the role of prayer in our spiritual programs, let us review what scientists have learned about intercessory prayer.

PRAYING FOR HEALING: A HEALTH-ENHANCING GIFT

The most famous and provocative scientific prayer study to date was conducted by Randolph Byrd, M.D., and published in 1988. To measure clinically the effects of intercessory prayer, Dr. Byrd carefully designed his study. In the coronary-care unit of the San Francisco General Hospital, 393 patients were randomly assigned to two groups. One group of 192 patients was prayed for by outside intercessors ("born-again" Christians from around the country), who were informed of the patients' names and clinical status and who committed to pray regularly for each patient until the patient's discharge. The second group of 201 patients, the control group, did not receive this experimental prayer, in order to provide a basis for comparison for the prayed-for group. All patients in the study knew they were participating in a study of prayer, but no patient knew to which group he or she had been assigned. Only the research nurse administering the study knew which patients were in which group; the doctors and nurses providing care had no such knowledge, so the study met the rigorous scientific criteria of double-blind, placebo-controlled clinical trials, the customary benchmark for testing new medicines and procedures. Both groups received standard medical care.

During the course of the patients' hospitalization, Dr. Byrd measured multiple clinical variables and complications of illness, including the numbers of patients who developed congestive heart failure, cardiopulmonary arrest, and pneumonia; the use of diuretic and antibiotic medications; and the use of intubation and mechanical ventilation to assist patients with respiratory failure. The presence of higher numbers of variables indicated more severe illness and/or complications; the absence of such variables indicated that the patient had a successful and uneventful recovery. The findings were statistically significant: patients in the control group were nearly twice as likely to suffer complications than were patients in the prayer group (27 percent as opposed to 15 percent).

The Byrd Intercessory Prayer Study

	Prayed-For Patients (n = 192)	Control-Group Patients (n = 201)
Episodes of congestive heart failure	8 (4%)	20 (10%)
Use of diuretics	5 (3%)	15 (7%)
Episodes of cardiopulmonary arrest	3 (2%)	14 (7%)
Episodes of pneumonia	3 (2%)	13 (7%)
Use of antibiotics	3 (2%)	17 (9%)
Intubation required	0 (0%)	12 (6%)

Is this study perfect? No—but, then again, no study is. How might we critique Byrd's study? We know nothing about the psychological status and spiritual beliefs and practices of the two groups before the study began. Since patients were randomly assigned to the groups, one may reasonably assume that the groups were similar after the randomization process with regard to these characteristics. But a confirmation of their similarity on these points would have been helpful in ensuring that the results did not simply reflect that the prayed-for group may have had greater belief in the power of prayer or greater devotion in their personal prayers for their own health. We also lack information about the amount, duration, or style of prayer practice among the outside intercessors.

To date, there are very few comparable studies of the effects of intercessory prayer; the Byrd study stands out because of its scientifically valid design and significant results. A 1969 study of intercessory prayer looked at life expectancy in eighteen children with leukemia. Eighteen is too low a number of subjects from which to draw reliable, statistically valid, and generalizable results, and the authors provided insufficient data on the clinical status of the patients before and after the prayer intervention, but this study also offered a tantalizing hint of prayer's possible effectiveness. Ten of the children were prayed for daily for fifteen months by prayer groups at a Protestant church in Washington; the eight children in the control group did not receive experimental prayer. At the end of the study period, seven of the ten prayed-for children were still alive, and only two of the eight children in the control group had survived—a 70-percent survival rate among prayed-for patients versus 25 percent among those who were not prayed for. Had similar results been found in a larger, more carefully documented study, the findings would have much greater scientific validity.

In addition to "distant" or "long-distance" prayer, studies have also shown the positive value of in-person intercessory prayer. For example, the practice of the laying on of hands, most frequently used today by Christians, has proved beneficial in helping people quit smoking, as discussed in chapter 1. But is the laying on of hands more or less effective than intercessory prayer at a distance? A Dutch study of people with hypertension evaluated these two types of intercessory prayer. Individuals with a systolic blood pressure of 140 millimeters of mercury (mm Hg) or higher, or a diastolic pressure of 90 mm Hg or higher, or both, were selected for the study. They continued taking medications prescribed by their doctors and following doctor-recommended diets during the course of the study. Two groups of forty patients each received different prayer "therapies:"

1. The laying on of hands was performed once weekly for fifteen weeks by healers trained in this procedure. (The study does not specify the faith background of the healers.)

2. "Positive intentions"—thoughts aimed to evoke healing—were directed at patients from trained healers in a room next to the experimental laboratory.

A third group of forty patients formed the control group; they received no prayer therapy. Blood pressure was lowered in all three groups to a similar degree, but the group that received laying on of hands reported a significantly greater sense of well-being than the patients in the other two groups. A greater sense of well-being is certainly a worthwhile outcome. The link between the laying on of hands and well-being in this study points to the importance of touch for human beings. Perhaps one day researchers will prove conclusively that adults need caring touch in order to get and stay well, just as babies cannot thrive without being held and cuddled.

No one knows how intercessory prayer "works." Is it a form of unseen energy, like electricity or radio waves, that has not yet been characterized? Are certain individuals better "transmitters" or "receivers" of healing messages? Are certain types of prayer more effective than others? In his book, *Healing Words,* Dr. Larry Dossey has written extensively about the possible mechanisms of prayer. Incorporating new models from the field of quantum physics, he proposes that intercessory prayer is "nonlocal"—i.e., a manifestation of the essential unity of human and divine consciousness that is not limited by space and time. Extrapolating from plant and animal studies, he proposes that certain types of prayer (for example, "nondirected" prayers like "May the best possible outcome prevail") may be more effective than others. Regardless of *how* it works and how best to test it, Dr. Dossey and I agree wholeheartedly that the effects of intercessory prayer are important and worthy of continued study.

I designed the Clearwater study of the effects of intercessory prayer on rheumatoid arthritis to expand our understanding in what I hope will be a significant way, and other researchers are working on similar studies. Perhaps by the new millennium, we will have more answers about the actual mechanisms of prayer in making people better.

REAPING THE BENEFITS OF HEALING PRAYER

Naturally, your approach to intercessory prayer will be guided by beliefs, experiences, and your faith tradition, and I would urge you to seek counsel from a clergy person or some other spiritual authority. I can, however, provide for your consideration some basic guidelines on how to incorporate the apparent benefits of intercessory prayer into your life.

1. *If you are sick, ask specifically for people's prayers for healing.* If you are sick or suffering in any way, I recommend that you ask others to pray for you. Many people find it particularly comforting to have their clergy visit and pray with them. A study of women with breast cancer demonstrated this clearly: among 103 members of breast-cancer support groups, who were members of various faiths, 93–98 percent of the women were highly satisfied with home and hospital visits from ministers and rabbis. The patients particularly valued clergy visits that included prayer, counseling, talking about the patients' families, and reading of the Bible.

If you are a member of a church or synagogue, you may be able to add your name to a prayer list or "prayer chain," which members use to pray for those in need. Even if you are not a member—and even if you're not at all religious—most congregations will happily add you to a prayer list if you ask for their help. Usually a church or synagogue secretary can add your name to the prayer list or pass it along to a clergy person or another prayer minister, so a simple phone call will suffice. It does not appear to be necessary for people to know you personally in order to pray for you effectively; the patients in the Byrd study never met the intercessors who prayed for them, but the prayer appeared to make a difference in the patients' health.

Also, ask your family and friends to pray for you; even those who are not overtly religious may be perfectly willing to say a prayer for you on a regular basis.

2. *Pray for your own healing.* Sometimes people will tell me that they feel uncomfortable asking God to make them better. My patient Monica, a devout older woman with fibromyalgia, a painful, debilitating rheumatic disorder, was in this camp. Retired from a career as a medical secretary, Monica spent at least an hour each day praying for people in her congregation who were on the prayer list, and she had strong convictions about the propriety of certain kinds of prayer.

"Dr. Matthews, I feel it is somehow disloyal to ask God to heal me," she told me. "It is all right for *you* to ask him on my behalf, but I cannot. You see, I believe he knows what I need, and that if he believes that I need this illness, I should simply ask him for the strength to endure it."

Knowing Monica's profound love for her children, and knowing that we shared similar Christian beliefs, I drew on one of Jesus's parables to help her explore this issue.

"Monica, when your children were little, if they asked you for a piece of candy, would you give them some broccoli?" I queried.

"Certainly not!" she retorted.

"And if they asked for a toy, would you give them a lecture?" I continued.

"What are you getting at, Doctor?" she asked, with a puzzled look.

"May I read you a passage from the Bible, Monica, to illustrate my point?" I asked. When she nodded, I read from the Gospel of Luke:

" 'Is there anyone among you who, if your child asks for a fish, will give a snake instead of a fish? Or if the child asks for an egg, will give a scorpion? If you then, who are evil, know how to give good gifts to your children, how much more will the heavenly Father give the Holy Spirit to those who ask him?' " [LUKE 11:11–13.]

"Monica, I believe God wants to give us good gifts," I told her, "just as you wanted to give your children wonderful things when they were little, and relieve them of any pain or discomfort. And I believe the Bible tells us to ask for what we need from our Heavenly Father. Would you consider studying some Bible verses on this?"

"Yes," she said. "I guess I didn't want to admit that I need God's help—I wanted to 'tough it out' on my own. It's hard for me to ask for help, from people *or* from God. Maybe it's a type of pride—spiritual pride."

"I understand that," I said, "but the Lord invites us to turn to him with all our troubles. He wants us to depend on him for everything. And scientists are showing that people who pray for themselves when they are ill cope better than those who don't. So, from the Biblical *and* the medical points of view, I hope you will decide to pray for your own recovery."

"I'll give it a whirl, Doctor," Monica said. She left the office with a prescription for medication and a list of Bible passages. At her next office visit, she told me that both prescriptions were helping. The anti-inflammatory medication had eased her pain and stiffness. The Bible verses had opened up new possibilities for prayer.

"I never realized just how often the Bible tells us to pray for everything we need," she marveled. "My upbringing trained me to grin and bear it, no matter how hard things were, so I thought that's what God wanted me to do, too—to just be a good girl and keep a stiff upper lip. It turns out all along I could have been saying, 'Okay, God, you know I need your help with this!' "

We laughed together that day, and closed our session with a prayer of thanksgiving. Like most patients with fibromyalgia, Monica has had many ups and downs with her illness, suffering exhaustion and extreme muscle pain for weeks or even months at a time, then enjoying a brief remission. Though there is no known cure for fibromyalgia, she has found that praying for her recovery gives her a more hopeful attitude and a greater sense of closeness to God.

"Now that I know that God wants me to ask him for the things I need, I find that I like him a lot better! Well, that may be an inappropriate way to speak of the Almighty," she said, quickly resuming her normal attitude of formality and propriety. "Of course, I *love* God, but now I feel more like he's my friend."

3. *Seek out healing services.* Many Christian churches offer opportunities to receive prayer for healing, but the nature and format of these opportunities vary widely. Some television evangelists and revivalists have raised a great deal of skepticism through their practices of healing, particularly because these theatrical and sometimes frightening-looking healing services are often accompanied by pleas for money. The very phrase "healing service" brings to mind for many the movie *Leap of Faith,* in which Steve Martin plays a revival preacher who literally stages phony healings in order to "rake in the dough" from unsuspecting sufferers. Also, many faith healers have undermined their own credibility by making extravagant claims for their healing ministries which are not borne out by visible or lasting results.

Some self-proclaimed preachers and healers do exploit believers' desires for healing, but most healing services bear absolutely no resemblance to this popular media image. For example, healing services at the Washington National Cathedral follow a structured Episcopal liturgy, including celebration of Holy Communion. Participants who wish to receive prayer for healing kneel at the altar rail; the priest or lay minister lays hands on each person's head and prays silently for his or her healing. The service is calm, formal, and devoid of requests for contributions. In other church healing services, prayer for healing may involve two or more prayer ministers

working with each supplicant, and they are likely to pray aloud, in a colloquial style, with specific requests for God's healing touch in the person's
life. Such services are characterized by an atmosphere of love and peace,
not melodrama.

If you are a church member, consult your clergy person about the possibility of participating in healing services. If there are no healing services
at your church, ask your pastor or other church members for information
about healing services in other parishes. Because the laying on of hands is
modeled on the healing ministry of Jesus and his disciples, and because
the scientific literature reports that patients find it effective, I recommend
participating in a service or healing-prayer group where this ancient practice is used. You may also wish to consult a national healing ministry, such
as Christian Healing Ministries, the organization providing prayer teams
for the Clearwater Rheumatoid Arthritis Study. (See the list of resources
at the end of this book for more information.)

Some Jewish congregations are now offering healing services. Consult
your rabbi, or call the National Center for Jewish Healing (see Resources),
to learn if such services are offered in your area.

4. *Pray persistently.* Judith and Francis MacNutt of Christian Healing
Ministries advocate an approach to healing prayer known as "soaking
prayer." They believe it is important to pray, and to lay on hands, for
more than just a moment or two. For the patients in the Clearwater
study, the prayer-team members conducted "hands-on prayer" for an
hour or more at a time, with two or more prayer sessions per day. Even if
you are not devoting large amounts of time to praying for yourself, do
keep praying until you are better. Most leaders in the healing-prayer
movement are quick to say that God doesn't always heal instantly; healing may happen through faithful prayer over days, weeks, months, or
even years.

When we keep praying regardless of apparent results, we express our
faith in God's goodness. I believe that this is important theologically *and*
psychologically. The Bible gives us many examples of persistent prayer,
including Moses, who prayed continually for the people of Israel as he led
them on a forty-year journey out of slavery in Egypt to the Promised
Land, and the prophetess Anna, who for many years "never left the temple but worshiped there with fasting and prayer night and day" (Luke

2:37), and who praised God when the Child Jesus was brought to the temple for his presentation. In his first letter to the Thessalonians, the apostle Paul urges them to "pray without ceasing" (1 Thessalonians 5:17). Centuries later, a Russian peasant wanted to discover what this instruction really meant; he set out on foot, without possessions, on a pilgrimage of prayer, attempting to pray continually. His book, *The Way of a Pilgrim,* introduces a form of prayer known as Hesychasm, or prayer of the heart. In the pilgrim's case, he prayed constantly a prayer known as the Jesus prayer: "Lord Jesus Christ, Son of the living God, have mercy on me, a sinner." According to the anonymous pilgrim, when one repeats this prayer consciously as often as possible over a long period of time, it becomes part of the body's rhythm, aligning itself with the heartbeat—thus literally becoming a prayer of the heart, a mystical response to the mysterious, seemingly impossible injunction to "pray without ceasing."

Whatever form our persistent prayer takes, when we pray continually, we benefit emotionally by reminding ourselves that we can and do count on God to help us and to heal us. Our continuing prayer is an expression of our faith and our hope, and that is good for our relationship with God *and* for our morale.

5. *Pray for others who are suffering.* Since I have studied and witnessed personally the scientifically documented power of prayer in improving health, I take intercessory prayer very seriously. On request, I pray for my patients—with them or in private, according to their preference. I pray also for any special needs of my family members, and for friends and colleagues who are in need. Unlike my patient Monica, I do not spend an hour or more in intercessory prayer every day. I use a form of prayer known as "arrow prayers," quickly "shooting up" brief prayers for others to God when the opportunity arises. For my patients, this may be in the examining room, or between appointments or rounds in the hospitals. For my family and friends, I frequently pray while driving to and from the hospital, or while doing chores at home like mowing the grass.

If you have not already done so, you will find your own times—even in the busiest of schedules—for brief but heartfelt prayers on behalf of others. A friend told me recently that her intercessory prayer consists of an adapted version of the ancient Jesus prayer; my friend prays, "Lord Jesus Christ, have mercy on Fred and relieve his suffering."

When your schedule permits, however, you might try longer prayers of intercession, praying at length for all your concerns about each person on your prayer list. You might also dedicate times of meditative prayer to the well-being of someone in need, perhaps accompanied by fasting. Some Christians in sacramental traditions will silently dedicate their participation in the Eucharist on behalf of another who cannot take part in the sacrament.

You will find a great deal of guidance in praying for healing within the Bible's pages (please see chapter 10 for an extended discussion of Biblical accounts of healing). Whatever your approach, I hope you will pray for others, because they may benefit from your prayers, and you may, too, as you observe how God responds to your intercessions. Often, I believe, you will see your prayers answered. You will have a real cause for thanksgiving, *and* your faith in God will grow. When you pray for people you know personally, you may also find that you come to care more deeply for them; as the eighteenth-century Anglican mystic William Law wrote, "There is nothing that makes us love a person so much as praying for him."

STYLES OF PRAYER

As we have seen, praying for others, and receiving others' prayers, may help us recover from illness faster and cope with sickness more effectively. In some cases, complete recoveries may follow prayers for healing. We cannot know, or control, the outcome of our prayers for healing, any more than we can know in advance how our medical, surgical, or psychiatric therapies will work, but we do know—from the scientific data—that such prayers often make a positive difference in the lives of patients.

But there is another way in which prayer affects health, and that is as a mechanism for deepening our relationship with God. As we have discussed previously, people with an intrinsic, or deeply felt and personally authentic, faith orientation do better medically than those with an extrinsic orientation. To cultivate an intrinsic orientation, or to continue to walk on the path towards intrinsic religiosity, we must develop a regular habit of prayer. Just as you cannot expect to have a good marriage, a close friendship, or a loving relationship with your children unless you communicate with them regularly and sincerely, you cannot grow in knowledge and love of God without devoting time frequently to speaking with—and listening to—him.

In chapter 6, I mentioned sociologist Margaret Poloma's research on the effect of different types of prayer on well-being. Given Dr. Poloma's findings, I will concentrate on the two types of prayer that she has found to produce greater happiness and well-being: colloquial prayer and meditative prayer.

Colloquial Prayer

People who pray colloquially, says Margaret Poloma, report greater happiness than those who pray more formally or meditatively. By "colloquial," we mean an informal, honest, self-revealing kind of prayer that we "make up as we go along," just as we do in conversations with people who are close to us. Our manner of addressing God reflects how we feel about him, and colloquial prayer presupposes an intimacy with God that may not be present for people who need to follow a written format or ritual pattern when they pray.

Praying colloquially allows us to talk over the events of our lives, our feelings, and our desires with God, much as we would with a spouse or trusted friend. If you have been raised in a more formal liturgical tradition, this may seem awkward to you at first, but I hope you will try it. I like to pray colloquially because I feel a greater sense of familiarity and friendship with God when I communicate this way. I don't need to "dress things up" for him; he already knows me through and through.

If you find praying colloquially to be awkward at first, I encourage you to consider a slightly different approach. Write God a letter—a spontaneous, truthful letter in your usual style, simply telling him how you feel about what's going on in your life. Thank him for the good things and ask for his help with the difficult things. Tell him honestly how you feel about him, even if you're angry or alienated. As Martin, my patient with AIDS who was profiled in chapter 7, learned, "God's a big guy—he can take it!"

Sometimes writing can help us get past the embarrassment we feel when speaking, either in our minds or aloud, to God informally. A letter written to God on a regular basis may become a prayer journal, a wonderful resource that will help you see how your relationship with him is developing.

Many people find that joining a prayer group helps their prayer life grow exponentially, and this is certainly true for people who pray colloquially aloud together. In my experience, the most effective prayer groups are small, with perhaps five to seven members who agree on the group's purpose, schedule, and prayer method. I also recommend finding a group in which confidentiality is a ground rule, so that members feel free truly to open up to one another. Meeting with a prayer group weekly can be a tremendous boost to spiritual growth. Hearing others' prayers gives us insight into how they relate to God. Being prayed for is also beneficial, and close supportive relationships often spring up between prayer-group members. At first, you may feel shy, but I encourage you to overcome your hesitation and to try this wonderful aid to faith.

Colloquial prayer expresses an intimacy with God and a continual confession of our need of and love for him. But there is another aspect to our relating to God. Though he is the loving shepherd who tends his sheep, he is also a transcendent mystery, not fully knowable to mortals. This reality engenders the need for a different approach to prayer.

Meditative Prayer

Margaret Poloma's research on well-being and types of prayer revealed that people who prayed meditatively enjoyed an increased sense of existential well-being. They felt more secure about their reason for being; they were more likely to feel they understood their place in the world and in the world to come. In our time, when perceptions of meaninglessness and randomness pervade the culture, having a high degree of existential well-being is a tremendous advantage to your mental and physical health.

In meditative prayer, we focus on listening to God, on perceiving his movements within us and within our lives. We await the "still small voice within" so valued by the Quakers and others in contemplative traditions. To listen to God's voice, we must enter into silence. Whereas colloquial prayer consists primarily of talking to God, meditative prayer consists primarily of listening to him. Meditative prayer can also include or grow out of adoration, one of the five primary purposes of prayer outlined below, as we consider God's attributes as revealed to us in scripture.

Meditative, or contemplative, prayer exists in all the great religious traditions of the world; it has been and continues to be practiced by all the great mystics. But it is not easy to find its adherents in the pews of your church or synagogue. You might say meditative prayer is a minority approach; few people seem to have the patience for twenty to thirty minutes of silent stillness every day. But those who *do* learn to "be still and know that I am God" (Psalm 46:10) reap tremendous benefits, spiritually and in terms of health. When practiced according to certain guidelines, meditative prayer will evoke the Relaxation Response we discussed in chapter 2, putting the pray-er into a state of deep relaxation which aids the body and the mind. Here, from Dr. Herbert Benson's book, *Timeless Healing,* are the steps he recommends for evoking the Relaxation Response:

Step 1. Pick a focus word or short phrase that's firmly rooted in your belief system.

Step 2. Sit quietly in a comfortable position.

Step 3. Close your eyes.

Step 4. Relax your muscles.

Step 5. Breathe slowly and naturally, and as you do, repeat your focus word, phrase, or prayer silently to yourself as you exhale.

Step 6. Assume a passive attitude. Don't worry about how well you're doing. When other thoughts come to mind, simply say to yourself, "Oh, well," and gently return to the repetition.

Step 7. Continue for ten to twenty minutes.

Step 8. Do not stand immediately. Continue sitting quietly for a minute or so, allowing other thoughts to return. Then open your eyes and sit for another minute before rising.

Step 9. Practice this technique once or twice daily.

This technique can easily be made into meditative prayer by choosing a religiously significant word or phrase as your focus point. For example, Christians might choose "Jesus" or "Hail Mary," or Jews might choose "Shalom" or the Shema. Your prayer word or phrase may be uniquely yours, significant for reasons only you understand, and it may change from time to time just as your relationship with God will change.

The primary difficulty with meditative prayer comes in the form of distractions. By recommending a passive attitude toward distractions, Dr. Benson echoes the advice of many great spiritual teachers; if we react to distractions by getting irritated with ourselves, we will only make matters worse. Accept distractions as part of the reality of meditative prayer. You are not alone: people who have engaged in contemplative prayer daily for many years still experience distractions. Even a spiritual giant like the seventeenth-century Anglican priest and poet John Donne struggled with them:

> I throw myself down in my chamber, and I call in, and invite God, and his Angels thither, and when they are there, I neglect God and his Angels, for the noise of a fly, for the rattling of a coach, for the whining of a door.

Because it is so easy to give up in the face of multiple distractions, try to continue your meditative prayer practice daily *no matter what* the results may appear to be. It usually takes a few weeks—and some faith!—before you begin to see the benefits, among which may be a calmer and more centered approach to life, lessened anxiety, easier sleep, greater energy—not to mention the most important benefit, an increased sense of intimacy with God.

There are many excellent books on contemplative prayer, and you may find it helpful to join a prayer group led by an experienced instructor. More and more churches and other religious organizations are offering such groups today; consult with your clergy person or with one of the organizations in the resource list at the back of this book for possible referrals to a meditative-prayer group. Some leaders will offer *guided meditations,* in which participants are asked to follow their own inner images at the prompting of the leader. This is the kind of prayer Martin (in chapter 7) took part in when he encountered Jesus at the well of tears in his prayer experience.

If you find yourself drawn to contemplative prayer, you might consider "going on vacation with God" by making a *retreat.* There are many retreat houses throughout the United States where you can go for a day, a week, or longer, to experience real quiet and to be in an atmosphere that is supportive of prayer and meditation. Most retreat facilities offer such opportunities to individual retreatants; many also offer programs for groups that focus on contemplative prayer or scripture study. Often, retreat houses are located in beautiful environments—the mountains, the seashore, or by a river—and many will provide a room, three meals, and access to a library and chapel for a surprisingly small amount of money. Retreats provide a wonderful opportunity for a time-out in our busy lives, a time when we can truly listen for God's voice speaking to us from deep within. In making a retreat, we follow the Biblical examples of Moses, Elijah, Jesus, and Paul, who, at critical junctures in their lives and in preparation for ministry, withdrew to quiet places so they could pray, fast, and discern God's will for them.

Engaging in the ancient practice of *spiritual direction* can also help your prayer life grow. In every faith tradition, wise spiritual leaders have taught disciples who were less experienced in the faith; spiritual direction, or, as it is more frequently known today, spiritual guidance or friendship, formalizes such a relationship. Growing from the Christian Desert tradition of the third and fourth centuries, spiritual direction was long a staple of the Christian spiritual life but fell into disuse, except among Roman Catholic priests, monks, and nuns, until approximately twenty-five years ago, when a revival of this wonderful practice began to take root.

Contemporary spiritual directors do not so much *direct* someone who comes to them as they *listen with the person to discern God's movements in his or her life.* The director may offer advice, such as a book to read, a retreat to take advantage of, a prayer practice to try; he or she may hold the "directee" accountable to a discipline the two had agreed upon. But the practice as it is most widely undertaken today is more like a spiritual companionship or mentoring than an authoritarian relationship of director and directee. Usually, people see their spiritual directors on a monthly basis for about an hour. It is important to choose the right person as your spiritual director or guide, and there are a number of good books on this subject to help you do so (see Resources for several suggested titles).

Whether you choose to pray colloquially or meditatively—and I hope you will do both—it's most important simply to pray regularly, both in worship settings and on your own, just as you are, not worrying too much about whether you're "doing it right."

FIVE PURPOSES OF PRAYER

Theologians and saints have used hundreds of terms to describe types of prayer, but we can understand our most common reasons for praying simply by defining five main purposes for prayer, well known in all three of the great Western religious traditions. A well-balanced, complete prayer life will include prayers that serve each of these five purposes.

Praise and Adoration: Responding to the Glory and Grandeur of God

> One thing I asked of the Lord,
> that I will seek after:
> to live in the house of the Lord
> all the days of my life,
> to behold the beauty of the Lord,
> and to inquire in his temple.
> [PSALM 27:4.]

When we examine the evidence left to us by ancient cultures, we see that people have always praised the being (or beings) they perceived to be divine. For the person who loves God, praise is uplifting and joyful, drawing us closer to the Divine Lover and defining our relationship with him. It is because adoration is so important to our well-being that I named it Remedy No. 4 of the twelve remedies that make up the faith factor. Praising God is particularly beneficial to human beings when we include our whole beings—body, mind, and spirit—by using music and movement as well as words in our worship.

In the Judeo-Christian tradition, praising God with words and music forms the basis for many of the Bible's Psalms. The Book of Psalms, often referred to as "the prayer book of the Bible," contains songs composed expressly for worship, and many are accompanied by musical directions. Contemporary worshipers may choose from thousands of hymns, chants, and songs; they may also choose among worship styles, from highly formal liturgies to celebrations including jazz, rock-and-roll, or gospel music. Liturgical dance has also become popular among some congregations, offering participants an opportunity to move their bodies joyfully in worship, as David did when he "danced before the Lord" (2 Samuel 6:14).

Religious art, too, is often inspired by adoration. In the Eastern Orthodox branch of Christianity, the making of icons, or paintings of religious figures or scenes, is often undertaken only after days of prayer and fasting; the artist may dedicate himself or herself wholly to the task of contemplating God's glory and being a vehicle for that glory through the act of painting, which is also known as "icon writing."

My patient Susan, a middle-aged woman suffering from depression and chronic fatigue syndrome, makes adoration part of her daily prayer time. From there, she enters a meditative state in which she experiences God's presence. This practice came naturally to her, she believes, because of her religious upbringing.

"I was born a Quaker, and so 'Be still and know that I am God' is in my roots," she told me, when I asked her about her prayer practice. "Even in a praise-and-worship service, after the first few songs I get very quiet and go into a presence. I can't clap or dance or speak or sing in that. It's just personal and very special, just the silence and awe of it all."

Starting with active praise in the form of songs, Susan taps into "the peace which passes all understanding," becoming quiet and centered as she contemplates God's grandeur.

I recommend reciting one of the praise-centered Psalms (for example, Psalms 100 and 150), or singing a favorite hymn, as a satisfying way to adore and praise God. I recommend it, not only because it makes us feel better, but because I believe that God deserves our adoration. When we focus on the greatness of God, we remember that we can trust this merciful, generous Lord. Fortunately, that mental focus is also good for our health.

Thanksgiving:
Acknowledging the Giver of All Good Gifts

> O give thanks to the Lord, for he is good,
> for his steadfast love endures forever.
> O give thanks to the God of gods,

for his steadfast love endures forever.
O give thanks to the Lord of lords,
for his steadfast love endures forever. . . .
[PSALM 136:1–3.]

It is easy to confuse adoration and thanksgiving, but they are different, though certainly related to one another. Adoration might be likened to the feeling lovers have for one another as they gaze into each other's eyes, or the emotion that overcomes a parent when a newborn is placed in his or her arms. Thanksgiving is a conscious recounting of the blessings God has given us, and a deliberate act of recognizing his work in our lives. I think of thanksgiving simply as giving credit where credit is due—to the God who gives us life and breath. In the process of giving thanks, we remind ourselves that God is trustworthy, that he cares about us, and that we do not struggle through this life alone. In so doing, we activate Remedies 10 and 11 of the faith factor—"Trust—'Letting Go and Letting God' " and "Transcendence—Connecting with Ultimate Hope."

We need no elaborate methods in order to give thanks; it is perhaps the simplest type of prayer to list the many good things in our lives and to thank God for them. Often, our spirits will lift as we enumerate our blessings and our blessedness. Ultimately, as we grow in faith, we may be able to follow the instructions of the apostle Paul to the church at Thessalonica:

Rejoice always, pray without ceasing, give thanks in all circumstances; for this is the will of God in Christ Jesus for you. [1 THESSALONIANS 5:16–18.]

Though it does not come naturally, thanking God for the difficult things in our lives reinforces our faith that God will provide for us in all things, even when we cannot see at the present moment how this will happen. When we sincerely try to thank God for our challenges as well as our joys, we may find that our attitudes and outlooks change markedly for the better, thus making it easier to bear our burdens.

Confession: Admitting Our Failings and Asking for Pardon

When deeds of iniquity overwhelm us,
you forgive our transgressions
[PSALM 65:3.]

Because we do not like to admit our shortcomings, we often neglect prayers of confession, but in so doing, we deprive ourselves of the joyous freedom of absolution. This process constitutes Remedy No. 5 of the faith factor, "Renewal—Confessing and Starting Over." Carrying the burdens of our misdeeds can literally make us sick, so it is important to find time in our prayers to confess to God our specific failures to live according to his ways. Having done so, we can receive assurance of God's forgiveness through scriptural passages, including:

He does not deal with us according to our sins,
nor repay us according to our iniquities.
For as the heavens are high above the earth,
so great is his steadfast love toward those who fear him;
as far as the east is from the west,
so far he removes our transgressions from us.
As a father has compassion for his children,
so the Lord has compassion for those who fear him.
[PSALM 103:10–13.]

In some Christian denominations, confession is regarded as a sacrament that takes place between penitent and priest. The priest hears the person's confession, then grants absolution from sin. Confession of sin and pronouncement of God's pardon is also part of corporate worship for many Christians and Jews. Jews observe a yearly Day of Atonement, Yom Kippur, with fasting, attendance at temple services, and personal self-examination and confession. Some Christian denominations encourage a similar time of penitence during Lent, the forty days preceding Easter. Fasting, confession, alms-giving, and works of charity characterize these times of communal soul-searching, repentance, and renewal.

Prayers of confession are found in many prayer books, but perhaps the most heartfelt confessions will be in our own halting words as we realize that we have fallen short of the mark. If you find it difficult to get started on your prayers of confession, it may be helpful to consider the following words from Augustine's *Confessions:*

> The house of my soul is too small for you [God] to come to it. May it be enlarged by you. It is in ruins; restore it. In your eyes it has offensive features. I admit it, I know it; but who will clean it up? Or to whom shall I cry other than you? "Cleanse me from my secret faults, Lord, and spare your servant from sins to which I am tempted by others." [PSALM 31:5.]

Confessing to God is an essential element of a relationship with him as our omnipotent, omniscient, loving Creator. Even if you feel awkward and strange praying your confession, I hope you will try to do so on a regular basis, so that you will not continue to carry the burdens of guilt and shame that our misdeeds cause for us.

Petition: Asking God to Take Care of Us

> Incline your ear, O Lord, and answer me,
> for I am poor and needy.
> Preserve my life, for I am devoted to you;
> save your servant who trusts in you.
> [PSALM 86:1–2.]

Can we be bold enough to ask God for the things we need and want? The great figures of the Bible certainly did so. To give just one example from the Hebrew Bible, Daniel, looking death in the face in the lion's den, prays for deliverance and receives it (Daniel 1:8–16). In the New Testament, Jesus teaches that we are to ask God for everything we need, and he demonstrates God's willingness to help us by healing thousands of persons who came to him for help. In the Gospel of Mark, Jesus asks blind Bartimaeus, "What do you want me to do for you?" (Mark 10:51.) Bartimaeus says, "Rabbi, I want to see," and his desire is granted; Jesus restores his sight.

Prayer that asks for these things is known as *petition*. Though many faithful people feel, as my patient Monica did, that they shouldn't ask for things for themselves, the Bible tells us that God wants us to ask specifically for what we want, as long as we have the right motives (James 4:2–3).

When we ask God for what we need, we are employing faith-factor Remedy No. 10, "Trust—'Letting Go and Letting God.' " We acknowledge that we are not totally in control of everything in our lives, and we express our confidence in a God who can care for us when we ourselves cannot. When people are sick, using petitionary prayer to ask for God's help seems to come naturally, as we have seen in the scientific literature. A study of two hundred women found that their most frequent coping response to medical problems was prayer, with 91 percent reporting the use of prayer when facing illness. Other studies show that older people in particular use prayer to cope with illness; one study found that 72 percent of the elderly people surveyed prayed privately once a day or more.

Our prayers, of course, may not be answered in the ways we would prefer. Theologians have written volumes on how to understand this reality, and I will not attempt to summarize their findings. For me, it is helpful to remember what C. S. Lewis wrote about unanswered prayer in a letter to a friend: "If God had granted all the silly prayers I've made in my life, where should I be now?"

Spiritual maturity involves trusting that God will answer our prayers according to our *real* needs as he sees them, and not as *we*, with our limited vision, see them. Our task is to "let go and let God." We can let go of the idea that we know best what we need and how to meet our needs, and let God be in charge of determining and providing for those needs. Our petitionary prayer should not be an attempt to control God but, rather, to relinquish control of our problems and to acknowledge God's presence and activity in our lives. After all, the ultimate goal of prayer is not to get our needs met or to get what we want; it is to draw us nearer to God.

Petitionary prayer, then, is an important part of a sound spiritual program, but it should not be the *only* form of prayer used. In her prayer study, Margaret Poloma found no relationship between the exclusive use of petitionary prayer and well-being; this type of prayer neither boosted nor depressed people's life satisfaction. From a medical point of view, therefore, I would advise using petitionary prayer *in conjunction with*, not instead of, the other forms of prayer discussed here.

Intercession: Asking God to Help Others

O save your people, and bless your heritage;
be their shepherd, and carry them forever.

[PSALM 28:9.]

As discussed above, intercession is petitionary prayer on behalf of others. When we pray for others, we ask God to do what needs to be done for them, rather than falling into the misguided notion that we can solve our loved ones' problems all by ourselves. We know, too, from the scientific literature (including the Byrd study and several others) that praying for others may have a real and positive physical effect; with this knowledge in hand, we may decide to devote more time and attention to our intercessory prayer.

As with petitionary prayer, it is important to remember that the answers to our prayers may not be what we had hoped for. Having faith in God means recognizing that he alone has the omniscient view of our lives, and that his solutions to our problems are by definition far better than our own. At the same time, people who pray in the Bible ask for what they want quite specifically. Daniel does not equivocate when asking to be delivered from the lions' den; blind Bartimaeus does not say to Jesus, "I'd like my sight to return, but, then again, you are the Lord, so you do what you think best." For me, the Lord's Prayer helps clarify the relationship between accepting God's will and asking for what we want, both in praying for myself and in praying for others:

Our Father, who art in heaven, hallowed be thy name. *Thy kingdom come, Thy will be done,* on earth as it is in heaven. *Give us this day our daily bread.* . . . [MATTHEW 6:9–11.]

In teaching his disciples how to pray, Jesus gave them this prayer that puts doing God's will *before* fulfilling our needs, but Jesus *does* instruct his followers, here and elsewhere, to ask God to fulfill their particular needs.

Our prayers will not always be answered as we like. At times, it is the task of faith to trust that God's plans for us are more beneficial than our own desires or expectations. I hope you will feel free to pray for the needs of others, given the potential importance of such prayer to health and well-being, trusting in God's generosity to all of us, and yet remaining ready to accept answers to prayer that do not fulfill our initial wishes or make sense to us from our limited perspective.

"PRAYER 101"

There is value in starting small in prayer. Jesus tells his disciples that it takes only a very small amount of faith in order to do great things:

> The apostles said to the Lord, "Increase our faith!" The Lord replied, "If you had faith the size of a mustard seed, you could say to this mulberry tree, 'Be uprooted and planted in the sea,' and it would obey you." [LUKE 17:5–6.]

In our enthusiasm, we may start out praying for a cure for all cancers, or for world peace, and certainly those are worthy goals. But I advise my patients to focus on the smaller things; faith will grow as we continue to pray. Doctors in training to become surgeons begin by cutting small benign lesions from the skin. Once these simple procedures are mastered, they move on to taking out diseased appendices, then to gallbladders. Some go on to more complex types of surgery on the heart and brain. We would not expect a medical student to make critical decisions about people in intensive care, or a surgical intern to remove a brain tumor. There is a natural growth process as students, interns, and residents learn and develop more skills.

The same is true in the spiritual life. We begin with simple prayers and regular worship attendance. Then we may wish to learn about different kinds of prayer. We might seek out a spiritual director or a prayer group. Retreats, pilgrimages, and engagement in ministry to others may follow. Each sincere seeker of faith will grow naturally, in a pattern ordained for him or her by God. But no matter how spiritually sophisticated we may become, it is important always to remember that prayer, ultimately, cannot be done "wrong." As the Quaker writer Richard Foster says:

> God receives us just as we are and accepts our prayers just as they are. In the same way that a small child cannot draw a bad picture so a child of God cannot offer a bad prayer.

Prayer does not have to be complicated or frightening. Ultimately, it is very simple—a means of communication between the Divine Lover and his beloved creatures. Wherever you are in your faith journey, I hope you will establish or strengthen a commitment to a daily time of prayer, following the dictates of your faith tradition and seeking God's guidance in developing your spiritual practices.

CHAPTER 10

The Riches of the Bible:
A Handbook for Healing

The Bible is the best-selling and most influential book in the history of the world. Bibles are *everywhere:* missionaries distribute pocket versions on street corners and at bus and train stations; most lodgings have one in every room (courtesy of the Gideons); every bookstore carries at least one or two of the myriad editions and translations. In 1996, twenty-nine million Bibles were sold in the United States, and 1.8 *billion* Bibles were distributed overseas, translated into over two thousand languages.

Given the pervasive presence of "the Good Book," we can hardly overestimate its influence on our civilization. Biblical images have inspired countless masterpieces of art, architecture, music, and literature. Biblical concepts form the basis of our philosophical, ethical, and legal systems and treatises. And many of the Bible's stories resound throughout our culture; for example, even nonreligious people and children know about Noah, the man who built the Ark and saved the animals.

But although the Bible is the recognized cornerstone of Western civilization, its value as a handbook for healing and healthy living is less well known. As a physician, I have seen repeatedly that the Bible can have a healing effect in my patients' lives. By engaging with the Bible's stories and wisdom, many patients have found new ways to interpret their illnesses and cope with their problems. They have sought—and found—

new outlooks and new solutions. Some have even experienced physical healings after praying about scriptural stories of healing and making those stories their own.

Few scientific studies have measured scripture-reading alone as a health-inducing factor. It is more frequently measured as a marker of the degree of one's religious commitment, for all the world's great religious traditions advocate the study of holy scriptures, and regular scripture-reading is a vital part of devotional life and worship for most religious people.

I acknowledge the value and respect the wisdom found in the holy scriptures of all religions. However, I am unqualified to comment on their use as a health-promoting measure, because I am not sufficiently familiar with them. By contrast, even though I am not a theologian or a trained Biblical scholar, my knowledge of the Bible's healing effects has come from years of observing my patients' experiences and through my own personal spiritual journey, which has included a program of daily Bible-reading for much of the past thirty years.

The Bible's role in healing is not something I learned about in medical school. The state licensing boards require that we learn to interpret chest X-rays and electrocardiograms; they don't require us to interpret scripture. For many doctors, talking about the medical benefits of Bible-reading is far less comfortable than talking about the medical benefits of antihypertensive medication or smoking cessation. But for me, talking about the Bible comes naturally, because my experience has shown me that the Good Book is one of the most valuable—and powerful—medicines in my black bag.

HOW SCRIPTURE "WORKS" AS MEDICINE

If your doctor prescribed a new medication for you, you might ask a series of questions: "What dose do I need to take, and how often?" "How much does it cost?" "What are the possible side effects?" "How long will I have to take it?" "How does it work?" Since I am advising the use of the Bible as a specific, health-boosting "medicine," it is reasonable to answer such questions, acknowledging, of course, that the Bible is far grander, more complex, mysterious, and transcendent than "just a pill."

How much do I take? I recommend a daily "dose" of Bible reading. Many have found that reading at the same time each day is the most useful approach. I've found the early morning to be the best time, because it allows me to prepare myself for the day by grounding myself in God and finding sustenance to help buffer life's stresses. As for the amount of scripture to read daily, it may be helpful to know that many devout persons read for fifteen to twenty minutes or more per day. You can "overdose" on Bible reading if you are thereby avoiding other obligations; it is important to find a healthy balance between Bible-reading, prayer, community and family activities, and work.

How much does it cost? Using the Bible costs almost nothing except time. If you do not already own a Bible, you can borrow one from any library or buy one very inexpensively—which is not the case with many pharmaceuticals!

What are the possible side effects? No "side effect" of Bible-reading is likely to make you physically ill, but problems do arise. One danger to avoid is giving up on Bible study when we hit a chapter or verse that is difficult to understand. Some Biblical passages have spawned centuries of scholarship and debate, and still do not easily yield their meanings. For the novice, such passages can lead to discouragement and to quitting the Bible-reading regimen. Using resources like Bible commentaries and participating in study groups can help us avoid this "side effect."

We can also go astray by misusing the Bible, by distorting and misinterpreting it to meet our personal needs. Some problematic approaches to the scripture include "proof-texting," or taking a single scripture verse out of context in order to prove a point, and interpreting the Bible in an overly literal way. Again, group study of the Bible can often prevent such distortions, as can consultation with a pastor or spiritual director.

How long do I have to take it? I recommend that my patients eat a balanced diet, exercise regularly, and get enough sleep daily for the rest of their lives, because these habits are vital to health. Similarly, Bible-reading should be continued indefinitely.

How does it work? In terms of scientific knowledge, we cannot definitively say how the Bible "works" as medicine, because so few studies have been undertaken to evaluate the specific health effects of scripture-reading. We *do* know from the studies that regular Bible-reading often goes hand in hand with a deeper devotional life and frequent church attendance, so we might say that Bible-reading is a key component of the religious lifestyle that produces good health effects.

From my own observations, I believe the Bible helps people get better because it helps them *reframe* their problems in a more helpful and spiritually healthy way. For example, by remembering and placing herself within the Bible story of the woman with hemorrhages who was healed by Jesus, Barbara (the cancer patient mentioned in chapter 3) symbolically reached out for healing at her church's altar rail. She received a deep sense of peace that sustained her throughout her cancer treatment, replacing the anxiety that had plagued her for weeks, and her thyroid cancer has not returned since treatment ended years ago.

How did Barbara overcome her anxiety? Was it a psychological event, brought about by a change in her belief structure? Was it a physiologic event, triggered by alterations in the levels of endorphins, serotonin, cortisol, or other neurochemical substances? Or was it a supernatural event, evidence of the influence of divine healing energy on the tissues of a human being? Scientifically, we do not know the answer to this question. As a person of faith, I believe God granted Barbara's prayer request, whatever the associated psychological, physiologic, or supernatural mechanisms of that healing may be. As a physician, I am eager to see more patients enjoy the healing benefits of regular Bible-reading, because I am convinced that any negative consequences of Bible study are far outweighed by its good effects on health.

Let us look now at how we might approach the Bible as a book about healing and a book that can bring healing.

FOUNDATIONS FOR BIBLICAL HEALING

In this book, we are examining the Bible through a medical lens, looking specifically for the ways it speaks to us about health and well-being. But, drawing back from that lens to take a larger view, we see that the Bible is the story of God's relationship with his people. We need to place the Bible's healing miracles and "medical" wisdom into this larger context. From my study of the Bible, I believe we can best understand the "why" of Biblical healing when we take into account three profound Biblical realities:

1. *God is love.* The very nature of God is love, according to the Bible: "God is love, and those who abide in love abide in God, and God abides in them" (1 John 4:16).

2. *God loves us.* The Bible tells us that God loves us as parents love their children. He yearns for us, broods over us, delights in us—even when we neglect or reject him. As the late Catholic priest Henri Nouwen wrote, our very identity is as God's beloved; we are the objects of God's passionate and undying love.

3. *God wants to heal us.* Because God loves us so much, he wants to give us gifts, including health and well-being. Healing is so much a part of God's nature that the Hebrew word *rapha,* which means "to cure, to heal, to restore health," is one of the words used to describe God in scripture; Yahweh-Rapha is a name for God as healer. In the New Testament, the same Greek word, *sozo,* is used for both "healing" *and* "salvation," thereby linking earthly healing with our heavenly destination.

According to the Bible, God is in the business of restoration through directly healing his people and through giving healing power to those who honor his name. As we read the Bible, we witness God healing people of every kind of problem, from leprosy to epilepsy, from paralysis to hemorrhages, from blindness to snakebite. In some cases, the Bible gives us excellent preventive medicine advice, as we will see in the section below. It is important to note, however, that, though the Bible has much to say about healing, it is not a textbook with cut-and-dried treatment modalities for various physical and mental problems. The Bible's principles of healing are encoded in its stories and sayings, and it is from these that we must draw out Biblical lessons on health and wholeness.

We can gain much from studying the Bible as a handbook for healing. But studying it is not enough. To understand and benefit from the Bible's messages about healing, we must experience a living encounter with the Word of God.

THE BIBLE AS A REMEDY FOR ILLNESS

When I look at the Bible from a medical perspective, I see its passages on health and healing as belonging to two categories:

1. *Wisdom.* In this category, we find the poetry of the Psalms and the Song of Songs, the impassioned prophecies and warnings recorded by the Hebrew prophets, the medical advice of books like Proverbs and Deuteronomy, and the instructions on living found in the New Testament Epistles, the letters from the apostles to the newly founded churches.

2. *Stories.* From Adam and Eve in the Garden of Eden (Genesis) to the depiction of the angels praising God in heaven (Revelation), the Bible contains hundreds of narratives. We see the history of an entire nation of people, the people of Israel, told over the course of centuries in the Old Testament. We follow the life of Jesus from his conception through his healing ministry, crucifixion, resurrection from the dead, and ascension into heaven. But in addition to major narratives like these, we find stories of spiritual giants like Abraham, Moses, Elijah, Peter, and Paul; stories of ordinary folks like Ruth and Boaz, Esther and Mordecai, Anna and Simeon; and stories of characters who, though unnamed, may have a profound influence on our lives, as the woman with hemorrhages did for Barbara.

Whether we use Biblical wisdom or stories (or both) for healing, we will benefit by encountering the Bible's words with openness and expectation. Let's look in a bit more depth at how we might approach the two major categories of Biblical healing literature.

Wisdom:
Words of Admonishment and Comfort

Generically speaking, wisdom appears throughout the Bible. Here I am using the term "wisdom" as a category for the Bible's advice about healing, healthy living, and our right relationship to God. I frequently use passages of this type to help my patients find courage, meaning, and forbearance in their struggles.

Within the larger category of the Bible's wisdom, we find a number of health precepts, written thousands of years ago, that hold up well under twentieth-century scientific scrutiny. We might think of these writings as "prescriptions" from the Bible. In chapter 7, we presented evidence indicating that Orthodox Jews are healthier and live longer than secular Jews. In part, their health advantages might be credited to following scriptural admonitions regarding health and well-being:

Physical Illness: Prevention and Recovery. The Old Testament offers both general and specific guidelines about avoiding illness and recovering from it. Perhaps the broadest prescriptive statement comes in the Book of Exodus, where God speaks to his people:

> "If you listen carefully to the voice of the Lord your God and do what is right in his eyes, if you pay attention to his commands and keep all his decrees, I will not bring on you any of the diseases I brought on the Egyptians, for I am the Lord, who heals you." [EXODUS 15:26.]

This healing covenant with God's people makes the vital link between the obedience of a nation and physical health, or between disobedience and disease (specifically, the plagues visited upon the Egyptians because their pharaoh did not release the Hebrew people).

Is God promising perfect health in return for perfect behavior? This literal interpretation seems unlikely. First, no human being will ever be able to behave perfectly. Rabbinical tradition identified 613 individual statutes of the law that needed to be kept—a monumental—and impossible—task. The apostle Paul reported that he was a strict Pharisee and follower of the law, but, despite his zeal, he couldn't keep the Tenth Commandment: "You shall not covet . . ." Thus, we cannot proclaim this covenant as a formula for avoiding sickness by behaving without sin, because, like Paul, "all have sinned and fallen short of the glory of God" (Romans 3:23); all have broken the healing covenant outlined in Exodus 15:26. Second, the covenant was made with the nation of Israel, not individuals. Third, the weight of scripture and human experience indicates that righteous men and women *do* get sick.

Nor does it seem likely that God is saying all illness is the result of sin. Though a number of Biblical passages, including this one, state that there is a link between disobedience to God and illness, other passages imply there are additional reasons for sickness. When Jesus's disciples ask him about the cause of a man's congenital blindness, he not only heals the man but also dismisses the idea that the disability was caused by sin, a popular idea at that time:

> His disciples asked him, "Rabbi, who sinned, this man or his parents, that he was born blind?" Jesus answered, "Neither this man nor his parents sinned; he was born blind so that God's works might be revealed in him." [JOHN 9:2–3.]

The causes of illness laid forth in the Bible, then, are several, and we cannot always attribute illness to sinful behavior. But it *does* appear that we will be healthier if we obey God's laws. For example, by loving God with our whole beings, as we are instructed to do in Mark 12:30, we demonstrate an intrinsic religious orientation, one that activates the faith factor's remedies in our lives and, as we have seen, greatly enhances our chances for better health and greater well-being.

More specifically, we can prevent some kinds of physical illness by following Biblical injunctions. For example, you have doubtless heard that limiting dietary fat intake is good for your health, preventing atherosclerosis, gallstones, and breast and colon cancer. The writer of the Book of Leviticus knew this thousands of years before modern scientific method was established: "You shall eat no fat of ox or sheep or goat" (Leviticus 7:23). Scientific studies have proved the wisdom of limiting the intake of animal fats. As we have seen in previous chapters, a series of studies has shown that Seventh-Day Adventists, many of whom follow a low-fat diet, live longer, have lower blood pressure, and develop fewer cases of cancer than individuals in the general population. Though most Jews and Christians do not interpret scripture as calling for a strict vegetarian diet, science has proved that we would do well to follow the warning of Leviticus 7:23 to avoid eating unnecessary fat.

In Biblical times, before the discovery of antibiotic medicines, preventing the spread of infectious diseases was literally a matter of life and death. Speaking through scripture, God gave the Israelites an effective means of infection control: use of quarantines. "He shall remain unclean as long as he has the disease; he is unclean. He shall live alone; his dwelling shall be outside the camp" (Leviticus 13:46). Quarantines have been effectively used throughout history to combat various infections—smallpox, polio, tuberculosis. We still use infection-control methods to safeguard healthy patients from diseased individuals and to protect patients with depressed immune systems from contamination by other patients. This Biblical injunction, written thousands of years before Pasteur, has remained an important and successful means of preventing illness, including sexually transmitted diseases. The sexual transmission of disease could also be stopped entirely through universal obedience to another Biblical edict, the Seventh of the Ten Commandments, "You shall not commit adultery," since such diseases do not occur in a setting of lifelong monogamy between husband and wife.

Avoiding Addiction and Living a Balanced Life. No contemporary account of alcoholism's miseries could improve upon this accurate and concise description written thousands of years ago:

> Who has woe? Who has sorrow? Who has strife? Who has complaining? Who has wounds without cause? Who has redness of eyes? Those who linger late over wine, those who keep trying mixed wine. Do not look at wine when it is red, when it sparkles in the cup and goes down smoothly. At the last it bites like a serpent, and stings like an adder. Your eyes will see strange things, and your mind utter perverse things. You will be like one who lies down in the midst of the sea, like one who lies on top of a mast. "They struck me," you will say, "but I was not hurt; they beat me, but I did not feel it. When shall I awake?" [PROVERBS 23:29–35.]

The writer of this proverb wisely advised readers to avoid wine—or at least "lingering over" wine, consuming too much of it. Indeed, in other books of the Bible, we see that wine is valued by the Hebrew people and used in Passover celebrations. In the New Testament, Jesus turns water into wine at a wedding. Later, he likens wine to his own blood the night before his crucifixion, and the apostle Paul advises Timothy to "take a little wine for the sake of your stomach and your frequent ailments" (1 Timothy 5:23).

But moderation is important; Paul writes to the Ephesians, "Do not get drunk with wine, for that is debauchery; but be filled with the Spirit" (Ephesians 5:18).

The Bible seems to advocate a balanced approach to alcohol, neither abstinence nor overconsumption. Scriptural passages also advise against extremes in work and rest. We are commanded not to indulge in workaholism, which, though not a classic addiction, is an unhealthy pattern of living; the establishment and maintenance of the Sabbath is a strong preventative against workaholism:

> Remember the sabbath day, and keep it holy. Six days you shall labor and do all your work. But the seventh day is a sabbath to the Lord your God; you shall not do any work. . . . [EXODUS 20:8–10.]

At the same time, the Bible warns against idleness:

> Anyone unwilling to work should not eat. For we hear that some of you are living in idleness, mere busybodies, not doing any work. Now such persons we command and exhort in the Lord Jesus Christ to do their work quietly and to earn their own living. [2 THESSALONIANS 3:10–12.]

Finding a balance between wholesome work and needed rest requires that we confront another ill the Bible warns against—idolatry, in which we put other things before God. In Old Testament times, God warned against the creation of physical idols, "gods" made of precious metals, such as the golden calf the Israelites made while Moses was on Mount Sinai receiving the Ten Commandments (Exodus 32):

> Do not make any gods to be alongside me; do not make for yourselves gods of silver or gods of gold. [EXODUS 20:23.]

Our idols today are not so easily identified. Instead of gods of silver and gold, we make idols out of something that in itself may be laudable, like professional achievement, social acceptability, or earning money, by distorting its importance. Idolatry endangers our physical *and* spiritual health. For example, if achievement and money are more important to us than anything else, we are likely to work ourselves into the ground, neglecting health habits like exercise, good nutrition, and adequate sleep. Mental health may well decline as we neglect vital relationships with loved ones in favor of overwork. If our false god is status among our peers, we may take up addictive habits like smoking cigarettes, drinking too much, and using illicit drugs to be one of the crowd. Relying on any false god threatens our well-being, as does turning to sources other than God for guidance and help:

> You shall not practice augury or witchcraft. . . . Do not turn to mediums or wizards; do not seek them out, to be defiled by them: I am the Lord your God. [LEVITICUS 19:26, 31.]

The Bible tells us to look to God alone for our guidance, not to depend on human beings who claim to have esoteric knowledge or special powers of predicting the future.

In these warnings against workaholism and idolatry, the Bible tells us to stay in balance, with God at the center of our lives. As we have seen in numerous scientific studies, such a balance, as reflected in frequent church or synagogue attendance (a major part of regular Sabbath observance) and a regular program of prayer, scripture-reading, and fellowship with other believers, is related to better health.

Preventing Depression and Anxiety. To ward off depression, anxiety, and despair, the Bible gives us passages like these to hold in our minds:

> The cheerful heart has a continual feast. Better a little with the fear of the Lord than great wealth with turmoil. Better a meal of vegetables where there is love than a fattened calf with hatred. [PROVERBS 15:15–17.]

> Be still before the Lord and wait patiently for him; do not fret when men succeed in their ways, when they carry out their wicked schemes. Refrain from anger and turn from wrath; do not fret—it leads only to evil. [PSALM 37:7–8.]

Throughout the Bible, we are repeatedly told to focus on God as a means for quelling anxiety and depression. As we have seen in chapter 4 on mental illness, contemporary research confirms this Biblical advice: religious involvement has been repeatedly shown to protect against the development of mental illness.

The Bible also helps prevent mental illness by issuing injunctions against sexual abuse within families, which many scientific studies have shown to have long-term psychological and physical effects. The Old Testament clearly proscribes incestual sexual abuse:

No one is to approach any close relative to have sexual relations. I am the Lord. [LEVITICUS 18:6.]

Disobeying this directive results in great emotional suffering. Sexual abuse has also been linked to a variety of diseases, including irritable bowel syndrome, pelvic pain, somatization disorder, and infertility. Here again, the wisdom of a book written thousands of years ago is as fresh and important today as it was in the time of Moses.

These ancient preventive measures have proved to be remarkably effective catalysts for enhancement of health, reflecting the wisdom of the Great Physician. With the Psalms, prophetic books and passages, the teachings of Jesus, and the exhortations in the Epistles, they constitute the Biblical writings we are calling "wisdom"—a body of literature that offers help, hope, and instruction for all who seek healing and a more vibrant, fulfilling life.

The Power of Story

All Biblical texts have much to offer us, but it is in the Bible's stories that we will most readily understand healing. Stories—narratives that allow us to experience vividly a "slice of life" lived by another—have a special power, and Bible stories seem especially charged with meaning. As Episcopal priest and monk Martin Smith writes in his book, *The Word Is Very Near You:*

Of all the means available to God for drawing us into relationship and setting us free through the truth, stories are among the most powerful. . . . The [Bible] stories themselves are indispensable sacramental means of encounter with the Word which became flesh. . . . Stories are the chief way human beings make sense of their experience.

Just as we would read a romantic novel to understand the unfolding of a love relationship between a man and a woman, we can read the Bible to understand the love relationship between God and his people. As we enter into the lives of men and women like Abraham and Sarah, Moses and Miriam, Mary, Martha, and Lazarus, their stories become our own. Through them, we learn about God and we come to see our personal stories in the context of our relationship with him.

To gain this intimate spiritual knowledge from Bible stories, we must be open to the stories intellectually and emotionally. We must engage in the same willing suspension of disbelief that allows us to enjoy a movie without constantly thinking, "Now, wait a minute—why am I getting excited? This isn't real, it's just a movie!" We should not approach Bible stories armed with skepticism, but in an honest search for the truth.

When we start with a receptivity to the movement of God in our lives, we will grow in our relationship to scripture, and our capacity to receive healing through the Bible will grow as well. The requirement for this growth is simple: a regular commitment to prayerful, faithful Bible-reading. Once we have set out on this path, we can expect to come to our own very personal understandings of their meanings. Let's consider two stories of my patients from previous chapters in which Biblical stories aided recovery:

• In order to accept a diagnosis of depression and receive appropriate treatment, my patient Ron (chapter 4) needed to reflect on the stories of Biblical heroes who became depressed, including Jonah and Elijah. Once Ron could reframe his experience of depression, understanding it not as a failure on his part but as a difficulty he shared with great men of faith, he could let go of his feelings of shame and proceed with treatment.

• Louisa (chapter 5), a recovering alcoholic, learned also from the story of the prophet Elijah that God could speak to her in a still, small voice; she concluded that, in order to hear God's whisper, she needed to make time for quiet contemplation every day. By comparing herself to Elijah and learning from his experience, Louisa modified her lifestyle in a way that would bolster her recovery, both from alcoholism and from depression.

These are just some of the ways my patients have made the Bible's stories their own. Just as they have done, you will find your own unique insights in the Bible's pages. Some of the stories' lessons will be idiosyncratic, with unique meanings given to you by God's spirit moving through the Bible's words and into your soul. But the stories also hold other lessons that serve as common ground for all who value the Judeo-Christian tradition. Going from the particular to the general, we can now extract some of the Bible's guidelines for healthy living and recovery from illness from its stories about healing.

Biblical Healing Lessons for the Community of the Faithful

Lessons from the Hebrew Bible. In drawing out the Bible's lessons about healing that can be applied to us all, we will start in the beginning, with the Hebrew Bible or Old Testament. This collection of books provides a sweeping chronicle of God's relationship with his people, the Israelites. A treasure-house of spiritual wisdom, it is regarded by Jews and Christians alike as the Word of God. Healing stories in the Hebrew scriptures demonstrate how God reaches out to his people in their experiences of illness and recovery. These stories have a number of key lessons to teach us. Let us examine some of the major healing themes of the Old Testament and the stories through which they are communicated.

1. *God wants to heal us, and our desire for healing is important to God.* In 2 Kings 20, we read of King Hezekiah, who becomes ill and is told by the prophet Isaiah that he will die. Hezekiah prays for recovery, reminding God of his long-standing faith and obedience:

"Remember now, O Lord, I implore you, how I have walked before you in faithfulness with a whole heart, and have done what is good in your sight." Hezekiah wept bitterly. [2 KINGS 20:3.]

Immediately, Isaiah returns with a word from the Lord: Hezekiah will be healed, and fifteen years will be added to his life. From this story, we can infer that God longs to make us well, but he also wants us to ask for healing. By responding once we have prayed for help, God invites us to be partners in the healing process.

In Hezekiah's healing, we also see faith and medicine working together: Hezekiah prays, and Isaiah orders that a poultice of figs be made: "Bring a lump of figs. Let them take it and apply it to the boil, so that he may recover" (2 Kings 20:7). The sick king gets better because of the prayer *and* the poultice, not just one or the other. God's healing power can come to us directly, or mediated through a poultice of figs, or in both ways. Hezekiah's approach is one of several Biblical instances of "prayer-and-Prozac" medicine.

2. *You don't have to be perfect to receive God's healing touch.* The Bible tells us of several instances in which God healed people who had ignored or rejected him. In 1 Kings 13:4–6, the hand of the evil King Jeroboam is withered when he tries to harm a man of God who prophesies against him. But Jeroboam pleads with this same man of God:

"Entreat now the favor of the Lord your God, and pray for me, so that my hand may be restored to me." [1 KINGS 13:6.]

The man of God prays for the king, and God heals Jeroboam's hand. Similarly, King Nebuchadnezzar, an idol-maker and oppressor of the Hebrew people, is healed of madness after his confession of humility before God (Daniel 4:34–36).

In this and other scripture stories we find an encouraging message: though God is never pleased when we commit sins, we can be protected and healed in spite of them.

3. *Illness can have redemptive purposes.* Strangely, illness and the factors that cause illness can contain the seeds of healing and growth. We see this in Numbers 21:4–9, where the entire tribe of Israel is punished for its rebelliousness:

The people spoke against God and against Moses, "Why have you brought us up out of Egypt to die in the wilderness? For there is no

food and no water, and we detest this miserable food." Then the Lord
sent poisonous serpents among the people, and they bit the people, so
that many Israelites died. [NUMBERS 21:5–6.]

Moses pleads to God on behalf of his tribe, and God provides a remarkable antidote:

And the Lord said to Moses, "Make a poisonous serpent, and set it on
a pole; and everyone who is bitten shall look at it and live." [NUMBERS
21:8.]

The snake, the symbol of evil, death, and disobedience, the embodiment of Satan and the plague of human beings since the Garden of
Eden, had now been transformed into an instrument of life and healing.
From this story, a new and hopeful theme emerges: paradoxically, illness
and its causes can contain healing power, helping people overcome sickness and/or grow emotionally and spiritually. Many of my patients confirm this, saying that illness is a teacher, and that they have learned more
from their suffering than they could have learned through any other
means.

   4. *To be healed, we must submit in obedience to what the healing process
requires.* Doctors are always concerned about issues of patient compliance: Will our patients take their medicines as instructed, or quit smoking
or drinking? Often, the answer is "no," and the progress of healing is
retarded. We can see the importance of complying with the prescribed
healing regimen in the story of Naaman, the Syrian general (2 Kings 5).
Despite his unmatched prowess in battle, this great general suffered from
leprosy. When Naaman sought healing from the Hebrew prophet Elisha,
he was insulted that the prophet simply sent back a message through an
intermediary rather than meeting with him personally. Naaman had specific ideas about how his healing should happen:

But Naaman became angry and went away, saying, "I thought that for
me he would surely come out, and stand and call on the name of the
Lord his God, and would wave his hand over the spot, and cure the leprosy!" [2 KINGS 5:11.]

Instead, Elisha had issued a prescription: "Go, wash in the Jordan seven times, and your flesh shall be restored and you shall be clean" (2 Kings 5:10). Naaman protests this prescription, saying that the Jordan River is nothing special, and that surely the rivers in his native country would be more suitable. Finally, Naaman's servants point out that their master was ready to do anything in order to be healed; why not go ahead and wash in the Jordan River? Swallowing his pride, Naaman complied with Elisha's prescription, and "his flesh was restored like the flesh of a young boy, and he was made clean" (2 Kings 5:14).

When I visited the Jordan River on a recent pilgrimage to the Holy Land, I understood Naaman's skepticism about the special properties of this particular body of water: it is little more than a stream, not the mighty river described in spirituals and hymns as "deep and wide." Still, accounts from the Bible as well as contemporary experience tell us that this *is* a special place. The Episcopal priest who led my pilgrimage group, Father Terry Fullam, told us of a healing effected by the waters of the Jordan River just a few years ago. A skeptically inclined chemist named Don participated in one of Father Fullam's pilgrimages. While on a boat anchored off the coast of Israel, the engineer fell and gashed his arm. The large cut was treated, and Don was able to continue with the group to the next destination, the Jordan River, which, Father Fullam explained, though not a magical place where all diseases are cured, was an appropriate place to receive healing prayer. Father Fullam prayed for Don as he immersed his body in the water. Don was amazed when his arm emerged completely healed. "His flesh became like a young boy's, smooth and perfect," Father Fullam told me.

We can learn from Naaman's—and Don's—experiences. Even though many actions required for healing may seem foolish to us, we can "wash in the Jordan" by being obedient. Our doctors may ask us to take medicines, to cut fat from our diets, to take up walking as a form of exercise. God may ask us to confess our sins and amend our behavior. We can hasten our healing by following "doctor's orders" and turning to God with a willing heart.

Lessons from the Healing Ministry of Jesus. Healing plays an important role in the Old Testament, but it is of paramount significance in the New Testament. The casual reader of the Bible may not be aware of the centrality of healing to Jesus's ministry. The Christian Gospels (the books of

Matthew, Mark, Luke, and John in the Bible) record forty-two accounts of healing by Jesus, and nearly a quarter of the Gospels is devoted to healing. We can learn a number of important lessons from an overview of the New Testament accounts of healing.

1. *All illnesses can be healed, and illness in itself carries no stigma.* Jesus confronted the worst afflictions known to the world of his time. Throughout his ministry, he reached out to individuals possessed by demons, who may have manifested various types of physical or mental illness. (Modern scientists and theologians can only speculate as to the diseases attributed to demon possession in the Bible. Were these people actually overcome by evil spirits, or were they suffering from mental illnesses like schizophrenia or neurologic illnesses like epilepsy?) Jesus was not repelled by the demon-possessed, nor did he turn away from those with leprosy and other skin conditions, which rendered sufferers ritually unclean according to Hebrew law.

In several instances, Jesus healed blind, deaf, mute, and physically handicapped people. These disabilities bring plenty of hardship today, but in Jesus's time they were even more devastating, for there was no hope of cataract surgery, corrective lenses, hearing aids, or speech or physical therapy. Furthermore, the disability was often seen as a moral failing on the part of the sufferer. Shunned by their peers, handicapped individuals would live in a world of isolation, poverty, and fear. Jesus stood against the prejudice of the time, demonstrating only acceptance and caring for those who were suffering.

2. *All types of people can be healed; holiness is not a prerequisite for healing; sinners can still apply.* In his ministry, Jesus healed every kind of illness and every kind of person, including those considered unworthy of help by the religious establishment of the time.

3. *All methods of healing can be employed; there is no single formula.* Just as a modern physician would choose the best remedy from among those available, Jesus employed various healing methods, apparently selecting the most effective treatment for the individual "patient" before him. His healing methods included:

The word of command. In some cases, Jesus literally ordered disease and death to relinquish their grip on people. He restored to life three individuals: Jairus's daughter, Lazarus, and the son of the widow of Nain:

> Soon afterwards he went to a town called Nain, and his disciples and a large crowd went with him. As he approached the gate of the town, a man who had died was being carried out. He was his mother's only son, and she was a widow; and with her was a large crowd from the town. When the Lord saw her, he had compassion for her and said to her, "Do not weep." Then he came forward and touched the bier, and the bearers stood still. And he said, "Young man, I say to you, rise!" The dead man sat up and began to speak, and Jesus gave him to his mother. [LUKE 7:11–15.]

Touch. Jesus frequently touched the sick person, as he did with a woman who had been beset by orthopedic problems for eighteen years:

> Now he was teaching in one of the synagogues on the sabbath. And just then there appeared a woman with a spirit that had crippled her for eighteen years. She was bent over and was quite unable to stand up straight. When Jesus saw her, he called her over and said, "Woman, you are set free from your ailment." When he laid his hands on her, immediately she stood up straight and began praising God. [LUKE 13:10–13.]

Sometimes the sick person touched Jesus, as the woman with hemorrhages did (Luke 8:43–48).

Ancient forms of medicine. As previously mentioned, saliva was thought to have medicinal qualities in Biblical times. By using saliva to make a paste to treat blind and deaf individuals, Jesus validated the use of the medical technology of his time. Jesus also demonstrated a positive attitude toward the medical establishment by telling the ten lepers he healed to visit the priests—the doctors of that era—to verify their healing (Luke 17:11–19).

Even for Jesus, healing was not always easy or straightforward. In the healing of the man who was born blind, Jesus encountered some resistance:

> Some people brought a blind man to him and begged him to touch him. He took the blind man by the hand and led him out of the village; and when he had put saliva on his eyes and laid his hands on him, he

asked him, "Can you see anything?" And the man looked up and said, "I can see people, but they look like trees, walking." Then Jesus laid his hands on his eyes again; and he looked intently and his sight was restored, and he saw everything clearly. [MARK 8:22–25.]

Knowing that Jesus needed two steps to complete this healing, we can conclude that not all healings will come instantly; many will be gradual. We are on firm Biblical ground when we pray for instant healing, but God may have a lengthier process in mind for us.

In fact, an overview of Jesus's healing methods shows that we may expect healing to occur in many forms.

4. *Having faith will help us be healed.* Whichever healing methods he employed, Jesus responded to people who had great faith. Sometimes, Jesus healed in response to the faith of the sick person himself. At other times, he healed in response to the faithful entreaties of the sick person's loved ones. This is perhaps most remarkably seen in the following story of a paralytic:

One day, while [Jesus] was teaching, Pharisees and teachers of the law were sitting nearby . . . and the power of the Lord was with him to heal. Just then some men came, carrying a paralyzed man on a bed. They were trying to bring him in and lay him before Jesus; but finding no way to bring him in because of the crowd, they went up on the roof and let him down with his bed through the tiles into the middle of the crowd in front of Jesus. When he saw their faith, he said, "Friend, your sins are forgiven you" . . .

He said to the one who was paralyzed—"I say to you, stand up and take your bed and go to your home." Immediately he stood up before them, took what he had been lying on, and went to his home, glorifying God. [LUKE 5:17–20, 24–25.]

In direct response to the extraordinary faith of the paralyzed man's friends, Jesus forgave the paralytic's sins and restored him to wholeness.

The effect of faith's absence is seen when Jesus visits his hometown, where he was received with skepticism and disrespect by those who had known him from childhood:

Then Jesus said to them, "Prophets are not without honor, except in their hometown, and among their own kin, and in their own house." And he could do no deed of power there, except that he laid his hands on a few sick people and cured them. And he was amazed at their unbelief. [Mark 6:4–6.]

The people's lack of faith restrained Jesus's healing power.

Given faith's importance, we might attempt to manufacture it, to "fake it" by manifesting a confidence in God that we do not really feel. I believe it is more effective simply to pray for more faith as the disciples did when they beseeched Jesus, "Lord, increase our faith" (Luke 17:5). Even if our reserves of faith are low, healing is available to us through the prayers of others—and through our own prayer to God for greater faith.

In reviewing Jesus's approach to healing, we find a message of hope: divine healing can come to us in many forms, regardless of our rectitude or the nature of our illness; and when we (or our loved ones) have faith, the potential for healing increases. Turning now to a question Jesus posed to a man seeking healing, let us gather together some of the Bible's advice to anyone who wants to get well.

"Do You Want to Be Healed?"

How can we prepare ourselves for healing? What steps can we take to remove any blockages to healing?

1. *First, admit you are sick.* The Psalmist speaks frankly about his illness:

Be merciful to me, Lord, for I am faint; O Lord, heal me, for my bones are in agony. [Psalm 6:2.]

We, too, will benefit from truthfulness about our suffering. In a culture that values self-sufficiency, it can be difficult to acknowledge illness, even to ourselves. But denial of reality will not help us get better, nor will keeping a "stiff upper lip." Honesty allows us to proceed with the healing process, admitting our need for help from God, our doctors, and our loved ones.

2. *Know and ask for what you want.* The Bible shows us the importance of desiring healing and asking for it, as well as believing in God's power to heal. Though it may seem that any sick person would want to be healed, this is not always so. Sometimes the sickness is serving a deeper purpose for the sufferer. Some of us don't want to give up our old patterns of behavior in order to gain health. By asking people "What do you want?" and "Do you want to be healed?," Jesus let us know that we *will* need to break away from those old patterns and that we *do* need to establish our desire as a prerequisite for healing.

3. *Confess your sins and pray for the healing of others.* The apostle James gave members of the new churches instructions on how to help the sick:

> Are any among you sick? They should call for the elders of the church and have them pray over them, anointing them with oil in the name of the Lord. The prayer of faith will save the sick, and the Lord will raise them up; and anyone who has committed sins will be forgiven. Therefore confess your sins to one another, and pray for one another, so that you may be healed. The prayer of the righteous is powerful and effective. [JAMES 5:14–16.]

James links the confession of sins to healing, pointing to the negative impact of guilt and anxiety on our physical, emotional, and spiritual health. He also links praying for *each other,* and not just for ourselves, to regaining health.

4. *Remember that God is the healer.* Physicians, nurses, therapists, pharmacists—we all have our roles in the healing process. But from the Bible's perspective, we act only as instruments of God's healing power. God does the healing; human beings assist in the process. As God says in the Book of Exodus, "I am the Lord who heals you" (Exodus 15:26). Speaking through Moses, God also says:

> See now that I, even I, am he; there is no god beside me. I kill and I make alive; I wound and I heal; and no one can deliver from my hand. [DEUTERONOMY 32:39.]

So, though we work faithfully with our human healers, we need to remember that our healing powers are limited, but God's are not. Yahweh-Rapha, the God who heals, deserves the thanksgiving and the glory when we are well again.

✢

Now that we have explored the treasury of lessons about healing in the Bible's pages, and examined the power of Biblical wisdom and story, how best can we approach this great "book of books" to gain its many benefits? I would like to offer several simple suggestions that have been helpful to me and to my patients.

ENCOUNTERING GOD'S WORD: A SHORT GUIDE TO BIBLE STUDY

If you have not studied the Bible on a regular basis, you may feel overwhelmed at the prospect of approaching this mighty tome. Perhaps you started such a study with the best intentions, but became discouraged when you hit a patch of incomprehensible text. Try not to let such difficulties interrupt your Bible-reading discipline. Even when some of what we read remains unclear, we can learn much from what *is* clear. How do we begin?

1. *Start slowly.* The Bible is an enormous book—really a library in itself—and it can be overwhelming. Generally, I do not recommend beginning at the beginning with the intent of reading straight through. Instead, make use of a guide that provides a calendar of daily Bible readings. (Several Bible-reading guides are listed in the Resources section at the end of this book.) Whatever plan you choose, remember to look upon your Bible-reading as a gradual process. When you start an exercise program, you don't expect results the first day but, rather, a slow, steady improvement over time. Similarly, in the spiritual life, it's the regular practice of reading the Bible that has value.

2. *Choose a Bible translation that is comfortable for you.* There are many different translations of the Bible, from the Shakespearean language of the seventeenth-century King James Version to the contemporary idiom of the New Revised Standard Version. You may dislike one version intensely, finding it hard to understand, but find a different version to be

poetry to your ears. Ask your clergy person to recommend a version, or do some research yourself by visiting a library or bookstore and reading a familiar passage—Psalm 23 or Paul's "love chapter" (1 Corinthians 13), for example—in several different translations.

It can also be helpful to use a Bible that includes a *concordance*—a keyword index that will help you find Bible passages—or other study guides. There are many Bible editions to choose from, each offering different benefits. Start with the one that catches your eye (or use the Bible you have at hand), then consider other versions and editions later.

3. *Learn with others.* Consider joining a Bible-study group in your congregation or community. The instruction and companionship of others in the discipline of scripture study can add a great deal to your learning, and the accountability of regular group meetings will help you stay on track. If you cannot find a suitable Bible-study group, you can benefit from the guidance provided by books—commentaries, dictionaries, and interpretive works.

4. *Pray for guidance and inspiration.* Start your Bible-reading time with a simple prayer, asking God to show you the meaning of the passages you are about to read, and to open your mind and your heart to the scripture. Keep a pen and notebook handy to jot down any particularly significant messages you find in your daily readings. Looking back over such a journal can give you great insight into the course of your spiritual journey.

5. *Use scripture as a basis for other forms of prayer.* I described meditative prayer in chapter 9, and suggested using a significant word or phrase as part of this kind of prayer. The Bible offers a limitless supply of beautiful and significant phrases. You can deepen your knowledge of the Bible by incorporating Bible passages into meditative prayer, prayerful journal-writing, and an ancient Christian practice known as *lectio divina,* or "holy reading." In *lectio divina,* we prayerfully focus on one short scripture passage, waiting for a word or phrase to engage us and draw us into contemplative prayer.

When you are reading Biblical stories of healing, consider using imaginative prayer for a deeper encounter with the story. In imaginative prayer, we attempt to place ourselves in the midst of the story so that we experience it as a participant—either as the person being healed or as an observer. Try imagining what it would feel like to be in that setting.

Praying imaginatively is easier when you are listening to a scriptural passage being read aloud slowly. You might ask someone to read the story to you, or make a tape yourself. Start your imaginative-prayer time with a prayer for God's guidance, then relax and see how you can become part of a story that is thousands of years old yet as meaningful today as it was at the time of its occurrence.

6. *Make your practice regular.* It stands to reason that daily doses of scripture will transform and renew our minds more steadily than an occasional Bible-reading splurge. But however often you decide to read the scripture, make your practice intentional. Decide what will be best for you for the next three months or so, then ask God's help in staying with your commitment. It may be helpful to decide upon a specific time and place for your Bible-reading, too, choosing a quiet time and a comfortable spot to which you return regularly, creating a "hallowed ground" on which to seek the presence of God. This helps build a consistent, comforting routine and reinforces the idea that you are dedicating this portion of your life to your relationship with God.

7. *"Just do it!"* As the familiar motto indicates, sometimes it is best to plunge ahead without thinking too much about what you're doing, because thinking too much about it can destroy momentum. I advise patients not to wait until they feel like doing something beneficial, like exercising; scripture-reading is the same. We cannot wait until we feel enthusiastic in order to build up a spiritual discipline like reading the Bible; rather, we must set time aside for it and make a commitment that overrides the occasional "down," sleepy, or irritated mood.

If you are not currently reading the Bible on a regular basis, I hope you will try it as an experiment. Find a Bible-reading plan, or simply start reading—a chapter a day is an easy way to approach it—with an open mind and heart, and see what you think. I believe that, if you embark on a regular, faithful study of this book, you will become "hooked," and that you will sense that a deep hunger in your heart is being filled.

CHAPTER 11

⬩⬩⬩

Spiritual Community:
Living Together in Love

"Doctor, I've come to terms with my illness. I'm at peace with God. I have only one fear: I just don't want to die alone," said Francesca, a middle-aged woman with terminal cancer.

"My life feels so—I don't know—*empty,* I guess, since the divorce," admitted Bert, a thirty-five-year-old man whose wife retained full custody of their three children. "When I go home to an empty apartment at night after work, I can't help but feel despair."

"My children and grandchildren live so far away, I almost never see them," confided Rose, a seventy-four-year-old woman with hypertension and diabetes. "I'm glad I can stay in my own home, but all the neighbors are young working people and they're busy, so I never see anybody. Life has gotten so lonely. My only companion is the television. Sometimes I feel like I'm the only person left on earth!"

Any doctor who has the time and willingness to listen will hear many tales of loneliness, a problem that can afflict people of all ages and all walks of life. This problem is on the rise as our society becomes ever more transient and ever less community-oriented. So often, neighbors don't know each other, relatives live hundreds of miles apart, and even parents and children are too busy to spend significant time together as families. Loneliness will increase if the current trend toward working from in-home offices ("telecommuting") continues to grow; many workers will no longer enjoy face-to-face socializing at coffee breaks and during lunch hours. We may grow more isolated, more lonely, and, as a consequence, also less able to resist infection and recover from illness. Many studies have demonstrated the relationship between social support and health. In a 1997 study published in the *Journal of the American Medical Association,* researchers at Carnegie Mellon University reported that individuals who had a greater variety of social relationships were more able to resist infection with the common cold virus. Researchers assessed the number of different types of relationships each of the study's 276 subjects regularly took part in (with a spouse, parent, child, close family member, classmate, church member, employee, and others). They also assessed the subjects' health habits, including smoking, quality of sleep, diet, exercise, and consumption of alcohol. Next the subjects were exposed to a cold virus, then observed while in quarantine. The results could be plotted on a straight-line graph: 62 percent of the subjects who had three or fewer social roles or relationships got colds, whereas 43 percent with four or five types of relationships became infected, and only 35 percent of those with six or more types of relationships became sick.

Resisting cold viruses is always desirable, but the advantages of social support extend to far more serious health issues, like cancer and mortality. Researchers at Stanford University and the University of California, Berkeley, found that women with breast cancer who took part in support groups lived an average of *eighteen months longer* than patients who did not. The support groups employed self-hypnosis for pain control as well as group therapy. Researchers performed a second study of these patients to determine if the longevity difference could be explained by medical causes—differences in courses of treatment or causes of death. The follow-up study showed only insignificant differences in treatment and cause of death between the two groups, suggesting that support-group participation alone was the determining factor.

In addition, a nine-year study (discussed in more detail in chapter 7) of almost seven thousand residents of Alameda County, California, showed a marked decrease in mortality rates for men and women who had strong social networks.

We do not know *how* having many and frequent social contacts might boost the immune system, but these studies offer the possibility that social support is one of the main building blocks of health. A number of studies support this hypothesis. One found that people who have experienced negative life events, in particular the loss of personal relationships, are more susceptible to a variety of illnesses. This finding held true for a number of illnesses and among several patient populations.

Just as we human beings appear to be "hard-wired for God," in the words of Dr. Herbert Benson, it also seems we were built to interact with one another. Our need for contact with other human beings is vital. The importance of caring touch was demonstrated scientifically during the nineteenth century, when many babies in orphanages died of an illness known as *marasmus,* which we now call "failure to thrive." To counteract this problem, doctors instituted "mothering," instructing staff to follow a regimen of holding, carrying, and rocking the babies several times a day. Once mothering was introduced at Bellevue Hospital in New York, infant mortality rates dropped precipitously, from around 35 percent to under 10 percent. The famous primate experiments of Harry Harlow a half-century ago demonstrated conclusively that young monkeys deprived of maternal affection at birth wither and die at an alarmingly high rate, and that baby monkeys value being touched and held above receiving milk from their mothers. The contemporary practice of recruiting volunteer "huggers" for neonatal intensive-care units is based on the findings of early-twentieth-century orphanage doctors and researchers like Harry Harlow. The ministrations of the "huggers" are not just nice—they are physically necessary for the healthy development of the infants.

Numerous scientific studies have shown the importance of social support to health and well-being. These data prove scientifically what we instinctively know: We need good relationships with relatives and friends in order to thrive in the world. Conversely, if such relationships are missing, as when we lose a loved one to death, or broken, as in the case of divorce, people are at greater risk of illness and death. The importance of having a functioning social network increases in times of stress, such as illness and aging, when social support often includes not only emotional sustenance but also practical assistance, like rides to the doctor's office and help with strenuous household chores.

Religious Versus Secular Community:
Is There a Difference in Terms of Health?

The studies showing the health benefits of social support have often focused on nonreligious measures of social networks. For example, researchers have looked at membership in community organizations, participation in volunteer activities, and number of contacts with family and friends per week. But in the last few decades, researchers have also started looking at membership and involvement in religious communities as an important measure of social support. The results indicate that participation in religious congregations or groups can deliver *more* health benefits through social support than participation in nonreligious organizations, and that both the quantity and quality of social interactions tend to be greater among religiously active people.

M. E. O'Brien's study of the role of religious faith in the lives of long-term hemodialysis patients, which I discussed in greater detail in chapter 6, found that weekly church attenders had more social contacts with others; they were more successful at avoiding the depressing isolation that often accompanies frequent hemodialysis. In the 1997 study of 6,928 residents of Alameda County, California, conducted by W. J. Strawbridge and colleagues, which showed significant differences in mortality rates between religious and nonreligious individuals (see chapter 7), individuals who attended religious services once a week or more were significantly more likely than less frequent attenders or nonattenders to enjoy strong connections with others and to increase their social connectedness over time. And researchers examining the relationship between religious involvement and social support among 2,956 respondents in North Carolina found that frequent church attenders had more ties to individuals outside the family, and enjoyed more visits and phone calls with their friends and family; their quality of social support was markedly higher than non–church attenders or infrequent attenders.

But the most striking scientific demonstration of this phenomenon comes from a study of Israelis living in religious and nonreligious kibbutzim, which I mentioned in chapter 7. This study traced mortality rates over fifteen years among two groups—2,123 members of eleven secular kibbutzim and 1,777 members of eleven religious kibbutzim. Studying these individuals, who were similar in terms of demographic characteristics such as age and education, allowed researchers to compare accurately the health benefits of religious and nonreligious community life. The results showed a dramatic difference, with 192 deaths among the secular-kibbutzim members (8 percent) and only 69 deaths among the religious-kibbutzim members (4 percent). Secular kibbutzim members died at a greater rate from all causes of death—coronary-artery disease, circulatory conditions, cancer, accidents, and suicide—so the health benefit enjoyed by the religious-kibbutzim members has a protective effect across the whole spectrum of health problems.

What can we conclude from these findings? Why do the religious kibbutzim members live longer? I believe several factors account for their increased longevity:

1. *Religiously observant people have better health habits (Remedy No. 2, Temperance: Honoring the Body as a Temple of the Spirit)*. Other studies have shown that religiously observant Jews are less likely to smoke, to drink alcohol, or to have high cholesterol levels (although, interestingly, they are more likely to develop diabetes, for unknown reasons). Smoking, drinking, and high cholesterol levels are clearly associated with higher mortality rates, particularly for cancer and heart diseases.

2. *Religious-kibbutzim members attend worship services more frequently.* As we have seen, numerous studies have linked better health with frequent worship-service attendance, the only single activity that incorporates all twelve remedies of the faith factor. Though the kibbutzim study did not measure frequency of worship attendance per se, it may be safely assumed that religious-kibbutzim members attended worship regularly as part of their community activities, and certainly much more frequently than members of the nonreligious kibbutzim (many of whom were atheists or agnostics), thus accruing to themselves all the health-boosting advantages of worship-service attendance.

3. *Religious-kibbutzim members enjoy stronger marriages and other forms of social support.* This finding echoes the studies mentioned above which demonstrate the higher quality of social support enjoyed by religious people. The study found that divorce is *eleven times more common* among members of the secular kibbutzim. The greater number of stable

marriages in the religious kibbutzim could in itself account for some of the difference in mortality rates between the two groups: being married has been linked to lower mortality rates, especially among men, by several studies, including the Alameda County study cited above and in chapter 7.

4. *Religious-kibbutzim members may have a stronger sense of purpose and meaning.* Secular-kibbutzim members may also be highly idealistic and committed to a lifestyle that supports their country's development as well as the health and happiness of their companions, but it is possible that the members of religious kibbutzim find an even greater sense of fulfillment and purpose because they share a coherent world view, a unity of vision, that grows out of shared religious beliefs. Their regular, shared participation in ritual strengthens this unity of vision. The members of the secular kibbutzim, though united around some principles, are likely to bring a greater diversity of viewpoints and motivations to their new community than those who join for religious reasons.

All four of these contributing causes of greater longevity are favorable "side effects" of religious life lived in community; they are less likely to be replicated, particularly in combination, in a nonreligious setting. Like church attendance, membership in a religious community or congregation offers unique health benefits; it is an essential part of any spiritual program. How can *you* tap into the benefits of religious-community membership, which include decreasing your chances of contracting serious illness, boosting your sense of well-being and purpose, avoiding addiction and mental illness, and even living longer?

WHAT EXACTLY IS A RELIGIOUS COMMUNITY?

The world's great religious traditions have long recognized the importance of how we relate to one another as individuals and as members of a community. In the Judeo-Christian tradition, the quality of our relationships is crucial to our spiritual identity. For Jews, a person's individual faithfulness cannot be divorced from life in the congregation of believers. In one Jewish commentary on the scriptures, *Ethics of the Fathers,* theologians state the importance of the connection to other believers unequivocally: "Do not separate yourself from the community." In fact, spiritual community is essential to prayer and ritual in Judaism; for example, many Orthodox rites cannot be carried out without the presence of ten adult Jewish men, a *minyan*.

With its basis in Judaism, the New Testament is equally emphatic about the importance of community. As in Judaism, most rituals of Christianity can be practiced *only* when "two or three are gathered together" (Matthew 18:20), including baptism, confession, communion, and rites of healing and unction. Jesus leaves no doubt as to the importance of our connectedness to others when he summarizes the Hebrew laws with the two great commandments: "You shall love the Lord your God with all your heart and all your soul and all your mind, and you shall love your neighbor as yourself" (Mark 12:30–31).

The Bible urges us not just to get along peaceably with our fellow humans, but to *love* them deeply and unconditionally, to live so closely connected to them that we might be thought of as different parts of the same body, to forgive them repeatedly when they offend or harm us. This is a tall order indeed, but it is at the very heart of the spiritual life. As a popular saying goes, there are no Lone Ranger Christians, and the same could certainly be said for Jews, since the Hebrew Bible tells the story of the formation, deliverance, and dispersion of a community of people called Israel whom God has chosen for his own. Scriptural teachings lead us to relate more closely to others, and to serve them, rather than to withdraw into an individualistic spirituality that isolates us.

Monasteries, one of the most intense forms of spiritual community, showcase the great benefits and the great difficulties of living this intimately linked life with fellow believers. The monastic tradition is full of teachings on the importance of loving that brother monk who has the irritating table manners or the sister nun who sings loudly but off-key. Much of the spiritual growth of monastics comes not from transcendent personal prayer, but from dealing with feelings of irritation, competition, envy, and resentment toward other members of the community.

Most of us will never live in a monastery; religious community for us comes as members of a church or synagogue. We may not share the same household with our fellow believers, but we still have the opportunity to get to know them, to love them and be loved by them, and to help them and be helped by them. "The rubber meets the road" in the spiritual life when we interact with those close to us; we are often put to the test when we establish community with others, but we also receive rewards, including remarkable benefits to our health.

RELIGIOUS COMMUNITY FOR "REGULAR FOLK"

For the vast majority of people who do not join a formal religious community like a kibbutz or a monastery, religious community is more difficult to define, but no less essential to health and well-being. There are two main forms of religious community for nonmonastics: marriage and family, and membership in a religious congregation.

Marriage and Family

Marriage and family forms the primary spiritual community. God himself created the institution of marriage: In the Book of Genesis, God made Adam, the first man. Then, saying, "It is not good that the man should be alone; I will make him a helper as his partner" (Genesis 2:18), God created Eve, a mate for Adam. God blesses the married couple with children, who are seen as a gift from God throughout scripture. Together, the married couple and their children participate in the most meaningful and intimate relationships human beings can know.

Many scientific studies of the health of single, married, and divorced people have proved the importance of successful marriage to physical and emotional well-being. Even more dramatically, studies of divorced people and their children demonstrate the negative consequences of fractured marriages and families. David B. Larson, M.D., has studied the fallout from our nation's divorce epidemic extensively, reviewing over three hundred peer-reviewed scientific studies on the subject.

"There's really very little good that can be said about divorce," he said recently. "It's devastating for men, women, and children. People who divorce have an increased risk anywhere from two to four times as high for physical, psychiatric, and addiction problems as do those who stay married."

For example, as Dr. Larson and his colleagues, Susan Larson and Jim Swyers, state in their research-based book, *The Costly Consequences of*

Divorce, men who are separated or divorced receive hospital psychiatric care nearly twenty times more frequently than married men. Divorce is also the number-one factor linked with suicide in large American cities. Perhaps even more alarming, studies show that the risk of getting cancer and other illnesses skyrockets for men who have been divorced; the increase in cancer risk is equivalent to the risk associated with smoking a pack or more of cigarettes per day! Though divorce's negative health impacts are most devastating for men, women suffer similar consequences at heightened rates: divorced men are likely to lose up to ten years from their normal life span, women up to five years.

Children of divorce experience far more problems than those whose parents remain married. "Children who have experienced a divorce often score worse on measures of self-esteem and psychological adjustment, along with more critical real-life outcomes, including academic achievement and emotional and behavioral problems, than do children living in intact families," said Dr. Larson. "They are much more likely to abuse alcohol and drugs, to become involved in delinquent behavior, and, for girls, to become pregnant as teenagers."

In reviewing the extensive research data on divorce, Dr. Larson has hypothesized that it is the increased stress related to and caused by divorce that is linked with the dramatic negative consequences. "The research does not show such negative effects for people who have always been single," he noted. "It seems to be the breaking of the marriage and family bonds that wreaks the havoc. And it seems that the damage cannot be reversed by remarrying and creating 'blended' families. In fact, research is showing you might have more emotional and behavioral problems in a remarried family than if you're simply divorced."

Given the devastating consequences of divorce, on our children and ourselves, how can we avoid it? Putting this more positively, how can we reap the health *benefits* of stable marriages, for husbands, wives, and children? In study after study, we see one factor that emerges repeatedly: people of faith have happier, more stable marriages and happier, healthier children.

As I mentioned in chapter 1, a scientific study of 7,029 married men and women showed a strong relationship between frequency of worship attendance and marital stability; survey respondents attending church less than once a year had a divorce/separation rate of 34 percent, whereas the rate for those attending once a month or more was only 18 percent. Another study, of 997 men and 1,281 women, all married, assessed the significance of eight variables as predictors of marital happiness, including age, age at first marriage, family income, education level, occupation, wife's employment status, number of children at home, and frequency of church attendance. Church attendance proved to be the strongest of the variables in predicting marital happiness, and the only predictor of the eight that was common to both men and women. In a scientific study of couples married an average of fifty-three years, women named religion as the most important factor in marital happiness; men also said religion was very important to marital success, but ranked attitudes such as "it takes two to make a marriage work" as higher. (One might add that the values inherent in religious involvement would boost spouses' ability to be tolerant and loving toward one another.) Echoing the findings of other studies, a survey of 181 married Kansas couples found a positive correlation between marital satisfaction and the importance of church and religion.

Why is marriage so much better and more enduring between religious partners? Dr. Larson suggests that religious involvement should help spouses learn to forgive, to communicate more honestly, and to hold to their commitment, taking their marriage vows more seriously, since these vows, when made in a religious context, are made not only to their spouses but to God as well. In addition, he says, religiously involved people enjoy a large circle of friends who can provide support in times of stress, as well as mutual accountability for both partners in living up to their marriage vows. Being part of a religious congregation where marriage is recognized and upheld as a divinely sanctioned institution—and where divorce is not taken lightly and may be frowned upon—may also help marriages stay together, Dr. Larson believes.

Just as religiously involved couples enjoy happier, more stable marriages, their children appear also to be healthier and happier than children in nonreligious families, especially in the turbulent adolescent years. A 1983 study of 3,257 high-school students found that boys and girls who attended church regularly had a higher degree of self-esteem, faith in people, and family solidarity; they also had higher grades and participated more in leadership activities at school. (An earlier study that focused on adolescents' images of God found that high self-esteem was linked with images of a loving God; respondents who saw God as vindictive and damning did not enjoy higher levels of self-esteem.) In addition, as previously mentioned in chapters 1 and 5, researchers have repeatedly found lower levels of alcohol, tobacco, and marijuana use, as well as less involvement in premarital sexual activity and juvenile delinquency, among adolescents in families who participate in religious activities.

Marriage, family, and other close relationships form our spiritual communities in microcosm, but we must also consider how we relate as spiritual beings in a macrocosm, as members of a larger community. If we are all children of the same Heavenly Father, how do we best connect with and relate to the spiritual brothers and sisters God has given us?

Belonging to a Congregation

What does "active participation" in a religious community entail? In my opinion, the following components are essential to membership in a religious congregation.

1. *Weekly attendance at worship services.* Worship is the defining act of spiritual community. It is where we live out together, in rites and rituals, the relationship we have with God as individuals *and* as a community, where we hear together the words of scripture, listen to the teachings of our spiritual leaders, and take part in sacraments and ceremonies that symbolize our relationship with God, thus reaffirming and shoring up our faith as individuals. Worship is where "it all comes together," and as such, I believe it is the most important, indeed essential, component of church or synagogue membership.

2. *Regular participation in fellowship events with other church/synagogue members.* I define "fellowship" as activities focusing on the social aspects of life in the worship community; fellowship is play together, whereas ministry is work together. Possibilities include a broad selection of activities, starting with coffee hour after worship services, picnics, and potluck suppers, and extending to church softball leagues, singles groups, and trips taken together. Through fellowship activities, we build the social networks that so enhance our quality of life, may help prevent illness and lengthen life, and boost our ability to cope with difficulties.

Friendships in general are supportive of health and well-being, but spiritual friendships provide an added dimension, an intimacy based on the conscious and committed sharing of one's deepest values. When friends attempt to live by the same moral teachings of their faith tradition, their relationship may be enhanced by values such as tolerance, forgiveness, and commitment to one another as spiritual siblings—children of the same Father—a commitment that goes beyond the normal bounds of relationships between people who do not share spiritual values.

3. *Regular participation in ministry within the congregational framework.* In the Judeo-Christian tradition, we are called to serve those in need, and our religious community should provide many opportunities for service. To name just a few:

- singing in the choir or playing a musical instrument
- working in a food pantry, soup kitchen, or other program of outreach to the poor
- joining other members of the congregation in promoting religious convictions in the larger community (e.g., lobbying for better housing for the poor, promoting quality medical care for the dispossessed, working to diminish street violence, advocating the rights of victims of crime)
- teaching Sunday school
- helping to maintain the sanctuary grounds or building
- visiting and running errands for shut-ins and people who are hospitalized or in nursing homes
- leading a prayer group
- assisting with clerical tasks in the office

Truly, the options for service within a religious community are endless. We may also find ourselves called to serve within the context of our beliefs, but outside the confines of our religious community. For example, my work as a physician and a professor is my most important ministry, yet it has little direct connection to my church membership. I have directly served my church at various times (as deacon, youth leader, and Sunday-school teacher), but most of my ministry takes place at the hospital and in the clinic, at medical schools, and at conferences for physicians. To determine where we are called to serve, it helps to pray for guidance, evaluate our gifts, receive advice, and realistically appraise the time we can give.

A caution about ministry: too often, people throw themselves into a plethora of service activities; they start to "live at church," cutting back on family time, personal-prayer and Bible-study time, and self-care habits like exercise, all in order to "do more for God." Ministry is essential to our growth as believing people; it develops naturally out of our love of God, and it is good for us, providing meaning and purpose in life. But we must seek a balance. Overwork is overwork, no matter where it takes place, and service can become idolatry when it takes precedence over everything else. I have sometimes recommended that my patients cut back on their ministry activities so they can spend some time enjoying God through prayer and Bible study. It is important, too, to live fully as the human beings God created by participating in creative activities like playing a musical instrument or painting, and recreational activities like bird-watching and playing golf.

In short, if you find yourself working at the church or synagogue all weekend and several nights during the week, you may need to re-evaluate. Ministry does not have to be slavery in order to be significant and fulfilling, and it should not steal away the time we need to spend with our spouses, children, and other family members. On the other hand, if you have no time for ministry activities—for example, because of a demanding work schedule—this, too, needs re-evaluation. There should be time for God in every person's life—time for worship, time for rest in God (the Sabbath), time for individual Bible study and prayer, and time for service to others. Seeking a balance among the many demands of our lives, we may well need guidance from fellow believers, which brings us to the next component of active participation in religious community.

4. *Accountability to a pastor, spiritual director, and/or small group.* For independent-minded Americans, "accountability" can have an unpleasant ring. But in an authentic faith journey, there is no getting around the requirement for accountability, by which I mean a willing commitment to share, regularly and honestly, the course of our journeys as people of faith, under the guidance of a respected friend or mentor. Just as we need to seek God's will and be obedient to it, we need to be open to human support, feedback, and—yes—admonishment when it is needed. We must be willing to follow the apostle Paul's directive to "speak the truth in love" (Ephe-

sians 4:15) to one another, and to hear what our fellow believers have to say to us as well. This does not mean that we sit in judgment of each other, or that we present ourselves blindly to an authority figure who pronounces approval, condemnation, and "marching orders." Rather, we are well served when others who care about us hear our stories, encourage us in our strengths, and lovingly point out our need for growth.

In chapter 9, I mentioned spiritual direction as an important and useful practice to help us grow in our spiritual lives. You may also want to explore the possibility of joining a small group for regular prayer and discernment together.

One of the most successful Christian accountability and support-group structures is found in a renewal program called Cursillo—Spanish for "little course." Known as "a short course in Christianity," Cursillo started in Spain in the 1940s, when Catholic priests were searching for a way to bring men back into regular worship and a deeper participation in religious community. Proving its worth as a program for the renewal of faith, Cursillo migrated to the United States in the 1950s, and subsequently was adapted for use by Protestant denominations. Still known as "Cursillo" in the Episcopal Church, the program goes by other names as well: "Tres Dias" (Three Days) for Lutherans, "Walk to Emmaus" for Methodists, and "Rainbow Weekends" for some nondenominational churches.

Participation in the Cursillo movement starts with attendance at the "short course in Christianity," a three-day retreat that includes instruction, fellowship, and worship. Every participant has a sponsor who has already attended the weekend; the sponsor's duties include making sure the new "Cursillista" takes part in what is known as "the Fourth Day," the follow-up activities after the weekend that provide an excellent structure for support and accountability. The centerpiece of the Fourth Day is called "group reunion," a weekly meeting of several Cursillistas who follow a strict format, first praying for the guidance of the Holy Spirit, then each reviewing the week's spiritual activities in the following categories:

- *piety:* personal prayer, worship attendance, participation in spiritual direction
- *study:* Bible-reading, study of other faith-related works (books, videos, music), contemplation of God's creation

- *action:* ministry activities; what we have done to advance God's kingdom in the world

Group-reunion members form a covenant, pledging confidentiality and accountability through regular attendance and sincere participation in the group. People who have participated in such groups for a number of years find them to be a cornerstone of their faith development.

Cursillistas also participate in a larger monthly meeting, known as "Ultreya" (a medieval Spanish word meaning "forward," as a leader would encourage troops to keep climbing up a difficult slope). At Ultreyas, Cursillistas gather to hear a witness speaker, to participate in group reunion with people they normally do not "group" with, and to sing and pray together.

Just as the Twelve Step programs have provided an excellent support and accountability structure for people with addictions, Cursillo provides a template for those seeking to deepen their spiritual lives. Other programs using the small-group model, including Marriage Encounter, Promise Keepers, and Community Bible Study, provide similar benefits. For medical as well as spiritual reasons, I urge my patients to look for this kind of small-group structure, to anchor them emotionally and spiritually; the intimate sharing that goes on in such groups can be an important stress buffer. I can personally attest to the value of regular participation in a small group: meeting on a weekly basis with a group of men for sharing, fellowship, Bible study, and prayer has proved to be a valuable source of support, strength, and renewal for me.

5. *Financial commitment to the religious community.* The Bible tell us to return a portion of our income to God's work, setting the tithe, or 10 percent of total earnings, as the minimal standard for financial giving (Leviticus 27:30), in recognition of the belief that all money comes from God and belongs to God, and that we are privileged to be faithful stewards of the remaining 90 percent. Such giving, according to scripture, will be rewarded:

Bring the full tithe into the storehouse, so that there may be food in my house, and thus put me to the test, says the Lord of hosts; see if I will not open the windows of heaven for you and pour down for you an overflowing of blessings. [MALACHI 3:10.]

Church and synagogue members must determine the appropriate level of giving for them as individuals and families, but pledging support to a religious community is an important component of membership. The slang phrase "Put your money where your mouth is" applies to this aspect of spiritual community: if we say we are members of this family, if we say we believe in the creeds the family espouses, we need to act out these assertions by giving our time and talents (through ministry) and treasure (money) in support of the community.

SOME DIFFICULTIES WITH RELIGIOUS COMMUNITY

These five components of active participation in religious community outlined above serve to ground us in the Bible's teachings and anchor us in love—God's love, and the love of our fellow believers. Such participation is essential to authentic spiritual growth; isolation runs completely counter to faith development, except in the extremely rare cases of those called to the life of a hermit. (This call is considered so unusual that Thomas Merton, Trappist monk, mystic, theologian, and prolific writer, had to petition his abbot for decades before he was permitted to spend most of his time alone in a cinder-block hut in the woods!)

But despite the many benefits of spiritual community, there are certainly difficulties to contend with as well. These must be honestly faced and dealt with if we are to grow spiritually. I have addressed some of these difficulties before, in chapters 2 and 8, but I will reprise a few of them here. Let me phrase some of these difficulties in terms of what you, the reader, might be saying in response to what I've written thus far in this chapter.

"It sounds like a full-time job! I don't have that kind of time!" If you are not currently an active participant in a religious community, you may be wondering how in the world people find time for worship, fellowship, ministry, and accountability activities—in addition to personal devotions, not to mention all the other responsibilities facing us! Just as I have encouraged you to start small in prayer and Bible study, I recommend starting small in community life as well. You do not have to do everything at once, nor should you force yourself to do things that you are not sure

are right for you. Start with regular worship attendance; make that your main commitment. Then try adding one fellowship activity (like coffee hour after services) and one simple ministry activity (for example, volunteering once a month to deliver Meals on Wheels). Stay with these activities for a time (perhaps a few months or so), and then add to or change your ministry focus as needed.

Most important, listen to what God may be telling you and ask for his guidance as you grow as a community member. Most people do not accelerate from zero to sixty—from no church participation to major leadership roles—in one minute or one year. Spiritual growth in all of its aspects takes time, grace, discipline, and patience, and the path will vary for each of us. Don't be overwhelmed before you get started. Just put a toe in the water—the water of worship—once a week, and see what develops from there.

"My spouse/children won't go to church/synagogue with me. They'd rather stay home on Sunday morning and have a special breakfast together as a family. I feel torn: where are my priorities supposed to be?" Worshiping together as a family is the ideal, of course, but do not let your family members' unwillingness to participate prevent you from responding to God's call in your life. Move the special Sunday-morning breakfast to Saturday (or vice versa, if you are Jewish), explain gently that church is important to you, continue to invite family members to attend if that seems appropriate, and pray that one day you will be joined by them. Your participation in religious community will probably result in a deeper love for your family, even if they are not with you in church; most likely, they will come to appreciate and respect what your faith does for you—and for them.

You may feel lonely going to church or synagogue by yourself. This certainly can be painful, but take a look around: you're undoubtedly not the only one there without family members. Reach out and talk with the person next to you after the service. Seek out others at the coffee hour. Most important, remember that you are there because God loves you and you love God; truly, in worship you are never alone. It is all right to feel sad or bereft as you come to worship, and to bring all your feelings to God, who can heal and transform them.

"*I have a close-knit family and group of friends, I volunteer at the homeless shelter, and I pray on my own. Why do I need to go to church?*" Modern science, in the form of studies like those I have cited above, *and* the Bible and religious tradition together emphasize the importance of attendance at worship and membership in a religious community. It is certainly possible to lead a morally good and emotionally satisfying life without church membership and participation, but it appears that one is less likely to reap the full benefits of the faith factor without this corporate dimension of spirituality.

People who ask, "Why do I need to go to church?" may have had negative experiences of church that need to be explored and healed. If this is the case with you, I urge you to seek healing through work with a therapist, pastoral counselor, or minister; it is tragic to allow old hurts to prevent you from a full and vital spiritual life.

Such persons might also be unfamiliar with church or synagogue, raised in a nonreligious home and familiar only with media stereotypes about churchgoers that are inaccurate and incomplete. Though often portrayed as "holy rollers" or sanctimonious prudes, most worshipers are just people, with the usual assortment of positive and negative personality traits. The only difference, according to the scientific data, is that regular church attenders tend to be happier, to enjoy better health, to have happier marriages, and to find life more meaningful than nonchurchgoers. Far from being wild-eyed fanatics or judgmental prigs, they tend to be more emotionally fulfilled and balanced, not less.

Others who say, "Why do I need to go to church?" might have tried church a few times and found it lacking. As I wrote in chapter 8, it is important to keep trying, not only to find the right religious congregation for you, but to attend regularly with an expectation that worship and other activities will come to mean more to you as time goes on. Many relationships start slowly, and so it is with membership in religious community. You may fall in love with a church or synagogue on your first visit, or it may take a year of regular attendance before you really feel at home. For the sake of your mental, spiritual, and physical health, please do not give up easily.

Each person must find his or her own "right place" for spiritual community, just as we must each respond to God's call in ways that are authentic for us. It may take some time, some trial and error, and some effort that feels difficult or even artificial at first. Both as a medical doctor and as a person of faith, I hope you will find a welcome home in a religious congregation, thus completing the third goal—with your individual prayer and Bible-study disciplines—of your spiritual program.

PART III

Synthesis

CHAPTER 12

⊹

Medicine in the Twenty-first Century: Reconciling the Twin Traditions of Healing

Throughout this book, my focus has been on patients: how the faith factor has helped my patients and many others lead healthier lives, and how you, as an individual, might activate its power in your life by developing an effective spiritual program. But since most people turn to the medical profession for help in maintaining good health, we must now consider how my field—the field of medicine—needs to change—and is changing—in order to incorporate the spiritual dimensions of healing into clinical practice.

Most doctors recite (and health-conscious people already know) a litany of basic preventive health strategies, including: Eat a low-fat diet high in grains, vegetables, and fruits. Exercise regularly. Get enough sleep. Quit smoking, or don't start. Limit alcohol consumption, and if you drink, don't drive. The list goes on and on. But where on the list is the role of the faith factor? Given the strong scientific evidence presented in previous chapters, we know religious involvement can be important in maintaining physical and mental health, recovering from illness and injury, and improving the quality of life. But we do not commonly hear its virtues proclaimed in the medical journals, or in most doctors' offices—at least not yet.

Doctors have not often endorsed the benefits of healthy spirituality for three main reasons:

1. Some physicians are not yet aware of the data I have presented to you in this book, data I believe to be strong enough to warrant consideration by all health-care professionals. This situation, however, is changing rapidly, as opportunities for presenting this information to professional and general audiences continue to expand. A rapidly growing number of medical schools have developed courses to teach students about the faith-health connection, and recent conferences on the subject for physicians and other professionals have been well attended. The general public is becoming more familiar with the faith factor because it has received extensive coverage in the media over the last several years, including numerous stories in major newspapers and magazines.

2. Many doctors have been specifically instructed in medical school to keep religion out of their medical practices—not to mix science and faith. As discussed, this emphasis arose out of a concern that we might blur crucial professional and interpersonal boundaries and unduly influence, or even harm, the patient. However, now that the faith-factor data show that religion's benefits to health are a matter of science, not faith, more and more practitioners are looking anew at the relationship between medicine and spirituality.

3. The possibility of opening "Pandora's box" is unsettling for many physicians, for they are untrained to address patients' spiritual beliefs, practices, and experiences, and do not know how to proceed once they have identified a patient's particular spiritual problem. Until recently, modern medical science and education have failed to recognize the importance of spirituality to patient care. As medical-school courses and conferences proliferate, physicians' uneasiness in incorporating spirituality into clinical settings will, I hope, abate.

I believe we will begin to see a historic transformation, a reversal of centuries-old prejudices, and a re-uniting of spirituality and medicine. We need to expand our vision of science: To re-establish in medicine the importance of religion and spirituality to people's well-being, we must learn that the scientific method can be applied to studies of patients' individual experiences and beliefs. By definition, faith ultimately transcends the scientific method; for example, no scientist can conclusively prove, using conventional scientific "proofs," whether or not God exists. However, the health benefits of believing that God exists *can be* and *have been* measured, demonstrating conclusively that faith and religious involvement aid in maintaining health, boosting recovery, and enhancing well-being.

As doctors learn how to incorporate the spiritual dimension of healing in their medical practices, doctors and patients may develop new ways of working together. The "routine office visit" of the future will, I hope, offer patients new options—options that honor the spiritual dimensions of their lives and reflect the proven importance of religious involvement to whole-person medical care. Presenting yourself at the doctor's office, you might be seen initially by the nurse, who would take your vital signs and perhaps inquire about spiritual and emotional concerns as well as medical ones. In addition to examining you, talking with you, and prescribing medications, your doctor might identify spiritual problems you are facing, provide counseling and encouragement, and even pray with you for healing, if you so desire. Afterward, you might return to the nurses' suite for additional tests or procedures, and then move on to the staff chaplain or to volunteer prayer ministers for counseling support and healing prayer. If you are seeking a religious congregation or a pastor or spiritual director, the doctor, the nurse, or the chaplain might make a referral for you. Finally, you might add your name to a list of people desiring prayer by intercessors. Using Internet technology, your prayer request could be shared with willing intercessors locally, nationally, and internationally. Given the encouraging results of the relatively few intercessory prayer studies completed to date, we can only imagine the positive impact such prayer might have!

This vision of the future is exactly that: a vision, one not commonly witnessed today. However, you need not wait to create an approach to healing that combines medicine and spirituality. You will probably not find all the resources you need within the confines of your doctor's office, but many useful spiritual resources are available in most communities. Let's take a look at how you can get spiritually oriented medical care should you desire it, by considering the roles of various professionals in supporting your quest for physical, mental, and spiritual well-being.

DOCTORS AND FAITH: A NEW HORIZON

After a talk I gave about faith and medicine to a church group, a woman in the audience raised her hand with a question.

271

"This all sounds very nice," she said, "but my doctor is just not that kind of person. He barely seems to remember who I am most of the time, and I'm sure there's no way he's ever going to even think about praying with me!" Many of the other church members in the audience nodded vigorously. They could not imagine finding a doctor who would relate to them on a spiritual level.

To be frank, it may not be easy to find such a doctor. In addition to the effects of their training, which in most cases ignored religion or discouraged its use in the clinical setting, doctors have been shown in a number of studies to be significantly less religious than the general public. In one study, researchers T. A. Maugans and W. C. Wadland looked at how religious factors affect the practice of family medicine by surveying two groups: family-medicine doctors and patients of three family-medicine practices. They found that 91 percent of the patients believed in God, but only 64 percent of the physicians; patients were also more likely than doctors to use prayer (85 versus 60 percent) and to feel close to God (74 versus 43 percent).

Despite the doctors' lower levels of religiosity, 77 percent of them said they occasionally discussed religious matters with patients. However, most of the patients surveyed did not remember doctors' ever inquiring about religion. Doctors who spent two or more hours a week in formal religious activities (like worship) were most likely to talk with their patients about spiritual issues; nonreligious doctors said they never asked about religion in their intake interviews. Doctors were most inclined to address spiritual issues with patients who were facing terminal illness or decisions about abortion. These are appropriate times for the inclusion of the spiritual dimension, of course, but they are not the *only* such times.

Some doctors define and advertise their practices as incorporating religious and spiritual issues in treatment. If you are seeking a doctor who is attentive to your spiritual concerns, I recommend a visit to such a practice for a careful look. The prejudice against religion in medicine is so entrenched that prospective patients might worry that openly religious doctors lack medical credentials, skill, or experience, or that such doctors might inappropriately avoid using medications or medical procedures, tending to put greater emphasis on prayer or other spiritual practices. Throughout this book, I have proposed that the best medicine is one that combines up-to-date medical technology *and* spiritual practices, as appropriate for each patient. Are doctors who identify themselves as being religious practicing this type of medicine? A scientific study of Christian psychiatrists directed by Dr. David Larson found that they embraced both science and faith in their medical practice. In this study, researchers surveyed 193 psychiatrists and psychiatry residents who belonged to the Christian Medical and Dental Society, a professional organization of physicians and dentists dedicated to incorporating spiritual issues and principles in medical care. Unlike most mental-health professionals, these doctors were found to be somewhat more religious than the American general public. The respondents were given seven psychiatric diagnoses and asked to evaluate the probable effectiveness of three possible treatments: Bible-reading and prayer, insight psychotherapy, and psychotropic medications. For schizophrenia and mania, the psychiatrists favored pharmaceutical treatment, as would the majority of their non-Christian colleagues. For depressive neurosis (though not major depressive disorder), insight psychotherapy was considered most effective. For alcoholism, sociopathy, suicidal intent, and grief reaction, they rated use of the Bible and prayer as more effective than insight psychotherapy and pharmaceuticals, although they did not rule out using these methods in conjunction with Bible-reading and prayer for treating these difficult patients. The Christian psychiatrists demonstrated a professional approach to their medical practices; they were selective in their use of spiritual means to help their patients, and endorsed and employed standard medical methods whenever appropriate; but they also recognized the limitations of these approaches for certain troublesome clinical problems.

Though it may not be easy to find doctors who are comfortable discussing religious matters, it should not be impossible. I encourage you to seek advice from word-of-mouth sources, including members of local religious congregations and spiritual leaders. Of course, even if many patients would find it helpful to have a doctor who will pray with them, this is not absolutely necessary. Others—family members, ministers, chaplains, friends at church or synagogue—can pray with and for the patient. It *is* important, however, that doctors be aware of and respect their patients' spirituality, and even encourage it, if possible. Medicine is gradually embracing the whole-person model, recognizing the patient's physical, psychological, and social status as part of their health assessment. Now doctors are being urged to recognize another critically important aspect of patients' lives—their religious commitment and spirituality. Since many people say religion is the most important influence in their lives, doctors cannot hope to offer whole-person care if they neglect the spiritual dimension.

For several years, I have been teaching medical students and residents about how to incorporate the long-neglected spiritual dimension of patient care in their medical practice. As part of the "Faith and Medicine" program sponsored by the John Templeton Foundation through the National Institute for Healthcare Research, I have had the opportunity to witness and to encourage the development of exciting new educational programs by medical schools seeking to train the next generation of doctors to be sensitive to this domain. A simple approach to this area of medical education helps medical students and practicing doctors grasp the essentials. That is why my lectures continue to include this basic instruction: ask patients at least three fundamental questions during the initial (intake) interview:

1. *Is religion or spirituality important to you?* If the answer is "yes," the doctor can go on to ask in an open-ended way, "Tell me more about that." If the answer is "no," the doctor might ask, "Was religion or spirituality ever important in your life?" It may be important to know if a patient has rejected religion; he or she may harbor psychological pain that needs to be addressed. This is a genuine medical issue, since studies have indicated that the rejection of religion is correlated with a decline in happiness and higher rates of alcoholism. (See chapter 1 for discussions of these studies.)

2. *Do your religious or spiritual beliefs influence the way you look at your medical problems and the way you think about your health?* When patients answer "yes," doctors can ask them to describe their beliefs and how such beliefs influence the way they take care of themselves. Such information will be vital in determining the choice and course of medical therapy. A "yes" to this question leads the doctor directly to a third question.

3. *Would you like me to address your religious or spiritual beliefs and practices with you?* If the answer is "yes," the doctor needs to ask, "In what way?" Does the patient want the doctor to pray *with* him or her? To pray *for* him or her, either personally or as part of a "prayer chain"? The physician should, in turn, follow each patient's lead when determining the appropriate approach to meeting individual spiritual needs.

I believe every doctor should be able to ask these three questions and respond appropriately to the patients' answers. Not all doctors will wish to participate in prayer, scripture-reading, or other spiritual interventions with their patients. Doctors are free to practice the type of medicine they wish, within professional boundaries of clinical training and expertise. A doctor cannot and should not be forced to pray with patients, any more than a doctor can, or should, force patients to pray! For those who do not wish to delve deeply into the spiritual dimension with patients, asking these three questions when getting to know a patient, expressing interest in the patient's spirituality, and being respectful of the patient's religious convictions will be enough. (These physicians might also refer patients to others who can help them explore their spiritual needs more fully—chaplains and other clergy, for example.) Some doctors will go further, becoming proficient in spiritual interventions like praying with patients, spiritual counseling, and scripture-sharing.

When patient and doctor are of different faith traditions, the extent of religious sharing may be limited, given the significant differences in doctrine and practice between religions. However, doctors who wish to do so might develop a more generic spiritual approach to prayer in such instances. For example, one might choose to practice the Relaxation Response, select spoken prayer with inclusive references to "God" or "the Holy One" without mention of particular creeds or doctrines, or even suggest a moment of shared silence.

I hope doctors will encourage patients who are religious, but I believe that doctors should not "push religion" on patients or attempt to convert them to a particular faith. Doing so violates the trust so essential to this healing partnership. We should promote, not preach, endorsing the health value of authentic religiosity but respecting patients' choices about denomination and doctrine.

WALLS AND FENCES

As faith and medicine come together once again, we must be wary of delicate and crucial boundaries. But honoring those boundaries need not prevent us from going forward in our quest to combine the ancient twin traditions of healing. I have come to think of this balancing act in terms of two metaphors: walls and fences.

Twenty years ago, when I was in medical school, the wall between medicine and spirituality stood tall. I don't recall religious or spiritual issues ever being mentioned in lectures, other than in snide remarks. For example, a professor of obstetrics-gynecology once disparaged the rhythm method of birth control as "Vatican roulette"—at which a braver student than I promptly and rightfully took offense. Religion was indeed "the forgotten factor," a taboo subject among doctors and students. Although I had been a person of faith since childhood, I acquiesced to the secular model of training I saw around me and kept religion for sanctuaries and Sundays.

Yet something began to change in me by the time I was a medical resident. Seeing open and well-marked Bibles next to bedpans, watching sick people turn to faith to help them through chemotherapy, hearing family members in the intensive-care-unit waiting room pray for strength and support for their beloved and for themselves, I discovered what has now been firmly established by a number of researchers: issues of faith are important to patients. They don't want to check their beliefs at the sickroom door, and they don't want to be hemmed in by the artificial wall of separation between faith and medicine.

Should that wall, like the wall of Jericho, "come a-tumblin' down," as the old spiritual suggests? Or do "good fences make good neighbors," as a Robert Frost poem declares?

Both! The wall should come tumbling down, and be replaced by a fence.

Standing at the Berlin Wall, President Ronald Reagan challenged the Soviet premier: "Mr. Gorbachev, tear this wall down!" he cried. Today, many patients issue the same demand of their doctors. They want their spiritual needs discussed and met when they receive medical treatment. Doctors who choose to ignore religion and spirituality in medicine miss opportunities and resources for helping people in need.

If the wall is obsolete, what about a fence? Good fences *do* make good neighbors by marking boundaries, and we need to observe important boundaries between medicine and religion. Although many patients want their spiritual needs addressed by doctors, others do not, preferring to have these needs met elsewhere. Patient autonomy is a bedrock value in medicine, and it must be heeded in matters of religious beliefs and spiritual practices as much as in matters of choosing types of treatment for breast cancer. Physician autonomy in choosing whom to serve and how to do so is likewise imperative. All doctors don't perform surgery and psychotherapy; it is unlikely that all doctors will choose to pray with their patients.

Walls separate, fences demarcate. Walls between medicine and religion should come down, allowing free access. Fences between them should be respected, allowing proper boundaries. As doctors and patients travel in this newly mapped territory, both will benefit—and both will learn new lessons about how faith and medicine can work together.

A New Partnership: Doctors and Clergy

You might be wondering, "If my doctor is talking with me about my spiritual life and praying with me, then why do I need to see my pastor or a chaplain?" Physicians will not replace clergy; rather, medical and spiritual professionals should learn to work closely together to provide the best possible whole-person care. I have seen the power of this partnership a number of times, most memorably with my patient Serena, whom I mentioned in chapter 7; her father, a minister, and I joined hands to pray for her in her hospital room, creating a living symbol of the healing alliance clergy and doctors can form on behalf of their patients.

Many doctors will not want to embrace a spiritual-counseling role with their patients, but even those who do will face certain challenges. They will need additional training in order to deal appropriately with matters of the spirit. Almost all will face time constraints, given the strictures of current practices in the era of managed care. When limited to a ten-minute office visit, we doctors will do well simply to "touch base" with the patient on spiritual and emotional matters. Sadly, such limitations impede the development of an effective doctor-patient relationship, which requires time, and since this relationship is one of the key mediators of healing, I am extremely concerned that patient care and healing itself will be compromised in a medical system driven primarily by economic concerns. In such an environment, doctors may have to address spirituality with patients primarily by referring them to clergy members, just as today a primary-care practitioner refers patients to specialists for the definitive care of many problems.

Given the time limitations imposed on most doctors, the role of the clergy is more important than ever in assisting people who are facing serious health problems. But the clergy's role is separate and distinct from the doctor's: Ordained clergy have sacramental authority, the ability to hear confessions and pronounce absolution, to baptize, to bless, and to anoint. Ordained rabbis, priests, deacons, and ministers, as well as trained laypersons, will also teach the specific tenets of the faith traditions they represent and offer spiritual guidance based on those principles. In addition, most clergy persons represent congregations who may be enlisted to pray for or offer other assistance to the patient.

Scientific studies have shown that patients find great comfort and help in clergy visits. In a study I mentioned in chapter 9, women with breast cancer found visits from clergy members very helpful in dealing with their illness, particularly when the clergy persons used prayer, counseling, and Bible-reading in their visits. In another study, of 101 cancer patients and 45 parents of children with cancer, both groups derived comfort and help from clergy visits, particularly when these took place in the patients' or the parents' homes. Both the cancer patients and the parents of children with cancer found the clergy visits most helpful when they included the use of prayer and religious readings; they reported that they found secular approaches, like talking about the family, less valuable.

In the case of mental illness and emotional distress, clergy and other trained religious professionals also have a special role to play. Many spiritual directors, who may be ordained or lay, can offer directees a spiritual approach informed by insights from psychotherapy. A study comparing spiritual directors and psychotherapists found that spiritual directors were much more likely to use psychotherapeutic techniques with their clients than psychotherapists were to use spiritual approaches with theirs. Both professionals estimated that their clients spent about the same amount of time addressing psychological and physical concerns, but spiritual directors were more willing to use a wide array of techniques—psychotherapeutic as well as spiritual (prayer, meditation, silence)—than were psychotherapists. Interestingly, spiritual directors and psychotherapists were equally likely to have undergone psychotherapy themselves. But psychotherapists were much less likely to have experienced spiritual direction, and they rarely "crossed over" into spiritual dimensions with their clients.

The resources of religious professionals—clergy, pastoral counselors, and spiritual directors—may be especially important in helping people overcome mental illnesses like depression, since religious people may recover faster when their treatment includes a spiritual dimension. A study conducted by psychologist Rebecca Propst (mentioned in chapter 4) found that religious patients with mild to moderate depression were more likely to recover when the therapist conducting their therapy groups used religious imagery. In the group using religious imagery, only 14 percent of the patients remained depressed at the conclusion of the study, compared with 60 percent in the group using nonreligious imagery.

Despite the results of this study and others affirming the value of the spiritual dimension in treating emotional problems, finding a mental-health professional who is skilled at and comfortable with clients' spiritual experiences is not always easy. A survey of 409 psychologists found that only 40 percent believed in a personal, transcendent God; and only 18 percent valued organized religion as a source of spirituality—a significant finding, given that 43 percent of Americans attend worship services weekly, according to a Gallup poll. Though 53 percent of the psychologists believed that religious beliefs were helpful for most people, the majority thought it inappropriate to use religious scripture or prayer in psychotherapy (55 and 68 percent, respectively). One-third of the respondents believed they were personally competent to counsel clients regarding spiritual matters. The "religiosity gap" between psychologists and the general public is significant; however, this study shows that mental-health professionals have started to value religious commitment and practices as positive aspects of their clients' lives.

Not long ago, a similar group of psychologists would have been likely to dismiss religious involvement as a sign of neuroticism, so this study shows evidence of progress that will be enhanced significantly when training programs in clinical psychology include a more positive approach to spirituality in psychological practice. Recently, the American Psychiatric Association has developed guidelines to promote the inclusion of spirituality in psychiatric residency training, and a model curriculum for psychiatric residents has been created. These developments represent a major revolution in the field of psychiatry, whose founding father, Sigmund

Freud, denounced religious beliefs as illusions and universal neurotic fantasies which developed to ease deeply held anxieties. For many years, only members of the clergy provided a "safe place" for people to discuss their problems and their religious beliefs.

In the future, I see health and religious professionals working hand in hand to promote the physical, mental, and spiritual health of patients. This has occurred, of course, on the institutional level, with the inclusion of chaplains on the staffs of hospitals and other facilities, such as nursing homes. For outpatients, finding spiritual care can be more difficult, unless they are already connected to congregations. To close this gap in spiritual care, I envision rabbis, ministers, priests, and skilled lay pastoral caregivers becoming part of an interdisciplinary caring team, formal or informal, that brings different skills to bear on patients' problems.

The medical world is now considering the need for such changes in medical practice. These changes are coming about because patients are demanding them, and because more and more doctors are learning about the scientific studies demonstrating the positive impact of religious involvement on health and well-being. To continue reconnecting the twin traditions of faith and medicine, doctors will need to learn a great deal more about exactly how religiosity helps people stay healthier, recover from illness, live longer, and experience greater life satisfaction, and will need to be willing to incorporate a respect and sensitivity to spiritual values and practices in clinical care.

RESEARCH: DIRECTIONS FOR THE NEW MILLENNIUM

Building on the strong foundation created by numerous scientific studies of the faith factor in medicine, medical researchers can now go forward to examine in new depth its mechanisms. My Clearwater study of the effects of intercessory prayer on rheumatoid arthritis, mentioned in chapter 3, is one of a number of new studies currently under way on the effects of prayer. Given that most people use prayer in dealing with illness, we need many more similar studies that will look for answers to questions like these:

• For patients who pray for their own recovery from physical illness, what method or type of prayer brings the best results? Margaret Poloma's studies of prayer types indicate that the patients' approach to prayer may have a marked impact on its results in terms of health and happiness. This research question could be posed among patients suffering from a variety of physical, mental, and addictive disorders.

• How do frequency and duration of prayer affect medical outcomes?

• Do patient attitudes regarding the importance and effectiveness of prayer influence health outcomes?

• Do Randolph Byrd's findings showing the effectiveness of intercessory prayer for heart patients hold up in randomized controlled trials of patients with other conditions (like cancer and AIDS) and in other settings (primary-care clinics, emergency rooms, nursing homes)? If so, what are the implications for health-care policy?

• How can intercessory prayer best be used to help people heal? Who should pray?

Scholars of the faith-health connection are calling for more *longitudinal research studies*—studies that follow patients over a long period of time, rather than taking a one-time "snapshot" measurement of health and religious commitment factors. Longitudinal studies are more difficult and expensive to conduct, but they alone will answer questions about causality, such as "Do people who attend church weekly develop fewer cases of cancer than people who attend once a year or never?" The faith-factor data include results from relatively few longitudinal studies, but they are among the most significant results to date—for example, the study of individuals in religious and nonreligious kibbutzim in Israel, mentioned in chapter 11, followed patients for *fifteen years* to determine mortality rates among the two populations.

Frequency of church attendance has been an influential variable in assessing religiosity in many studies, but recognition of the complex, multidimensional nature of religious beliefs and practices is imperative for designing better studies in the future. For example, studies that use measures of intrinsic and extrinsic religiosity and patients' perceptions of the importance and effects of their beliefs are needed to evaluate the faith factor's impact more carefully.

ANSWERS TO SOME FREQUENTLY ASKED QUESTIONS

Whenever I speak to groups of people, ranging from medical students to church members, I can count on several key questions' being raised. Since you, too, may be wondering about the same issues, I thought it might be helpful to mention some of them here.

Q. *How can you say religious people are healthier when we all know religious people who have prayed fervently for healing yet have not been healed?*

A. Of course, not all people who are religious enjoy long, healthy lives; nor do all who pray for healing or receive intercessory prayer for healing recover from illness. In this respect, religious involvement and prayer are no different from standard medical treatment: neither can offer a guarantee. When you undergo surgery to remove a diseased gallbladder, chances are good that you will survive and experience few, if any, complications. But even under the best of circumstances, some patients *do* experience serious complications; a few die. Still, many patients undergo this procedure every day. They do not demand that the surgeon guarantee their safe and speedy recovery; if they did, the surgery could not be performed. Even the safest medical procedure carries some risk of failure, and so it is with religious involvement and healing prayer.

In a similar way, when we look at groups of patients, we see that religious involvement, including prayer, does appear to have significant health benefits, helping people recover faster, and with fewer complications, from serious illness, as well as helping them cope better with their illness. Looking at any one patient, however, we cannot make such a prediction. In recommending and undertaking the medical treatment of any individual patient, doctors operate on probabilities, not certainties; guarantees are not part of our practice. We draw our knowledge from research studies of groups of people, and such studies indicate that religion is good for your health—*not* that religion will prevent every instance of illness or prolong every life.

Q. *Are we trivializing religion by focusing on its pragmatic aspects?*

A. This is a real danger when we attempt to embrace religion only for its health benefits. Such an approach would exemplify an extrinsic religious orientation—engaging in religious activities primarily in order to gain nonspiritual advantages—and as we have seen in the research results, this attempt to manipulate God to gain health advantages will not produce the desired results. To me, documenting God's blessings through the use of scientific method does not trivialize religion; rather, it glorifies God, and has the potential to reveal God's truth to more people. Furthermore, the primary purpose of religion should always be to "love God with our heart, soul, mind, and strength" and to "love our neighbor as ourselves." We need not worry about trivializing God, whose mysteries will never be completely understood by science. If we engage in our research with an attitude of respect, even reverence, for the truth that will emerge, I believe we will avoid the risk of trivializing it.

Q. *Do we need to know how prayer works before using it medically?*

A. We have presented evidence for the generally positive benefits of prayer; negative effects are rare (for example, Margaret Poloma demonstrated that the exclusive use of ritual prayer is associated with depressed mood). Understanding the actual mechanisms of prayer's effects on health will probably take many years or even decades of research. To wait for such findings before using prayer to help sick people would hinder healing for many individuals who might benefit (with little risk) from prayer.

In many cases, the medical pioneers of past centuries went forward with effective treatments without proof of their physical mechanisms. In chapter 2, I wrote about Ignaz Semmelweis, the Austrian doctor who insisted the medical students wash their hands between the hospital autopsy room and patient wards, thus curtailing the spread of childbed fever. He did not know *why* hand-washing prevented infection; he simply observed that it did so, and, thanks to his courageous intervention, many lives were saved.

An eighteenth-century English country doctor named Edward Jenner took a similarly brave step. Jenner was struggling to find a way to prevent smallpox, which then claimed as many as forty-five thousand lives each year in Great Britain alone. Giving doses of the smallpox virus itself was the only preventive measure known. Though occasionally effective, it resulted in too many deaths to be useful.

Call it the workings of a scientifically trained mind, a flash of divine inspiration, or both, but Dr. Jenner observed that milkmaids rarely contracted smallpox. Constantly exposed to cows, the young women were also exposed to cowpox, a similar but much milder disease than smallpox. Were the young women immune to smallpox because of this exposure to cowpox? If so, Dr. Jenner hypothesized, cowpox might be used as an effective but much safer vaccine against smallpox.

In 1796, Jenner tested his observation by injecting a boy, James Phipps, with the cowpox virus from a milkmaid's lesions. After running a slight fever, James recovered fully. Two months later, Jenner gave James a potentially lethal injection of active smallpox virus—a measure that would probably be viewed as unethical by modern institutional review boards for research studies. Fortunately, the boy did not contract the disease. Jenner's hypothesis, based solely on observation, and not fully understood scientifically or accepted at the time by skeptical colleagues, was correct.

Unlike Edward Jenner, we do not have to risk the lives of patients in order to assess the effects of prayer or religious involvement on health. Like him, however, researchers in this field have often been met with skepticism and even scorn by their colleagues. This is changing, because of the strength of the faith-factor data. Given the relatively low risks of negative effects in the use of prayer and religious involvement, and given the strong possibilities of their positive effects, doctors are wise to proceed with the appropriate use of these resources, for the sake of patients' health, while waiting for, and encouraging the undertaking of, research studies to reveal exactly how they work.

Q. *If I don't get better, is it because I don't have faith?*

A. No. Faith *is* important to healing, but we cannot force God to do things our way, no matter how great our faith or how fervent our prayers. It is important to remember that we cannot manipulate or control the power of God for healing. The disposition of our illness will be determined by God, not simply by our level of faith. Also, we need to maintain an appropriate perspective; inevitably, whether or not we are healed, every day we come one step closer to our deaths.

Q. *Are you saying that all religions are the same?*

A. No. I *am* saying that the research to date has not shown that a commitment to any particular religion or denomination is more advantageous to health than any other. The research data suggests that the medical value of the faith factor depends more upon the intensity of our devotion and participation than upon the particularity of our preferred creed. However, religions vary greatly in terms of doctrine and practices and in their perspectives on life, death, and suffering. I believe that the choice of a particular faith tradition is a matter of utmost consequence, and should be based on one's perception of what constitutes truth, not what will give you better health.

Q. *If I go to my doctor with a sore throat, do I need to say a prayer with him or her in order to get better?*

A. Absolutely not. If your sore throat is caused by a strep infection, you need penicillin or a similar antibiotic. If you would *like* prayer as part of your treatment for a routine illness, and if your doctor is so inclined, prayer is always appropriate, but it is not necessary to make prayer or spiritual discussion part of every medical encounter.

Q. *Are you saying that physicians need to be "doctors of the soul"?*

A. No, but I believe doctors need to be sensitive to patients' beliefs concerning the soul's existence and its importance with regard to matters of health. Our primary role, given to us by society and for which we are trained, is to focus on health. Society has not given doctors the task of being spiritual teachers. But the spiritual realm *is* relevant for doctors, because it affects our assigned "territory"; as the faith-factor data have shown, there is a strong relationship between religious involvement and health. Doctors, then, can be expected to address spiritual issues in the context of the patient's health. Unless they have special qualifications, however, they would not be expected to provide spiritual guidance, to teach about doctrine, or to administer sacraments like baptism or reconciliation; these areas are the province of clergy and designated lay spiritual leaders.

In contrast, ministers, pastoral counselors, and spiritual directors are expected to deal with the spiritual in all of its aspects; their realm is not confined to the effects of spirituality on the health of the body and mind. Naturally, those trained to provide religious guidance do help people deal with medical issues. When a pastoral-counseling client is struggling with cancer, he or she will almost certainly want to talk with the counselor or minister about how the illness affects his or her spiritual life (and vice versa). But the pastor or counselor will *not* try to treat the cancer; that is the physician's realm.

If both doctor and patient so desire, they may share spiritual experiences like prayer and scripture-reading, just as the clergy person and the patient might share a discussion of medical decisions facing the patient. But the doctor will not pronounce absolution, and the clergy person will not prescribe medicine.

Q. *Personally, I would be offended if my doctor talked to me about religion.* Must *spirituality be part of medical care?*

A. If you are not religiously committed, it would certainly seem out of place for your doctor to "push" religion. Even if you are religious, you do not need to discuss your religious beliefs or pray with your doctor in order to reap the faith factor's many benefits. However, doctors do have an obligation to present research data that affect your health. To draw an analogy, if your doctor knows you are smoking two packs of cigarettes a day, he or she is duty-bound to tell you about your increased risk for cancer and cardiovascular disease due to your tobacco habit, whether or not you want to hear such bad news. Similarly, if your doctor learns that you have stopped going to worship services, he or she would be justified in stating the fact that your change in religious practice may have negative health consequences. This is a matter of medical knowledge, not a matter of religious preference or moral judgment. That is why it is important for doctors to ask basic questions (as outlined above) about your religious involvement in a sensitive, nonoffensive manner—because scientific studies have shown that religious commitment can make a difference to your health and well-being.

I hope you will feel comfortable discussing the broad outlines of your religious involvement with your physician, but you do not need to go into detail with your doctor about your religious beliefs, or accept any religious advice from him or her. As I have said, your boundaries—and your doctor's boundaries—should be respected as a basic principle of the effective doctor-patient relationship.

CROSSING THE FINAL FRONTIER IN WHOLE-PERSON MEDICINE

The taboos in medicine are changing. At one time, doctors withheld bad prognoses from seriously ill patients for fear of upsetting them and thereby limiting chances for recovery. Today, we doctors customarily tell patients everything we know about their conditions and the probabilities for recovery.

The next taboo to fall was the topic of death. Doctors used to avoid discussing death, even imminent death in intensive-care settings, with their patients. No one wished to "pull the plug" on patients with terminal illnesses; doctors instead chose to continue vigorous but futile attempts to preserve life. The works of Elisabeth Kübler-Ross and others, accompanied by the growth of the hospice movement, threw this issue into the open. Today, we discuss living wills and do-not-resuscitate orders with some patients judged to be terminally ill. (However, a recent national study indicates that much remains to be accomplished in this area. The Study to Understand Prognoses and Preferences for Outcomes and Risks of Treatments [SUPPORT] looked at the role of medical treatment at the end of life for 4,301 patients in the advanced stages of life-threatening illnesses. It found that the patients' instructions—including such important directives as "I don't want to be put on a machine"—were frequently ignored by their physicians. Even when special efforts were made by investigators to inform physicians of the patients' physical status and to facilitate communication between patients, families, and physicians, doctors often overlooked patients' wishes.)

Until recently, sexuality, like death, was taboo for discussion between patients and physicians, unless the patient specifically brought up a sexual problem or question. With the emergence of AIDS, details of sexual practices that I and other doctors would never have mentioned fifteen years ago are discussed routinely with increasingly (and surprisingly) little embarrassment.

The final taboo subject between doctors and patients, of course, is the spiritual realm. Revitalizing the spiritual dimension of medicine is *terra incognita*. There are few role models for doctors who want to meet the needs of the two out of three patients who long to discuss spiritual issues with their physicians. And yet incorporating the spiritual dimension into medical practice can be so natural, so obvious, that only centuries of prejudice could prevent us from seeing it: if we are to treat the whole person, we *must* consider the patient as a spiritual being as well as a biological, psychological, and social being.

But even as physicians start to embrace the spiritual dimension of medicine, the kind of doctor-patient relationship I have described is endangered by the managed-care revolution. Brought on by economic forces, this profound change in American medicine has turned physicians into "providers," and "managed care" has turned medical care into a commodity to be churned out at the lowest cost. When we measure our effectiveness by profit margins, medicine is endangered. Real listening cannot exist when the doctor is forced to end a patient visit every ten minutes in order to keep costs down. Doctors won't have the opportunity to develop that crucial "third ear," the listening skills that allow for confession of painful secrets and establishment of genuine empathy between doctor and patient. Managed care has the potential to squeeze the healing power of empathic listening right out of medicine, and I am deeply concerned about medicine's future as this trend continues to build momentum.

But there is hope. So many astonishing medical developments occurred so quickly in the last several decades; in my father's era in medical school, who would have thought that polio would be a thing of the past, and that some cancers would be curable, by the end of the century? We may see a similar explosion of our capacity for healing when we—doctors and patients—become more open to God's healing power.

"Where there is no vision, the people perish," says the writer of the Book of Proverbs (Proverbs 29:18, KJV); medicine, like people, can perish without a strong sense of direction for the future. We need to dream boldly as we approach this unknown territory which is exciting and full of potential; we may need to free ourselves of the constraints of old ways of thinking. Perhaps an entirely new model of medicine will emerge as faith and medicine reunite. We cannot predict what is going to happen, just as my father's generation of doctors could not possibly have predicted the radical change in medicine due to the development of the first antibiotics. But we can take our parts in this historic transformation eagerly, knowing that a reconciliation between faith and medicine may well help restore medicine by strongly affirming the primacy of the patient and the true vocation of the doctor.

✦

As society grows in its recognition of the need for spirituality in all dimensions of life, perhaps we will see a long-forgotten kind of medicine emerge anew, wherein the doctor's office truly can become a holy meeting ground between religion and medicine, the twin traditions of healing. When that transformation occurs, I believe we will witness a fuller flowering of the faith factor and greater opportunities for healing of mind, body, and spirit.

RESOURCES

─────────────── ✠ ───────────────

There are thousands of books, periodicals, audiotapes, and videotapes about the following subjects, and hundreds of organizations focusing on prayer, healing, and Bible study. We can offer only a small selection from this abundance of opportunities for learning and fellowship. We hope these are good places to start a quest for more information or support for your spiritual journey.

HEALING PRAYER

Organizations

Christian Healing Ministries
P.O. Box 9520
Jacksonville, FL 32208
(904) 765-3332

Publishes a newsletter, *The Healing Line,* and accepts requests for intercessory prayer. Staff members (including Francis and Judith MacNutt) will travel to speak and lead educational events nationwide. Produces training course materials, including videotapes, on healing prayer ministry.

Christian Medical and Dental Society
P.O. Box 5
Bristol, TN 37621
(423) 844-1000

A membership organization for Christian doctors, dentists, and public health professionals. Sponsors missionary trips, conferences, and a number of publications.

Resources

Institute for Christian Ministries
423 Martin Luther King Jr. Way
Tacoma, WA 98407-0384
(253) 274-8441
E-mail: JCMCENTRAL@aol.com

Roman Catholic organization with an ecumenical outreach; sponsors educational
programs for lay, clergy, and medical professionals wishing to incorporate healing
prayer into their work. Also makes referrals to trained prayer teams in the western
Washington/northern Oregon area.

Institute for Christian Renewal
New Creation Healing Center
148 Plaistow Road
Plaistow, NH 03865
(603) 382-0273

Offers conferences, seminars, and other teaching events on Christian healing; publishes a free monthly newsletter.

National Center for Jewish Healing
9 East 69th Street
New York, NY 10021
(212) 772-6601

Offers educational resources for the study and practice of healing within Judaism.

Books

Buckley, Michael. *His Healing Touch*. Mineola, N.Y.: Resurrection Press, 1987.
Finkel, Avraham, ed. *In My Flesh I See God: A Treasury of Rabbinic Insights About the
    Human Anatomy*. Northvale, N.J.: Jason Aronson, 1995.
Frankiel, Tamar, and Judy Greenfeld. *Minding the Temple of the Soul: Balancing Body,
    Mind, and Spirit Through Traditional Jewish Prayer, Movement, and Meditation*.
    Worcester, Vt.: Jewish Lights, 1997.
Kelsey, Morton. *Healing and Christianity: A Classic Study*. Minneapolis: Augsburg
    Fortress, 1995.
MacNutt, Francis. *Healing*. Notre Dame, Ind.: Ave Maria Press, 1974.
Schlemon, Barbara Leahy, Dennis Linn, and Matthew Linn. *To Heal as Jesus Healed*.
    Notre Dame, Ind.: Ave Maria Press, 1978.
Weintraub, Simkha, Rabbi, ed. *Healing of Soul, Healing of Body: Spiritual Leaders
    Unfold the Strength and Solace in Psalms*. Worcester, Vt.: Jewish Lights Press, 1995.

Resources

INTERCESSORY PRAYER MINISTRIES

The Upper Room
1908 Grand Avenue
P.O. Box 189
Nashville, TN 37202-0189
1-800-251-2468 (U.S. and Canada)
www.upperroom.org

Accepts prayer requests twenty-four hours a day, seven days a week, for its Living Prayer Center. See below for information on Upper Room publications.

Guideposts
39 Seminary Hill Road
Carmel, NY 10512
1-800-431-2344
E-mail: AtYourService@guideposts.org

Publishing organization that will include prayer requests in the staff's weekly prayer meeting on Mondays. Publishes a number of magazines and books, including *Guideposts,* an inspirational magazine ($13.97 for a one-year subscription). Interdenominational and interfaith.

National Prayer Center
1445 Boonville Avenue
Springfield, MO 65802-1894
1-800-4-PRAYER
E-mail: prayer@ag.org

The national prayer ministry of the Assemblies of God; will accept prayer requests by phone, e-mail, or fax.

INFORMATION ABOUT PRAYER IN GENERAL

Organizations and Periodicals

Shalem Institute for Spiritual Formation
5430 Grosvenor Road
Bethesda, MD 20814
(301) 897-7334
www.shalem.org

Offers programs on contemplative spirituality, information on spiritual direction, and quarterly newsletter, *Shalem News.*

Sacred Journeys
Fellowship in Prayer, Inc.
291 Witherspoon Street
Princeton, NJ 08542-3227
(609) 924-6863
www.fip.org

A bimonthly, interfaith journal of experiential articles on prayer and spirituality. Subscription is $16 per year.

Praying
The National Catholic Reporter Publishing Company, Inc.
P.O. Box 419335
Kansas City, MO 64141
1-800-333-7373

A bimonthly magazine on prayer from a Roman Catholic perspective.

Books

Donin, Hayim Halevy, Rabbi. *To Pray as a Jew: A Guide to the Prayer Book and the Synagogue Service*. New York: Basic Books, 1980.
Edwards, Tilden. *Living in the Presence: Disciplines for the Spiritual Heart*. San Francisco: HarperSanFrancisco, 1987.
Foster, Richard J. *Prayer: Finding the Heart's True Home*. San Francisco: HarperSanFrancisco, 1992.
Kaplan, Aryeh. *Jewish Meditation: A Practical Guide*. New York: Schocken Books, 1995.
Verman, Mark. *The History and Varieties of Jewish Meditation*. Northvale, N.J.: Jason Aronson, 1996.

SPIRITUAL DIRECTION

See also Shalem Institute for Spiritual Formation, above, which publishes a pamphlet about spiritual direction and sponsors an international training program for spiritual guides.

Books

Barry, William A., and William J. Connolly. *The Practice of Spiritual Direction*. San Francisco: HarperSanFrancisco, 1986.
Edwards, Tilden. *Spiritual Friend*. Mahwah, N.J.: Paulist Press, 1980.
Guenther, Margaret. *Holy Listening: The Art of Spiritual Direction*. Boston: Cowley Publications, 1992.
Leech, Kenneth. *Soul Friend: An Invitation to Spiritual Direction*. San Francisco: HarperSanFrancisco, 1992.
May, Gerald, *Care of Mind, Care of Spirit: A Psychiatrist Explores Spiritual Direction*. San Francisco: HarperSanFrancisco, 1992.

Resources

BIBLE STUDY GUIDES AND PLANS

Organizations

Bible Reading Fellowship
P.O. Box 380
Winter Park, FL 32790
(407) 628-4330
1-800-749-4331
E-mail: brf@biblereading.org

A nondenominational Christian ministry; publishes *Journey Through the Word,* a periodical offering a disciplined daily Bible-reading program, with scripture portions, commentary, and reflection questions. A one-year subscription costs $15.

Forward Movement Publications
412 Sycamore Street
Cincinnati, OH 45202
(513) 721-6659
1-800-543-1813
E-mail: forward.movement@ecunet.org

A publications ministry of the Episcopal Church. Publishes quarterly *Forward Day by Day,* a daily devotional guide to Bible reading. A one-year subscription costs $10. Large-print, Braille, and tape editions are available.

The Upper Room
1908 Grand Avenue
P.O. Box 856
Nashville, TN 37202-0189
1-800-972-0433
www.upperroom.org

An interdenominational Christian organization. Publishes *The Upper Room,* a bimonthly periodical offering daily Bible selections and devotions. Subscription costs $6.95 per year. Available in many languages and in a large-print edition.

American Bible Society
1865 Broadway
New York, NY 10023
(212) 408-1200
1-800-322-4253

Mail-order catalog offers numerous Bible editions. Pamphlets and publications for children are also available.

Presentation Ministries
3230 McHenry Avenue
Cincinnati, OH 45211
(513) 662-5378

Roman Catholic; publishes a pamphlet, *Through the Bible in One Year,* by Father Al Lauer, as well as other resources.

Project Genesis, the Jewish Learning Network
6810 Park Heights Avenue
Baltimore, MD 21215
(410) 358-9800
www.torah.org

On-line Jewish Bible study and other resources.

Books

A number of Bible editions include daily Scripture readings and commentaries. Call the American Bible Society (above) for a catalog or visit your local bookstore.

Freudmann, Lillian C. *What's in the Bible: A Concise Look at the 39 Books of the Hebrew Bible.* Northvale, N.J.: Jason Aronson, 1996.
Koester, Craig R. *A Beginner's Guide to Reading the Bible.* Minneapolis: Augsburg Fortress Publishing, 1991.
Phillips, Bob. *Daily Bible Reading Plan.* Eugene, Ore.: Harvest House, 1992.
Visotsky, Burton L. *Reading the Book: Making the Bible a Timeless Text.* New York: Schocken Books, 1996.

Lectio Divina (Meditative Bible Reading)

Hall, Thelma. *Too Deep for Words: Rediscovering Lectio Divina.* Mahwah, N.J.: Paulist Press, 1988.
Smith, Martin L. *The Word Is Very Near You: A Guide to Praying with Scripture.* Cambridge, Mass.: Cowley Publications, 1989.

NOTES

⊹

INTRODUCTION

Page 3: championed by Dr. George Engel in the 1950s: George Engel, "The Need for a New Medical Model: A Challenge for Biomedicine," *Science* 196 (1977): 129–36.

Page 4: According to polls: T. McNichol, "The New Faith in Medicine," *USA Today Weekend,* April 5–7, 1996; C. Wallis, "Faith and Healing," *Time,* June 24, 1996.

A study by Dr. Dana King: D. E. King and B. Bushwick, "Beliefs and Attitudes of Hospital Inpatients About Faith Healing and Prayer," *Journal of Family Practice* 39 (1994): 349–52.

Page 9: ". . . a deep understanding . . .": Henri J. M. Nouwen, *The Wounded Healer* (New York: Doubleday, 1972), 88.

"the University of Pain": David Biebel, *If God Is So Good, Why Do I Hurt So Bad?* (Grand Rapids, Mich.: Baker, 1989).

CHAPTER 1: THE FAITH FACTOR

Page 16: Several years ago: Dale A. Matthews, David B. Larson, and Constance P. Barry, *The Faith Factor: An Annotated Bibliography of Clinical Research on Spiritual Subjects* (Rockville, Md.: National Institute for Healthcare Research, 1993).

Page 19: A classic 1972 study of 91,909 individuals: G. W. Comstock and K. B. Partridge, "Church Attendance and Health," *Journal of Chronic Diseases* 25 (1972): 665–72.

Page 21: a 1991 study of 1,077 students: W. A. Oleckno and M. J. Blacconiere, "Relationship of Religiosity to Wellness and Other Health-Related Behaviors and Outcomes," *Psychological Reports* 68 (1991): 819–26.

295

Page 21: National Cancer Institute–funded studies: J. W. Gardner and J. L. Lyon, "Cancer in Utah Mormon Women by Church Activity Level," *American Journal of Epidemiology* 116 (1982): 258–65; J. W. Gardner and J. L. Lyon, "Low Incidence of Cervical Cancer in Utah," *Gynecological Oncology* 5 (1977): 68–80.

J. W. Gardner and J. L. Lyon, "Cancer in Utah Mormon Men by Lay Priesthood Level," *American Journal of Epidemiology* 116 (1982): 243–57.

Page 22: a 1983 study of Seventh-Day Adventists: J. Berkel and F. de Waard, "Mortality Pattern and Life Expectancy of Seventh-Day Adventists in the Netherlands," *International Journal of Epidemiology* 12, no. 4 (1983): 455–59.

A 1983 study of male Seventh-Day Adventists: O. M. Jensen, "Cancer Risk Among Danish Male Seventh-Day Adventists and Other Temperance Society Members," *Journal of the National Cancer Institute* 70 (1983): 1011–14.

A 1978 study of 355 men: T. W. Graham, B. H. Kaplan, J. C. Cornoni-Huntley, S. A. James, C. Becker, C. G. Hames, and S. Heyden, "Frequency of Church Attendance and Blood Pressure Elevation," *Journal of Behavioral Medicine* 1 (1978): 37–43.

A 1982 study of 2,754 men and women: J. S. House, C. Robbins, and H. L. Metzner, "The Association of Social Relationships and Activities with Mortality: Prospective Evidence from the Tecumseh Community Health Study," *American Journal of Epidemiology* 116 (1982): 123–40.

Page 23: conducted in 1995 by Thomas Oxman, M.D.: T. E. Oxman, D. H. Freeman, and E. D. Manheimer, "Lack of Social Participation or Religious Strength and Comfort as Risk Factors for Death after Cardiac Surgery in the Elderly," *Psychosomatic Medicine* 57 (1995): 5–15.

586 residents of Richmond, Virginia: D. M. Johnson, J. S. Williams, and D. G. Bromley, "Religion, Health and Healing: Findings from a Southern City," *Sociological Analysis* 46 (1986): 66–73.

Page 24: clinical depression affects over eleven million Americans annually: *Depression Is a Treatable Illness,* pamphlet published by the Agency for Health Care Policy and Research, United States Public Health Service, Silver Spring, Md., April 1993.

Page 25: a study from North Dakota State University in Fargo: D. Hertsgaard and H. Light, "Anxiety, Depression, and Hostility in Rural Women," *Psychological Reports* 55 (1984): 673–74.

A 1990 study of 451 African-American men and women: D. R. Brown, S. C. Ndubuisi, and L. E. Gary, "Religiosity and Psychological Distress Among Blacks," *Journal of Religion and Health* 29, no. 1 (1990): 55–68.

In a 1983 study of ninety-two families: J. A. Cook and D. W. Wimberley, "If I Should Die Before I Wake: Religious Commitment and Adjustment to the Death of a Child," *Journal for the Scientific Study of Religion* 22, no. 3 (1983): 222–38.

Christopher Rosik, Ph.D., surveyed 165 widows and widowers: C. H. Rosik, "The Impact of Religious Orientation in Conjugal Bereavement Among Older Adults," *International Journal of Aging and Human Development* 28, no. 4 (1989): 251–60.

Page 26: Researchers evaluated 275 African-American patients with schizophrenia: C. C. Chu and H. E. Klein, "Psychosocial and Environmental Variables in Outcome of

Black Schizophrenics," *Journal of the National Medical Association* 77, no. 10 (1985): 793–96.

A 1981 study: D. P. Desmond and J. F. Maddux, "Religious Programs and Careers of Chronic Heroin Users," *American Journal of Drug and Alcohol Abuse* 81 (1981): 71–83.

Page 27: A 1980 study of adult alcoholics: D. B. Larson and W. P. Wilson, "Religious Life of Alcoholics," *Southern Medical Journal* 73 (1980): 723–27.

Alcoholism expert Dr. William Miller: William R. Miller, "Spirituality: The Silent Dimension in Addiction Research," *Drug and Alcohol Review* 9 (1990): 259–66.

"You see, alcohol in Latin is *spiritus . . .*": C. G. Jung to William G. Wilson, Jan. 30, 1961, in G. Adler, ed., *Letters of Carl G. Jung,* vol. 2 (London: Routledge & Kegan Paul, 1975).

The data from a 1984 study: C. K. Hadaway, K. W. Elifson, and D. M. M. Peterson, "Religious Involvement and Drug Use Among Urban Adolescents," *Journal for the Scientific Study of Religion* 23, no. 2 (1984): 109–28.

Page 28: including a 1986 study: A. Y. Amoateng and S. J. Bahr, "Religion, Family, and Adolescent Drug Use," *Sociological Perspectives* 29, no. 1 (1986): 53–76.

Addiction to tobacco results in 340,000 premature deaths annually: Robert B. Mellins, "Chronic Lung Disease and Smoking," in *The Columbia University College of Physicians and Surgeons Complete Home Medical Guide,* 2d ed. (New York: Crown Publishers, 1989).

a startling study: M. Gmur and A. Tschopp, "Factors Determining the Success of Nicotine Withdrawal: 12 Year Followup of 532 Smokers After Suggestion Therapy (by a Faith Healer)," *International Journal of the Addictions* 22, no. 12 (1987): 1189–1200.

an estimated 2 percent success rate: M. Law and J. L. Tang, "An Analysis of the Effectiveness of Interventions Intended to Help People Stop Smoking," *Archives of Internal Medicine* 155, no. 18 (1995): 1933.

Page 29: a 1992 study conducted by the National Opinion Research Center: W. Feigelman, B. S. Gorman, and J. A. Varacalli, "Americans Who Give Up Religion," *Journal for the Scientific Study of Religion* 76, no. 2 (1992): 138–44.

This 1978 study of 2,164 American adults: C. K. Hadaway and W. C. Roof, "Religious Commitment and the Quality of Life in American Society," *Review of Religious Research* 19, no. 3 (1978): 295–307.

Page 30: A 1980 study of 7,029 individuals: W. Shrum, "Religion and Marital Instability: Change in the 1970's," *Review of Religious Research* 21, no. 2 (1980): 135–47.

A study of 2,278 Americans of all faiths: N. D. Glenn and C. N. Weaver, "A Multivariate, Multisurvey Study of Marital Happiness," *Journal of Marriage and the Family* 40 (1978): 269–82.

Researchers studying fourteen hundred tenth-graders: P. C. Higgins and G. L. Albrecht, "Hellfire and Delinquency Revisited," *Social Forces* 55 (1977): 952–58.

In a 1991 study: S. H. Beck, B. S. Cole, and J. A. Hammond, "Religious Heritage and Premarital Sex: Evidence from a National Sample of Young Adults," *Journal for the Scientific Study of Religion* 30, no. 2 (1991): 173–80.

Page 31: Even among students attending a religiously affiliated school: J. T. Woodroof, "Premarital Sexual Behavior and Religious Adolescents," *Journal for the Scientific Study of Religion* 24, no. 4 (1985): 343–66.

prominent gerontologist Dr. Harold Koenig: H. G. Koenig, "Religion and Older Men in Prison," *International Journal of Geriatric Psychiatry* 10, no. 3 (March 1995): 219–30.

Page 32: according to a 1997 study: B. R. Johnson, D. B. Larson, and T. C. Pitts, "Religious Programs, Institutional Adjustment, and Recidivism Among Former Inmates in Prison Fellowship Programs," *Justice Quarterly* 14, no. 1 (March 1997).

a 1994 study showed: S. C. Burgener, "Caregiver Religiosity and Well-Being in Dealing with Alzheimer's Dementia," *Journal of Religion and Health* 33, no. 2 (1994): 175–89.

A 1976 study of 272 patients: D. Blazer and E. Plamore, "Religion and Aging in a Longitudinal Panel," *Gerontologist* 16 (1976): 82–85.

Among the 1,170 respondents to a 1982 survey: R. F. Guy, "Religion, Physical Disabilities, and Life Satisfaction in Older Age Cohorts," *International Journal of Aging and Human Development* 15, no. 3 (1982): 225–32.

In a 1988 study: H. G. Koenig, L. K. George, and I. C. Siegler, "The Use of Religion and Other Emotion-Regulating Coping Strategies Among Older Adults," *Gerontologist* 28, (1988): 303–10.

Page 33: A 1982 study examined: M. E. O'Brien, "Religious Faith and Adjustment to Long-Term Hemodialysis," *Journal of Religion and Health* 21, no. 1 (1982): 68–80.

Researcher Susan D. Decker, Ph.D.: Susan D. Decker, and R. Schultz, "Correlates of Life Satisfaction and Depression in Middle-Aged and Elderly Spinal Cord–Injured Persons," *American Journal of Occupational Therapy* 39 (1985): 740–45.

A 1978 study of death anxiety: H. W. Gibbs and J. Achterberg-Lawlis, "Spiritual Values and Death Anxiety: Implications for Counseling with Terminal Cancer Patients," *Journal of Counseling Psychology* 25, no. 6 (1978): 563–69.

In another study of people with terminal cancer: D. K. Smith, A. M. Nehmkis, and R. A. Charter, "Fear of Death, Death Attitudes and Religious Conviction in the Terminally Ill," *International Journal of Psychiatry in Medicine* 13, no. 3 (1983–84): 221–32.

CHAPTER 2: TOO GOOD TO BE TRUE?

Page 37: over 75 percent of the 325 studies: D. A. Matthews, D. B. Larson, and C. P. Barry, *The Faith Factor: An Annotated Bibliography of Clinical Research on Spiritual Subjects,* vols. 1–4 (Rockville, Md.: National Institute for Healthcare Research, 1993–97).

Jeffrey S. Levin has posed three questions: J. S. Levin, "Religion and Health: Is There an Association, Is It Valid, and Is It Causal?," *Social Science and Medicine* 38, no. 11 (1994): 1475–82.

Page 39: according to researcher William J. Strawbridge: W. J. Strawbridge, R. D. Cohen, S. J. Shema, and G. A. Kaplan, "Frequent Attendance at Religious Services and Mortality over 28 Years," *American Journal of Public Health* 87, no. 6 (1997): 957–61.

Page 40: More carefully designed studies: See, for example, E. L. Idler and S. V. Kasl, "Religion, Disability, Depression and the Timing of Death," *American Journal of Sociology* 97, no. 4 (1992): 1052–79; H. G. Koenig, H. J. Cohen, D. G. Blazer, C. Pieper, K. G. Meador, S. Shelp, V. Goli, and B. DiPasquale, "Religious Coping and Depression Among Elderly Hospitalized Medically Ill Men," *American Journal of Psychiatry* 149, (1992): 1693–1700.

Page 43: In a 1975 book, Dr. Benson explained: Herbert Benson, M.D., with Miriam Z. Klipper, *The Relaxation Response* (New York: Avon Books, 1976).

"Practiced regularly, the relaxation response has proved beneficial: Herbert Benson, "Welcome and Introduction: The Genesis of the Course," conference paper from "Spirituality and Healing in Medicine—II," sponsored by Harvard Medical School and the Mind/Body Medical Institute CareGroup, Beth Israel Deaconess Medical Center, Boston, Mass., Dec. 15–17, 1996.

"The Relaxation Response has always existed": Herbert Benson, M.D., with Miriam Z. Klipper, *The Relaxation Response.*

Page 44: relaxation has been associated with: J. K. Kiecolt-Glaser, R. Glaser, D. Williger, et al., "Psychosocial Enhancement of Immunocompetence in a Geriatric Population," *Health Psychology* 4 (1985): 25–31.

Pages 44–45: "Studies have shown that music, for example: Charles Marwick, "Leaving Concert Hall for Clinic, Therapists Now Test Music's 'Charms,' " *JAMA,* January 24, 275 (1996): 267(2).

Page 45: Many surgeons listen to music: "Music and Blood-Pressure Reduction," *Harvard Heart Letter* 5, no. 7 (1995) (adapted from *JAMA,* Sept. 21, 1994).

Page 47: a study by Dr. Randolph Byrd: R. B. Byrd, "Positive Therapeutic Effects of Intercessory Prayer in a Coronary Care Unit Population," *Southern Medical Journal* 81 (1988): 826–29.

a study of medical students: J. K. Kiecolt-Glaser, W. Garner, C. E. Speicher, G. Penn, and R. Glaser, "Psychosocial Modifiers of Immunocompetence in Medical Students," *Psychosomatic Medicine* 46 (1984): 7–14.

and by a study showing that more isolated psychiatric patients: J. K. Kiecolt-Glaser, D. Ricker, J. George, et al., "Urinary Cortisol Levels, Cellular Immunocompetency, and Loneliness in Psychiatric Inpatients," *Psychosomatic Medicine* 46 (1984): 15–24.

Page 48: ". . . the brain retains a memory . . .": Herbert Benson, M.D., with Marg Stark, *Timeless Healing: The Power and Biology of Belief,* (New York: Scribner, 1996).

Page 49: "Man's search for meaning . . .": Victor Frankl, *Man's Search for Meaning* (New York: Simon & Schuster, 1984).

Page 53: researchers compared infant-mortality rates: C. Spence, T. S. Danielson, and A. M. Kaunitz, "The Faith Assembly: A Study of Perinatal and Maternal Mortality," *Indiana Medicine,* March 1984, 180–83.

Page 54: two basic types of religious orientation: Gordon W. Allport and J. Michael Ross, "Personal Religious Orientation and Prejudice," *Journal of Personality and Social Psychology* 5, no. 4 (1967): 432–43.

Page 55: In a 1991 study: V. Genia and D. G. Shaw, "Religion, Intrinsic-Extrinsic Orientation, and Depression," *Review of Religious Research* 32, no. 30 (1991): 274–83.

A 1989 study of bereavement: C. H. Rosik, "The Impact of Religious Orientation in Conjugal Bereavement Among Older Adults," *International Journal of Aging and Human Development* 28, no. 4 (1989): 251–60.

a study of death anxiety: B. Spilka, L. Stout, B. Minton, and D. Sizemore, "Death and Personal Faith: A Psychometric Investigation," *Journal of the Scientific Study of Religion* 16, no. 2 (1977): 169–78.

Page 57: obstetrician Ignaz Semmelweis: *The Encyclopedia Americana,* International Edition, vol. 24 (Danbury, Conn.: Grolier, 1997), 545.

CHAPTER 3: HEALING THE BODY

Page 60: St. Teresa of Avila: Carol Lee Flinders, *Enduring Grace: Living Portraits of Seven Women Mystics* (New York: HarperCollins, 1993).

Page 75: I mentioned previously the Swiss study: M. Gmur and A. Tschopp, "Factors Determining the Success of Nicotine Withdrawal: 12 Year Followup of 532 Smokers After Suggestion Therapy (by a Faith Healer)," *International Journal of the Addictions* 22, no. 12 (1987): 1189–1200.

a 1988 study in the Netherlands: J. J. Beutler, J. T. M. Attevelt, S. Schouten, J. A. J. Faber, E. J. D. Mees, and G. G. Geijskes, "Paranormal Healing and Hypertension," *British Medical Journal* 296 (1988): 1491–94.

A 1991 telephone survey of 325 Midwesterners: K. K. Trier, and A. Sufpe, "Prayer, Religiosity, and Healing in the Heartland, USA: A Research Note," *Review of Religious Research* 32, no. 4 (1991): 351–58.

Page 76: Twenty-one percent of respondents in a 1988 North Carolina study: D. E. King, J. Sobal, and B. R. DeForge, "Family Practice Patients' Experience and Beliefs in Faith Healing," *Journal of Family Practice* 27, no. 5 (1988): 505–8.

CHAPTER 4: HEALING THE MIND

Page 83: approximately 17.6 million Americans: D/ART Home Page, DEPRESSION Awareness, Recognition, and Treatment, Web site produced by the National Institute of Mental Health, Rockville, Md., Aug. 1997.

more than 23 million Americans: Anxiety Disorders Association of America Web site, "Launch of NIMH Anxiety Disorders Education Program," Anxiety Disorders Association of America," 11900 Parklawn Drive, Suite 100, Rockville, Md. 20852, Aug. 1997.

Page 84: The study of anxiety and depression among women in the rural Midwest: D. Hertsgaard and H. Light, "Anxiety, Depression, and Hostility in Rural Women," *Psychological Reports* 55 (1984): 673–75.

a national study of the causes of psychiatric illnesses: H. G. Koenig, L. K. George, K. G. Meador, D. G. Blazer, and P. B. Dyck, "Religious Affiliation and Psychiatric Disorder Among Protestant Baby Boomers," *Hospital and Community Psychiatry* 45, no. 6 (1994): 586–96.

In a study of Christian and Hindu patients in India: J. M. De Figueiredo and P. V. Lemkau, "The Prevalence of Psychosomatic Symptoms in a Rapidly Changing Bilingual Culture: An Exploratory Study," *Social Psychiatry* 13 (1978): 125–33.

Page 85: a 1992 study of 1,110 elderly male patients: H. G. Koenig, H. J. Cohen, D. G. Blazer, C. Pieper, K. G. Meador, S. Shelp, V. Goli, and B. DiPasquale, "Religious Coping and Depression Among Elderly Hospitalized Medically Ill Men," *American Journal of Psychiatry* 149 (1992): 1693–1700.

the psychological health of members of a Pentecostal church in Newfoundland: R. C. Ness and R. M. Wintrob, "The Emotional Impact of Fundamentalist Religious Participation: An Empirical Study of Intragroup Variation," *American Journal of Orthopsychiatry* 50, no. 2 (1980): 302–14.

a study of a hundred outpatients at a mental-health clinic: R. Stark, "Psychopathology and Religious Commitment," *Review of Religious Research* 12, no. 3 (1971): 165–75.

a 1974 study of suicidal feelings: E. S. Paykel, J. K. Myers, J. J. Lindenthal, and J. Tanner, "Suicidal Feelings in the General Population: A Prevalence Study," *British Journal of Psychiatry* 124 (1974): 460–69.

Page 86: A large 1972 community-based study: G. W. Comstock and K. B. Partridge, "Church Attendance and Health," *Journal of Chronic Diseases* 25 (1972): 665–72.

in a 1991 study: J. B. Ellis and P. C. Smith, "Spiritual Well-Being, Social Desirability and Reasons for Living: Is There a Connection?," *International Journal of Social Psychiatry* 37, no. 1 (1991): 57–63.

"I am in that temper . . .": Letter to Benjamin Bailey, Thursday 21 to Monday 25 May 1818, in Lionel Trilling, ed., *The Selected Letters of John Keats* (New York: Farrar, Straus and Young, 1951), 134.

A 1980 study measured the results: L. R. Propst, "The Comparative Efficacy of Religious and Nonreligious Imagery for the Treatment of Mild Depression in Religious Individuals," *Cognitive Therapy and Research* 4, no. 2 (1980): 167–78.

Page 98: "Researcher Harold Koenig assessed the relationship: H. G. Koenig, S. M. Ford, L. K. George, D. G. Blazer, and K. G. Meador, "Religion and Anxiety Disorder," *Journal of Anxiety Disorders* 7 (1993): 321–42.

CHAPTER 5: HEALING ADDICTIONS

Page 105: In most clinical studies: D. A. Matthews, D. B. Larson, and C. P. Barry, *The Faith Factor: An Annotated Bibliography of Clinical Research on Spiritual Subjects* vols. I–III (Rockville, Md.: National Institute for Healthcare Research, 1993–95).

In a 1995 study: L. T. Midanik and W. B. Clark, "Drinking-Related Problems in the United States: Description and Trends, 1984–1990," *Journal of Studies on Alcohol* 56 (1995): 395–402.

Page 106: A 1990 study of graduates of the Johns Hopkins University Medical School: R. D. Moore, L. Mead, and T. Pearson, "Youthful Precursors of Alcohol Abuse in Physicians," *American Journal of Medicine* 88 (1990): 332–36.

A significant body of research indicates: See, for instance, S. R. Burkett, "Religion, Parental Influence, and Adolescent Alcohol and Marijuana Use," *Journal of Drug Issues* 7, no. 3 (1974): 263–73; J. D. Hundleby, "Adolescent Drug Use in a Behavioral Matrix: A Confirmation and Comparison of the Sexes," *Addictive Behaviors* 12 (1987): 103–12.

A 1996 study of adolescents and their mothers: V. A. Foshee and B. R. Hollinger, "Maternal Religiosity, Adolescent Social Bonding, and Adolescent Alcohol Use," *Journal of Early Adolescence* 16, no. 4 (1996): 451–68.

a 1985 study: R. H. Coombs, D. K. Wellisch, and F. Fawzy, "Drinking Patterns and Problems Among Female Children and Adolescents: A Comparison of Abstainers, Past Users, and Current Users," *American Journal of Drug and Alcohol Abuse* 11 (1985): 315–48.

One study shows: D. Hasin, J. Endicott, and C. Lewis, "Alcohol and Drug Abuse in Patients with Affective Syndromes," *Comprehensive Psychiatry* 26, no. 3 (1985): 283–95.

Page 107: a 1991 study of alcoholics and drug addicts: H. P. Brown and J. H. Peterson, "Assessing Spirituality in Addiction Treatment and Follow-Up: Development of the Brown-Peterson Recovery Progress Inventory (B-PRPI)," *Alcoholism Treatment Quarterly* 8, no. 2 (1991): 21–50.

"Step One: We admitted . . .": Alcoholics Anonymous, 3d ed. (New York: Alcoholics Anonymous World Service, Inc., 1976).

Page 108: ". . . any sincere battle . . .": Gerald G. May, M.D., *Addiction and Grace* (San Francisco: Harper & Row, 1988).

As alcoholism expert Dr. William R. Miller notes: "Spirituality: The Silent Dimension in Addiction Research," *Drug and Alcohol Review* 9 (1990): 259–266; "Spiritual Aspects of Addictions Treatment and Research," *Mind/Body Medicine: A Journal of Clinical Behavioral Medicine* 2, no. 1 (1997): 37–43.

Page 113: Approximately forty-eight million American adults: Centers for Disease Control's Tobacco Information & Prevention Sourcepage, World Wide Web, Oct. 1, 1997.

Page 124: "Our hearts are restless . . .": Saint Augustine, Bishop of Hippo, *The Confessions* trans. Maria Boulding (Hyde Park, N.Y.: New City Press, 1997).

Page 125: four major ways in which A.A. helps: R. E. Hopson and B. Beaird-Spiller, "Why A.A. Works: A Psychological Analysis of the Addictive Experience and the Efficacy of Alcoholics Anonymous," *Alcoholism Treatment Quarterly* 12, no. 3 (1995): 1–17.

Page 130: the use of freebase or "crack" cocaine: J. F. Jekel, H. Podlewski, S. Dean-Patterson, D. F. Allen, N. Clarke, and P. Cartwright, "Epidemic Free-Base Cocaine Abuse: Case Study from the Bahamas," *Lancet,* March 1, 1986, 459–62.

CHAPTER 6: THE QUALITY OF LIFE

Page 135: A study in 1988 followed 1,650 individuals: F. K. Willits and D. M. Crider, "Religion and Well-Being: Men and Women in the Middle Years," *Review of Religious Research* 29, no. 3 (1988): 281–94.

A 1984 study of fifteen hundred Americans: A. St. George and P. H. McNamara, "Religion, Race, and Psychological Well-Being," *Journal for the Scientific Study of Religion* 23, no. 4 (1984): 351–63.

surveyed 750 Mexican-Americans in San Antonio: J. S. Levin and K. S. Markides, "Religious Attendance and Psychological Well-Being in Middle-Aged and Older Mexican-Americans. *Sociological Analysis* 49 (1988): 66–72.

One study focused on younger married women: K. Chamberlain, and S. Zika, "Religiosity, Life Meaning and Wellbeing: Some Relationships in a Sample of Women," *Journal for the Scientific Study of Religion* 27, no. 3 (1988): 411–20.

Page 136: A Canadian study of eighty-five individuals: B. Hunsberger, "Religion, Age, Life Satisfaction, and Perceived Sources of Religiousness: A Study of Older Persons," *Journal of Gerontology* 40 (1985): 615–20.

A 1982 study of 719 married or widowed women: L. J. Beckman and B. B. Houser, "The Consequences of Childlessness on the Social-Psychological Well-Being of Older Women," *Journal of Gerontology* 37 (1982): 243–50.

survey of 1,493 individuals aged sixty-five and over: L. Y. Steinitz, "Religiosity, Well-Being, and Weltanschauung Among the Elderly," *Journal for the Scientific Study of Religion* 19, no. 1 (1980): 60–67.

Researchers examined this link in 299 students: B. G. Frankel and W. E. Hewitt, "Religion and Well-Being Among Canadian University Students: The Role of Faith Groups on Campus," *Journal for the Scientific Study of Religion* 33, no. 1 (1994): 62–73.

Page 137: Margaret Poloma has defined four types of prayer: M. M. Poloma and B. F. Pendleton, "The Effect of Prayer and Prayer Experiences on Measures of General Well-Being," *Journal of Psychology and Theology* 19, no. 1 (1991): 71–83.

Page 138: the faith/well-being link among 1,481 respondents: C. G. Ellison, "Religious Involvement and Subjective Well-Being," *Journal of Health and Social Behavior* 32 (1991): 80–99.

In a 1990 German study: R. Schwab and K. U. Petersen, "Religiousness: Its Relation to Loneliness, Neuroticism, and Subjective Well-Being," *Journal for the Scientific Study of Religion* 29, no. 3 (1990): 335–45.

Page 140: students at Wilfred Laurier University: B. Hunsberger and E. Platonow, "Religion and Helping Charitable Causes," *Journal of Psychology* 120, no. 6 (1986): 517–28.

663 men respondents: L. D. Nelson and R. R. Dynes, "The Impact of Devotionalism and Attendance on Ordinary and Emergency Helping Behavior," *Journal for the Scientific Study of Religion* 15, no. 1 (1976): 47–49.

Page 142: a study of 114 adolescents: T. J. Silber and M. Reilly, "Spiritual and Religious Concerns of the Hospitalized Adolescent," *Adolescence* 20, no. 7 (1985): 217–24.

Pages 142–43: a research team led by Theresa Saudia: T. L. Saudia, M. R. Kinnery, K. C. Brown, and L. Young-Ward, "Health Locus of Control and Helpfulness of Prayer," *Heart and Lung* 20 (1991): 60–65.

Page 143: eighty women aged sixty-five and over: K. Conway, "Coping with the Stress of Medical Problems Among Black and White Elderly," *International Journal of Aging and Human Development* 21 (1985–86): 39.

"A 1990 study by L. B. Bearon and Harold Koenig: L. B. Bearon and H. G. Koenig, "Religious Cognitions and Use of Prayer in Health and Illness," *Gerontologist* 30 (1990): 249–53.

study of 586 patients: K. I. Pargament, D. S. Ensing, K. Falgout, B. Olsen, K. Van Haitsman, and R. Warren, "God Help Me (1): Religious Coping Efforts as Predictors of the Outcomes to Significant Negative Life Events," *American Journal of Community Psychology* 18, no. 6 (1990): 793–824.

Page 144: In a study mentioned in chapter 1: M. E. O'Brien, "Religious Faith and Adjustment to Long-Term Hemodialysis," *Journal of Religion and Health* 21, no. 1 (1982): 68–80.

Page 145: forty heart-transplant patients: R. C. Harris, M. A. Dew, A. Lee, M. Amaya, L. Buches, D. Reetz, and C. Colemen, "The Role of Religion in Heart-Transplant Recipients' Long-Term Health and Well-Being," *Journal of Religion and Health* 34, no. 1 (1995): 17–31.

patients with spinal-cord injuries: Susan D. Decker and R. Schulz, "Correlates of Life Satisfaction and Depression in Middle-aged and Elderly Spinal Cord–Injured Persons," *American Journal of Occupational Therapy* 39 (1985): 740–45.

For elderly women recovering from broken hips: P. Pressman, J. S. Lyons, D. B. Larson, and J. J. Strain, "Religious Belief: Depression and Ambulation Status in Elderly Women with Broken Hips," *American Journal of Psychiatry* 145 (1990): 758–60.

Page 149: "A 1994 study: C. R. Rutledge, J. S. Levin, D. B. Larson, and J. S. Lyons, "The Importance of Religion for Parents Coping with a Chronically Ill Child," *Journal of Psychology and Christianity* 14, no. 1 (1995): 50–57.

Page 150: caregivers of Alzheimer's and cancer patients: P. V. Rabins, M. D. Fitting, J. Eastham, and J. Fetting, "The Emotional Impact of Caring for the Chronically Ill," *Psychosomatics* 31, no. 3 (1990): 331–36.

Page 155: "a study assessing the value: K. I. Maton, "The Stress-Buffering Role of Spiritual Support: Cross-Sectional and Prospective Investigation," *Journal for the Scientific Study of Religion* 28, no. 3 (1989): 310–23.

one hundred recently widowed women: K. A. Gass, "The Health of Conjugally Bereaved Older Widows: The Role of Appraisal, Coping and Resources," *Research in Nursing and Health* 10 (1987): 39–47.

And in a study of epidemiological data: K. J. Helsing and M. Szklo, "Mortality After Bereavement," *American Journal of Epidemiology* 114 (1981): 41–52.

Researchers have found: R. Bartrop, E. Luckhurst, L. Lazarus, L. Kiloh, and R. Penny, "Depressed Lymphocyte Function After Bereavement," *Lancet* 1 (1977): 834–36; S. J. Schleifer, S. E. Keller, M. Camerino, J. C. Thornton, and M. Stein, "Suppression of Lymphocyte Stimulation Following Bereavement," *JAMA* 250 (1983): 374–77; M. Irwin, M. Daniels, T. L. Smith, E. Bloom, and H. Weiner, "Impaired Natural Killer Cell Activity During Bereavement," *Brain, Behavior, and Immunity* 1 (1987): 98–104.

CHAPTER 7: FAITH AND MORTALITY

Page 158: "In a carefully designed and executed 1997 study: W. J. Strawbridge, R. D. Cohen, S. J. Shema, and G. A. Kaplan, "Frequent Attendance at Religious Services and Mortality over 28 Years," *American Journal of Public Health* 87, no. 6 (1997): 957–61.

reaffirms the findings of a 1979 survey: L. F. Berkman and S. L. Syme, "Social Networks, Host Resistance, and Mortality: A Nine-Year Follow-Up Study of Alameda County Residents," *American Journal of Epidemiology* 109 (1979): 186–204.

In another noteworthy study: U. Goldbourt, S. Yaari, and J. H. Medalie, "Factors Predictive of Long-Term Coronary Heart Disease Mortality Among 10,059 Male Israeli Civil Servants and Municipal Employees," *Cardiology* 82 (1993): 100–121.

Page 159: Another study of Israelis: J. D. Kark, G. Shemi, Y. Friedlander, O. Martin, O. Manor, and S. H. Blondheim, "Does Religious Observance Promote Health? Mortality in Secular vs. Religious Kibbutzim in Israel," *American Journal of Public Health* 86, no. 3 (1996): 341–46.

a 1994 study of 2,956 individuals: C. G. Ellison and L. K. George, "Religious Involvement, Social Ties and Social Support in a Southeastern Community," *Journal for the Scientific Study of Religion* 33, no. 1 (1994): 46–61.

a 1992 study of 473 African-Americans: S. Bryant and W. Rakowski, "Predictors of Mortality Among Elderly African-Americans," *Research on Aging* 14, no. 1 (1992): 50–67.

Among 225 such elderly persons: D. M. Zuckerman, S. V. Kasl, and A. M. Ostfeld, "Psychosocial Predictors of Mortality Among the Elderly Poor," *American Journal of Epidemiology* 119 (1984): 410–23.

And in a 1981 study: D. K. Reynolds and F. L. Nelson, "Personality, Life Situation, and Life Expectancy," *Suicide and Life-Threatening Behavior* 11, no. 2 (1981): 99–110.

As mentioned in chapter 2: C. Spence, T. S. Danielson, and A. M. Kaunitz, "The Faith Assembly: A Study of Perinatal and Maternal Mortality," *Indiana Medicine,* March 1984, 180–83.

Page 160: "Among Seventh-Day Adventists: J. Berkel and F. de Waard, "Mortality Pattern and Life Expectancy of Seventh-Day Adventists in the Netherlands," *International Journal of Epidemiology* 12, no. 4 (1983): 455–459; J. E. Enstrom, "Health Practices and Cancer Mortality Among Active California Mormons," *Journal of the National Cancer Institute* 81 (1989): 1807–14; J. W. Gardner and J. L. Lyon, "Cancer in Utah Mormon Women by Church Activity Level," *American Journal of Epidemiology* 116 (1982): 258–65; J. W. Gardner, and J. L. Lyon, "Low Incidence of Cervical Cancer in Utah," *Gynecologic Oncology* 5 (1977): 68–80; J. W. Gardner and J. L. Lyon, "Cancer in Utah Mormon Men by Lay Priesthood Level," *American Journal of Epidemiology* 116 (1982): 243–57; O. M. Jensen, "Cancer Risk Among Danish Male Seventh-Day Adventists and Other Temperance Society Members," *Journal of the National Cancer Institute* 70 (1983): 1011–14.

Even in a broader slice of the population: N. H. Gottlieb and L. W. Green, "Life Events, Social Network, Lifestyle, and Health: An Analysis of the 1979 National Survey of Personal Health Practices and Consequences," *Health Education Quarterly* 11, no. 1 (1984): 91–105.

Page 161: A 1983 study of 1,428 Americans: V. Richardson, S. Berman, and M. Piwowarski, "Projective Assessment of the Relationships Between the Salience of Death, Religion and Age Among Adults in America," *Journal of General Psychology* 109 (1983): 149–56.

Page 162: attitudes about death among 260 older subjects: F. C. Jeffers, C. R. Nichols, and C. Eisdorfer, "Attitudes of Older Persons Toward Death: A Preliminary Study," *Journal of Gerontology* 16 (1961): 53–56.

Middle-aged male respondents: A. M. Downey, "Relationship of Religiosity to Death Anxiety of Middle-Aged Males," *Psychological Reports* 54 (1984): 811–22.

In a 1992 study: M. F. Highfield, "Spiritual Health of Oncology Patients: Nurse and Patient Perspectives," *Cancer Nursing* 15, no. 10 (1992): 1–8.

Page 163: In a study of twenty terminally ill patients: D. K. Smith, A. M. Nehmkis, and R. A. Charter, "Fear of Death, Death Attitudes and Religious Conviction in the Terminally Ill," *International Journal of Psychiatry in Medicine* 13, no. 3 (1983–84): 221–32.

In a 1978 study: H. W. Gibbs and J. Achterberg-Lawlis, "Spiritual Values and Death Anxiety: Implications for Counseling with Terminal Cancer Patients," *Journal of Counseling Psychology* 25, no. 6 (1978): 563–69.

Page 164: "The room was so crowded . . .": This and other quotes are from Bernardin, Joseph Louis, Cardinal, *The Gift of Peace* (Chicago: Loyola Press, 1997).

Page 167: Interestingly, religious patients and doctors: L. R. Seidlitz et al., "Attitudes of Older People Toward Suicide and Assisted Suicide: An Analysis of Gallup Poll Findings," *Journal of the American Geriatric Society* 43 (1995): 993–98; J. G. Bachman et al., "Attitudes of Michigan Physicians and the Public Toward Legalizing Physician-Assisted Suicide and Voluntary Euthanasia," *New England Journal of Medicine* 334, no. 5 (1996): 303–9.

CHAPTER 8: DEVELOPING A SPIRITUAL PROGRAM

Page 178: "Our brains are wired . . .": Herbert Benson, M.D., with Marg Stark, *Timeless Healing: The Power and Biology of Belief* (New York: Scribner, 1996).

Page 179: researchers gave a pregnant woman the drug ipecac: S. Wolf, "Effects of Suggestion and Conditioning on the Action of Chemical Agents in Human Subjects: The Pharmacology of Placebos," *Journal of Clinical Investigation* 29 (1950): 100–109.

Page 180: Until the late 1950s: E. G. Dimond, C. F. Kittle, and J. E. Crockett, "Comparison of Internal Mammary Ligation and Sham Operation for Angina Pectoris," *American Journal of Cardiology* 5 (1960): 483–86.

Page 182: The concepts I share here are one effort to synthesize this work: Physical Health Panel Report, Scientific Progress in Spiritual Research Conference. National Institute for Healthcare Research, Leesburg, Va., July 11–13, 1996.

Page 184: "In God you come up against something . . .": C. S. Lewis, *Mere Christianity* (New York: Macmillan, 1943).

Page 185: an overview of the research studies tracking the faith factor: D. A. Matthews, D. B. Larson, and C. P. Barry, *The Faith Factor: An Annotated Bibliography of Clinical Research on Spiritual Subjects* vols. 1–4 (Rockville, Md.: National Institute for Healthcare Research, 1993–97).

conducted by Thomas Oxman, M.D.: T. E. Oxman, D. H. Freeman, and E. D. Manheimer, "Lack of Social Participation or Religious Strength and Comfort as Risk Factors for Death after Cardiac Surgery in the Elderly," *Psychosomatic Medicine* 57 (1995): 5–15.

Page 186: As noted by epidemiologist Jeffrey Levin: J. S. Levin, "Religion and Health: Is There an Association, Is It Valid, and Is It Causal?," *Social Science Medicine* 38, no. 11 (1994): 1475–82.

Page 190: Over two million men: World Wide Web, www.promisekeepers.org, Oct. 2, 1997.

Page 195: St. Anthony of Egypt: James Bentley, *A Calendar of Saints: The Lives of the Principal Saints of the Christian Year* (New York: Facts on File, 1986).

CHAPTER 9: PRAYER

Page 198: "the great conversation": Peter Kreeft, *The Great Conversation: Straight Answers to Tough Questions on Prayer* (San Francisco: Ignatius Press, 1991).

A poll in 1996: Kenneth L. Woodward, "Is God Listening?," *Newsweek* 129, no. 13 (March 31, 1997): 56–57.

Page 199: conducted by Randolph Byrd, M.D.: R. B. Byrd, "Positive Therapeutic Effects of Intercessory Prayer in a Coronary Care Unit Population," *Southern Medical Journal* 81 (1988): 826–29.

Page 200: A 1969 study of intercessory prayer: P. H. Collipp, "The Efficacy of Prayer: A Triple-Blind Study," *Medical Times* 97 (1969): 201–4.

Page 201: A Dutch study of people with hypertension: J. J. Beutler, J. T. M. Attevelt, S. Schouten, J. A. J. Faber, E. J. D. Mees, and G. G. Geijskes, "Paranormal Healing and Hypertension," *British Medical Journal* 296 (1988): 1491–94.

Page 202: Dr. Larry Dossey has written extensively: Larry Dossey, M.D., *Healing Words: The Power of Prayer and the Practice of Medicine* (San Francisco: HarperSanFrancisco, 1993).

Page 203: A study of women with breast cancer: S. C. Johnson and B. Spilka, "Coping with Breast Cancer: The Roles of Clergy and Faith," *Journal of Religion and Health* 30, no. 1 (1991): 21–33.

Page 207: His book, *The Way of a Pilgrim:* Anonymous, *The Way of a Pilgrim,* trans. Olga Savin (Boston: Shambhala, 1996).

Page 208: "There is nothing . . .": Melanie Svoboda, "25 Quotations on Prayer," *Praying,* May–June 1992.

Page 209: Margaret Poloma's research: M. M. Poloma and B. F. Pendleton, "The Effect of Prayer and Prayer Experiences on Measures of General Well-Being," *Journal of Psychology and Theology* 19, no. 1 (1991): 71–83.

Page 211: "Step 1. Pick a focus word . . .": Herbert Benson, M.D., with Marg Stark, *Timeless Healing: The Power and Biology of Belief* (New York: Scribner, 1996).

Page 212: "I throw myself down . . .": John Donne, *Eighty Sermons,* no. 80, sect. 3 (1640; preached Dec. 12, 1626), as quoted in *The Columbia Dictionary of Quotations* (New York, Columbia University Press, 1993).

Page 218: "The house of my soul . . .": Saint Augustine, Bishop of Hippo, *The Confessions,* trans. Maria Boulding.

Page 219: A study of two hundred women: H. D. Koenig, D. O. Moberg, and J. N. Kvale, "Religious Activities and Attitudes of Older Adults in a Geriatric Assessment Clinic," *Journal of the American Geriatric Society* 36 (1988): 362–74.

one study found that 72 percent: K. Conway, "Coping with the Stress of Medical Problems Among Black and White Elderly," *International Journal of Aging and Human Development* 21 (1985–86): 39–48.

"If God had granted all the silly prayers . . .": C. S. Lewis, *Letters to Malcolm: Chiefly on Prayer* (New York: Harcourt Brace Jovanovich, 1963).

In her prayer study, Margaret Poloma: M. M. Poloma and B. F. Pendleton, "The Effect of Prayer and Prayer Experiences on Measures of General Well-Being," *Journal of Psychology and Theology* 19 (1991): 71–83.

Page 221: "God receives us just as we are . . .": Richard Foster, *Prayer* (San Francisco: HarperSanFrancisco, 1992).

CHAPTER 10: THE RICHES OF THE BIBLE

Page 223: In 1996, twenty-nine million Bibles: Figures from interview, Sidney Van Nort, librarian, American Bible Society, May 19, 1997.

Page 227: our very identity is as God's beloved: Henri J. M. Nouwen, *The Life of the Beloved* (New York: Crossroad, 1995).

Page 234: "Of all the means available . . .": Martin L. Smith, *The Word Is Very Near You* (Cambridge, Mass.: Cowley, 1989).

CHAPTER 11: SPIRITUAL COMMUNITY

Page 249: researchers at Carnegie Mellon University reported: S. Cohen, W. J. Doyle, D. P. Skoner, B. S. Rabin, and J. M. Gwaltney, Jr., "Social Ties and Susceptibility to the Common Cold," *JAMA* 277 (1997): 1940–44.

Researchers at Stanford University: D. Spiegel, J. R. Bloom, H. C. Kraemer, and E. Gottheil, "Effect of Psychosocial Treatment on Survival of Patients with Metastatic Breast Cancer," *Lancet* 2 (1989): 888–91.

Researchers performed a second study of these patients: M. M. Kogon, A. Biswas, D. Pearl, R. W. Carlson, and D. Spiegel, "Effects of Medical and Psychotherapeutic Treatment on the Survival of Women with Metastatic Breast Carcinoma," *Cancer* 180, no. 2 (July 15, 1997): 225–30.

a nine-year study (discussed in more detail in chapter 7): L. F. Berkman and S. L. Syme, "Social Networks, Host Resistance, and Mortality: A Nine-Year Follow-Up Study of Alameda County Residents," *American Journal of Epidemiology* 109 (1979): 186–204.

Page 250: people who have experienced negative life events: S. Cohen and S. L. Syme, eds., *Social Support and Health* (New York: Academic Press, 1985).

"hard-wired for God": Herbert Benson, M.D., with Marg Stark, *Timeless Healing: The Power and Biology of Belief* (New York: Scribner, 1996).

The importance of caring touch: Ashley Montagu, *Touching: The Human Significance of the Skin* (New York: Harper & Row, 1978).

The famous primate experiments of Harry Harlow: H. F. Harlow and M. K. Harlow, "Social Deprivation in Monkeys," *Scientific American* 207 (1962): 136–46.

Page 251: the role of religious faith in the lives of long-term hemodialysis patients: M. E. O'Brien, "Religious Faith and Adjustment to Long-Term Hemodialysis," *Journal of Religion and Health* 21, no. 1 (1982): 68–80.

In the 1997 study of 6,928 residents: W. J. Strawbridge, R. D. Cohen, S. J. Shema, and G. A. Kaplan, "Frequent Attendance at Religious Services and Mortality over 28 Years," *American Journal of Public Health* 87, no. 6 (1997): 957–61.

2,956 respondents in North Carolina: C. G. Ellison and L. K. George, "Religious Involvement, Social Ties, and Social Support in a Southeastern Community," *Journal for the Scientific Study of Religion* 33, no. 1 (1994): 46–61.

"But the most striking scientific demonstration: J. D. Kark, G. Shemi, Y. Friedlander, O. Martin, O. Manor, and S. H. Blondheim, "Does Religious Observance Promote Health? Mortality in Secular vs. Religious Kibbutzim in Israel," *American Journal of Public Health* 86, no. 3 (1996): 341–46.

Page 254: "Do not separate yourself . . .": Quoted in Rabbi Joseph Telushkin, *Jewish Wisdom: Ethical, Spiritual, and Historical Lessons from the Great Works and Thinkers* (New York: William Morrow & Company, 1994).

Page 255: David B. Larson, M.D.: D. B. Larson, S. S. Larson, and J. P. Swyers, *The Costly Consequences of Divorce* (Rockville, Md.: National Institute for Healthcare Research, 1996); interview with David B. Larson, M.D., May 23, 1997.

Page 256: Perhaps even more alarming: B. Bloom, S. Asher, and S. White, "Marital Disruption as a Stressor: A Review and Analysis," *Psychological Bulletin* 85 (1978): 867–94; L. M. Verbrugge, "Marital Status and Health," *Journal of Marriage and Family* 41 (1979): 267–85; J. K. Kiecolt-Glaser, S. Kennedy, S. Malkoff, L. Fisher, C. E. Speicher, and R. Glaser, "Marital Discord and Immunity in Males," *Psycho-*

somatic Medicine 50 (1988): 213–29; J. K. Kiecolt-Glaser, L. Fisher, P. Ogrocki, J. C. Stout, C. E. Speicher, and R. Glaser, "Marital Quality, Marital Disruption, and Immune Function," *Psychosomatic Medicine* 49 (1987): 13–34.

a scientific study of 7,029 married men and women: W. Shrum, "Religion and Marital Instability: Change in the 1970's," *Review of Religious Research* 21, no. 2 (1980): 135–47.

Page 257: Another study, of 997 men and 1,281 women: N. D. Glenn and C. N. Weaver, "A Multivariate, Multisurvey Study of Marital Happiness," *Journal of Marriage and the Family* 40 (1978): 269–82.

couples married an average of fifty-three years: M. J. Sporakowski and G. A. Hughston, "Prescriptions for Happy Marriage: Adjustments and Satisfactions of Couples Married for 50 or More Years," *Family Coordinator* 27, no. 4 (1978): 321–28.

"Echoing the findings: W. R. Schumm, S. R. Bollman, and A. P. Jurich, "The 'Marital Conventionalization' Argument: Implications for the Study of Religiosity and Marital Satisfaction," *Journal of Psychology and Theology* 10, no. 3 (1982): 236–41.

A 1983 study of 3,257 high-school students: H. M. Bahr and T. K. Martin, "And Thy Neighbor as Thyself: Self-Esteem and Faith in People as Correlates of Religiosity and Family Solidarity Among Middletown High School Students," *Journal for the Scientific Study of Religion* 22, no. 2 (1983): 132–44.

An earlier study: P. L. Benson and B. P. Spilka, "God-Image as a Function of Self-Esteem and Locus of Control," *Journal for the Scientific Study of Religion* 12, no. 3 (1973): 297–310.

Page 258: researchers have repeatedly found lower levels: On adolescent drug/alcohol abuse and religion, see E. M. Adlaf and R. G. Smart, "Drug Use and Religious Affiliation: Feelings and Behavior," *British Journal of Addiction* 80 (1985): 163–71; A. Y. Amoateng and S. J. Bahr, "Religion, Family, and Adolescent Drug Use," *Sociological Perspectives* 29 (1986): 53–76; S. R. Burkett, "Religion, Parental Influence, and Adolescent Alcohol and Marijuana Use," *Journal of Drug Issues* 7, no. 3 (1977): 263–73; R. H. Coombs, D. K. Wellisch, and F. Fawzy, "Drinking Patterns and Problems Among Female Children and Adolescents: A Comparison of Abstainers, Past Users, and Current Users," *American Journal of Drug and Alcohol Abuse* 11 (1985): 315–48; R. L. Dudley, P. B. Mutch, and R. J. Cruise, "Religious Factors and Drug Usage Among Seventh-Day Adventist Youth in North America," *Journal for the Scientific Study of Religion* 26, no. 2 (1987): 218–33; R. Guinn, "Characteristics of Drug Use Among Mexican-American Students," *Journal of Drug Education* 5, no. 3 (1975): 235–41; C. K. Hadaway, K. W. Elifson, and D. M. M. Petersen, "Religious Involvement and Drug Abuse Among Urban Adolescents," *Journal for the Scientific Study of Religion* 23, no. 2 (1984): 109–128; R. D. Hays, A. W. Stacy, K. F. Widaman, M. R. DiMatteo, and R. Downey, "Multistage Path Models of Adolescent Alcohol and Drug Use: A Re-Analysis," *Journal of Drug Issues* 16, no. 3 (1986): 357–69; J. D. Hundleby, "Adolescent Drug Use in a Behavioral Matrix: A Confirmation and Comparison of the Sexes," *Addictive Behaviors* 12 (1987): 103–12; M. D. Newcomb, and P. M. Bentler, "Cocaine Use Among Adolescents: Longitudinal Associations with Social Context, Psychopathology, and Use of Other Substances," *Addic-*

tive Behaviors 11 (1986): 263–73; R. P. Schlegel and M. D. Sanborn, "Religious Affiliation and Adolescent Drinking," *Journal of Studies on Alcohol* 40, (1979): 693–703. On sexual activity among adolescents, see S. H. Beck, B. S. Cole, and J. A. Hammond, "Religious Heritage and Premarital Sex: Evidence from a National Sample of Young Adults," *Journal for the Scientific Study of Religion* 30, no. 2 (1991): 173–80; S. V. Brown, "Premarital Sexual Permissiveness Among Black Adolescent Females," *Social Psychology Quarterly* 48, no. 4 (1985): 381–87; R. R. Clayton, "Religious Orthodoxy and Premarital Sex," *Social Forces* 47 (1969): 469–74; R. H. DuRant, R. Pendergrast, and C. Seymore, "Sexual Behavior Among Hispanic Female Adolescents in the United States," *Pediatrics* 85, no. 6 (1990): 1051–58; E. Fox and M. Young, "Religiosity, Sex Guilt and Sexual Behavior Among College Students," *Health Values* 13, no. 2 (1989): 32–37; P. Haerich, "Premarital Sexual Permissiveness and Religious Orientation: A Preliminary Investigation," *Journal for the Scientific Study of Religion* 31, no. 3 (1992): 361–65; E. S. Herold and M. S. Goodwin, "Adamant Virgins, Potential Nonvirgins, and Nonvirgins," *Journal of Sex Research* 17, no. 2 (1981): 97–113; A. Thorton and D. Camburn, "Religious Participation and Adolescent Sexual Behavior and Attitudes," *Journal of Marriage and the Family* 51 (1989): 641–53; J. T. Woodroof, "Premarital Sexual Behavior and Religious Adolescents," *Journal for the Scientific Study of Religion* 24, no. 4 (1985): 343–66. On juvenile delinquency, see S. R. Burkett and M. White, "Hellfire and Delinquency: Another Look," *Journal for the Scientific Study of Religion* 13, no. D (1974): 455–62; P. C. Higgins, and G. L. Albrecht, "Hellfire and Delinquency Revisited," *Social Forces* 55 (1977): 952–58; J. Rohrbaugh and R. Jessor, "Religiosity in Youth: A Personal Control Against Deviant Behavior," *Journal of Personality* 43, no. 1 (1975): 136–55 (also evaluates the relationship between religious involvement and premarital sex and marijuana use).

CHAPTER 12: MEDICINE IN THE TWENTY-FIRST CENTURY

Page 272: T. A. Maugans and W. C. Wadland looked: T. A. Maugans and W. C. Wadland, "Religion and Family Medicine: A Survey of Physicians and Patients," *Journal of Family Practice* 32, (1991): 210–13.

Page 273: researchers surveyed 193 psychiatrists: M. Galanter, D. Larson, and E. Rubenstone, "Christian Psychiatry: The Impact of Evangelical Belief on Clinical Practice," *American Journal of Psychiatry* 148 (1991): 90–95.

Page 274: This is a genuine medical issue: W. Feigelman, B. S. Gorman, and J. A. Varacalli, "Americans Who Give Up Religion," *Journal for the Scientific Study of Religion* 76, no. 2 (1992): 138–44; D. B. Larson and W. P. Wilson, "Religious Life of Alcoholics," *Southern Medical Journal* 73 (1980): 723–27.

Page 278: women with breast cancer found: S. C. Johnson and B. Spilka, "Coping with Breast Cancer: The Roles of Clergy and Faith," *Journal of Religion and Health* 30, no. 1 (1991): 21–33.

In another study, of 101 cancer patients and 45 parents of children: B. Spilka, J. D. Spangler, and C. B. Nelson, "Spiritual Support in Life-Threatening Illness," *Journal of Religion and Health* 22, no. 2 (1983): 98–104.

A study comparing spiritual directors and psychotherapists: M. A. Ganje-Fling and P. R. McCarthy, "A Comparative Analysis of Spiritual Direction and Psychotherapy," *Journal of Psychology and Theology* 19, no. 1 (1991): 103–17.

Page 279: A study conducted by psychologist Rebecca Propst: L. R. Propst, "The Comparative Efficacy of Religious and Nonreligious Imagery for the Treatment of Mild Depression in Religious Individuals," *Cognitive Therapy and Research* 4, no. 2 (1980): 167–78.

A survey of 409 psychologists: E. P. Shafranske and H. N. Malony, "Clinical Psychologists' Religious and Spiritual Orientations and Their Practice of Psychotherapy," *Psychotherapy* 27, no. 1 (1990): 72–78.

43 percent of Americans attend worship services weekly: George Gallup, *Religion in America: 1990* (Princeton, N.J.: Princeton Religious Research Center, 1990).

These developments represent a major revolution: D. B. Larson and S. S. Larson, *The Forgotten Factor in Physical and Mental Health: What Does the Research Show?* (Rockville, Md.: National Institute for Healthcare Research, 1994).

Page 281: the study of individuals in religious and nonreligious kibbutzim: J. D. Kark, G. Shemi, Y. Friedlander, O. Martin, O. Manor, and S. H. Blondheim, "Does Religious Observance Promote Health? Mortality in Secular vs. Religious Kibbutzim in Israel," *American Journal of Public Health* 86, no. 3 (1996): 341–46.

Page 283: Edward Jenner: Herman Styler, *The Plague Fighters* (Philadelphia: Chilton Co., Book Division, 1960).

Page 287: However, a recent national study: A. F. Connors, Jr., N. V. Dawson, N. Desbiens, W. Fulkerson, L. Goldman, W. Knaus, J. Lynn, and R. K., Oye, "A Controlled Trial to Improve Care for Seriously Ill Hospitalized Patients: The Study to Understand Prognoses and Preferences for Outcomes and Risks of Treatments (SUPPORT)," *JAMA* 274 (1995): 1591–98.

There are few role models for doctors: T. McNichol, "The New Faith in Medicine," *USA Today Weekend,* April 5–7, 1996; C. Wallis, "Faith and Healing," *Time,* June 24, 1996; D. E. King and B. Bushwick, "Beliefs and Attitudes of Hospital Inpatients About Faith Healing and Prayer," *Journal of Family Practice* 39 (1994): 349–52.

INDEX

✛

Absolution, 46
Accountability, 260–62
Acknowledgment of lack of control, 125
Addiction and Grace (May), 108
Addictions, 26–29, 105–33
  avoiding, 231–32
  change following conversion, 112–24
  recovery through spiritual community,
    124–33
  release from bondage, 108–12
  religiously observant people and,
    105–8
  Twelve Step programs and, 107–8
Adenoid cystic carcinoma, 70–71
Adolescent years, 30–31
Adoration, 45–46, 188, 210, 216
  prayer and, 214–15
Aesthetic "medicine," 44–45
African Americans, 146–49, 171–73
  mortality rates of, 159–60
  sense of well-being and, 135, 136
Afterlife, 141, 157, 163, 171, 173
Agape, 51–52
Aging, 32–33, 136
AIDS, 167–73
Al-Anon, 126, 127
Alateen, 129

Alcoholics Anonymous, 107, 111,
  124–30, 138
Alcoholism, 108–12, 120, 125–30
  Bible and, 231–32
  religiously observant people and,
    105–8
  Twelve Step programs and, 124–25
Alcohol use, abstinence from, 20–22,
  27–28, 105, 160
Alijani, Dr. Mohammad, 73–74, 81
Allen, Dr. David, 130–32
Allport, Gordon W., 54
Alzheimer's disease, 150
American Psychiatric Association,
  279
Ancient forms of medicine, 241–42
Anger, 169
Anorexia, 116
Anthony of Egypt, Saint, 195–96
Anxiety, 83–86, 97–104
  preventing, 233–34
Armstrong, Neil, 181
Arresting the progress of illness,
  68–74
"Arrow prayers," 207
Art and nature, 44–45, 187–88, 215
Assisted suicide, 166–67

313

Assurance of things hoped for, 181–82
Augustine, Saint, 124, 218

Balanced approach to life, 231–33
Beaird-Spiller, B., 125
Bearon, L. B., 143
Beauty, 44–45, 187–88
Bellevue Hospital, 250
Belonging to a congregation, 258–63
 accountability, 260–62
 fellowship events, 258–59
 financial giving, 262–63
 service to those in need, 259–60
 weekly attendance at services, 258
Benson, Dr. Herbert, 3–4, 18, 42–44,
  48, 178, 179, 211, 250
Bereavement, 25–26, 55, 153–56
Berkman, L. F., 158
Bernardin, Cardinal Joseph, 164–67
Bible, 11, 147, 150, 288
 addiction and, 130, 132
 Book of Psalms, 214–20
 caregiving and, 152
 faith and, 186
 healing the body, 62–64, 68, 80
 healing the mind, 87–95, 102, 103
 love and, 51–52, 191
 medical benefits of reading, *see*
  Medical benefits of Bible-reading
 mortality and, 157, 172–73
 pervasiveness of, 223
 prayer and, 206–7, 208
 study guide, 245–47
Biebel, David, 9
"Biopsychosocial model," 3
Bipolar disorder, 95–97
Bloodletting, 179
Body, healing the, 60–82
 arresting the progress of illness,
  68–74
 the Bible and, 62–64, 229–31
 Clearwater rheumatoid arthritis study,
  76–79
 coping with illness, 64–68
 mystery and potential, 81–82

remission or complete healing,
  75–76, 79–80
Body as a temple of the spirit, 44, 187,
  252
Brain injury, 150–53
Brain tumor, 146–49
Branch Davidians, 53
Breast cancer, 80, 203, 249
Broken hips, 145
Byrd, Dr. Randolph, 47, 199–200, 203,
  281

Cancer:
 healing and, 62–64, 70–71, 73–74,
  81
 lifestyle and, 20–22
 mortality and, 164–66
 see also types of cancer
Cardiomyopathy, 69–70
Caregivers, 146–53
Carnegie Mellon University, 249
Centers for Disease Control, 113
Charitable activities, 140
Charter, R. A., 163
Childbed fever, 57
Children's Hospital National Medical
  Center, 142
Christian Healing Ministries, 76, 77,
  206
Christian Medical and Dental Society,
  273
Chronic fatigue syndrome (CFS), 87
 bereavement and, 153, 154
 sense of purpose and, 139–40
Chronic illness, 32–33
Chu, C. C., 26
Churchill, Winston, 24
Clearwater Rheumatoid Arthritis Study,
  76–79, 202, 206, 280
Clergy, new partnership with doctors,
  277–80
Cocaine, 126, 130–32
Colloquial prayer, 137, 209–10
Coma, 150–53
Common cold, 249